Pediatric Oncology

Series Editors

Gregory H. Reaman
Center for Drug Evaluation and Research
U.S. Food and Drug Administration
Silver Spring, MD, USA

Franklin O. Smith
Medpace
Cincinnati, OH, USA

This series provides up-to-date information on important topics in pediatric oncology, from the diagnosis and treatment of particular forms of disease through to, for example, radiation oncology, supportive care, and survivorship. The entire spectrum of clinical management is covered with the aim of equipping readers with the latest knowledge relevant to daily practice. In addition, clinical, methodological, and research issues are addressed. The series benefits from homogeneous design and consistently high quality of illustrations. The volume editors are internationally renowned authorities and contributing authors have been selected for their expertise in the subjects discussed. *Pediatric Oncology* will serve pediatric oncologists, fellows, and residents both as a comprehensive source of information and as a quick reference. The series will also be of interest to pediatricians and general practitioners.

Jorge DiMartino
Gregory H. Reaman • Franklin O. Smith
Editors

Pediatric Cancer Therapeutics Development

Springer

Editors
Jorge DiMartino
Clinical Development
Kronos Bio
San Mateo, CA, USA

Gregory H. Reaman
Department of Pediatrics
George Washington University
Washington, DC, USA

Franklin O. Smith
Medpace
Cincinnati, OH, USA

ISSN 1613-5318 ISSN 2191-0812 (electronic)
Pediatric Oncology
ISBN 978-3-031-06356-5 ISBN 978-3-031-06357-2 (eBook)
https://doi.org/10.1007/978-3-031-06357-2

This Springer imprint is published by the registered company Springer Nature Switzerland AG
The registered company address is: Gewerbestrasse 11, 6330 Cham, Switzerland

Contents

History of Drug Development for Children with Cancer

1

Franklin O. Smith and Gregory H. Reaman

Contents

1.1 Introduction

It has been said that the profound improvement in the treatment and resulting overall outcomes of children with cancer represents one of the greatest achievements and success stories in all of medicine. As a result of decades of experimental approaches to the treatment of children pursued through clinical trials designed and conducted by dedicated scientists and clinicians, the willingness of children and their parents to participate in clinical research, the extraordinary increase in understanding the biologic basis of cancer, and the increasing ability to design therapies to target specific biologic processes, four out of five children diagnosed with cancer can now be cured of their disease (Smith et al. 2014; Howlander et al. 1975–2017). And in the most common childhood cancer, acute lymphoblastic leukemia (ALL), cure rates have risen to highs of 90–95% (Hunger and Mulligan 2015) (Fig. 1.1). Despite the impressive accomplishment, too many children experience recurrence of their disease during or upon completion of primary therapy, present with metastatic disease at diagnosis, or are inflicted with especially recalcitrant cancers and fail to experience favorable long-term outcomes. In addition, the

F. O. Smith (✉)
Medpace, Cincinnati, OH, USA

University of Cincinnati College of Medicine, Cincinnati, OH, USA
e-mail: f.smith@medpace.com

G. H. Reaman
Department of Pediatrics, George Washington University School of Medicine and Health Sciences, Washington, DC, USA

Oncology Center of Excellence, Office of the Commissioner, U.S. Food and Drug Administration, Silver Spring, MD, USA

J. DiMartino et al. (eds.), *Pediatric Cancer Therapeutics Development*, Pediatric Oncology,
https://doi.org/10.1007/978-3-031-06357-2_1

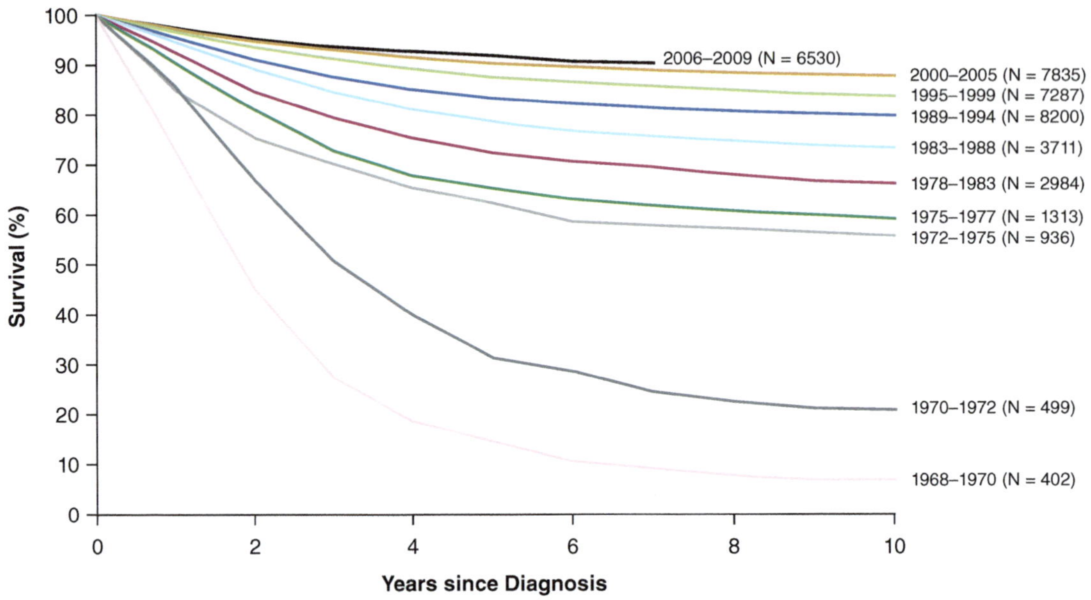

Fig. 1.1 Overall survival among children with acute lymphoblastic leukemia (ALL) who were enrolled in Children's Cancer Group and Children's Oncology Group clinical trials, 1968–2009. (Reproduced with permission)

cost of successful cancer therapy in terms of long-term or late-occurring toxicities associated with treatment provides a sobering reality to the successes achieved and provides the impetus for the search of optimally efficacious and safe therapeutic options for children with cancer.

In 2010, Siddhartha Mukherjee published the book *The Emperor of All Maladies,* a landmark achievement in the history of medicine (Mukherjee 2010). This elegantly written book is a self-described "biography" of cancer drug discovery and development. Interested readers are encouraged to read this complete history that traces therapeutic approaches from ancient to modern times. Instead of a similarly complete and epic tome on the scale of Mukherjee's book, this short chapter will instead focus on the advent of cancer chemotherapy from Sidney Farber's seminal investigations in the 1940s.

1.2 Initial Progress

By the 1930s, it was increasingly recognized that the use of surgery, pioneered in the nineteenth century, and radiation, pioneered in the early twentieth century, to treat cancer was limited to the local control of tumor masses, with neither effective in the treatment of children with leukemia. This led to the Roosevelt administration's passage of the National Cancer Institute Act of 1937 that created the National Cancer Institute (NCI) whose mission was to coordinate cancer research and education. In 1944, the NCI became a part of the National Institutes of Health (NIH).

In 1947, Sidney Farber used an antimetabolite, the antifolate, aminopterin, to first treat a child with leukemia (Fig. 1.2). His seminal work was based on George Minot's scientific work on B_{12} deficiency in patients with pernicious anemia and Lucy Mills identification of folic acid as essential for cell division in patients with nutrition-related anemias. Between 1948 and 1952, Farber's use of methotrexate to treat children with leukemia resulted in a median survival of 8 months, in striking contrast to median survivals of 1–3 months prior to Farber's experimental approach. The addition of purine antagonists, mercaptopurine, to these antifolates further increased the median survival to 1 year by the mid-1950s.

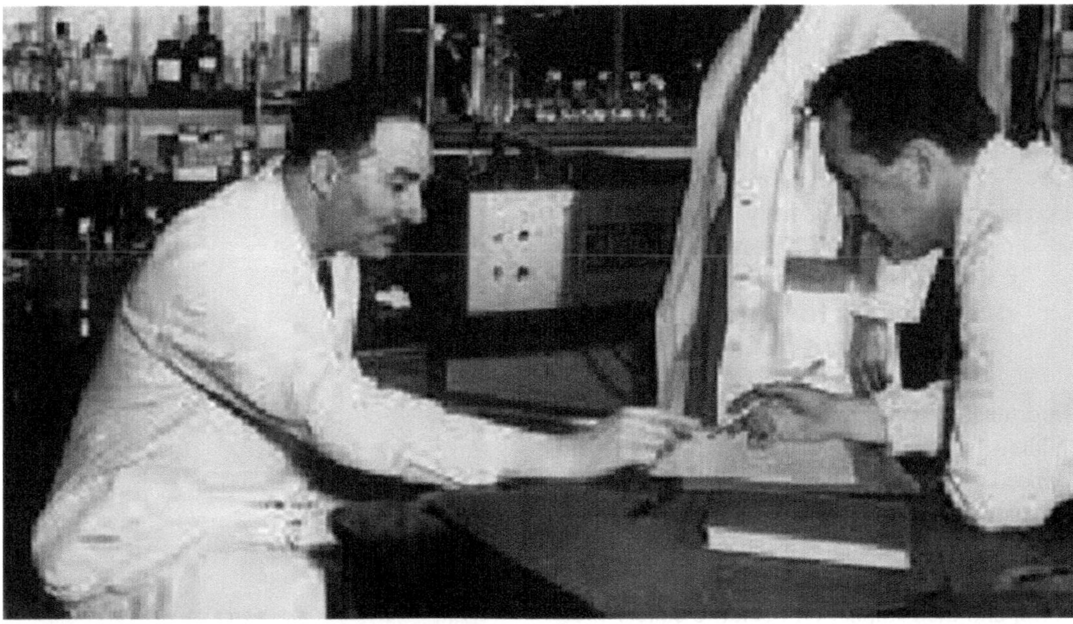

Fig. 1.2 Sidney Farber

1.3 Rise of the Cancer Cooperative Groups

Given the rarity of leukemia and other cancers in children, and the recognition of the need to work collaboratively across multiple institutions, the concept of cooperative groups emerged from the work related to the investigational approach to pediatric leukemias, and later several adult cancers. This led to the establishment of the Cancer Chemotherapy National Service Center at the NIH in 1955 (O'Leary et al. 2008). This innovative and paradigm shifting group had as its primary mission to study antileukemia agents in children. The clinical trials developed by this group were conducted by the Acute Leukemia Chemotherapy Cooperative Group A (ALCCSGA). The ALCCSGA initially included eight member sites, all children's hospitals, and pediatric cancer programs. The cooperative group's first clinical trial was a comparison of 6-mercaptopurine versus 6-mercaptopurine plus azaserine (Heyn et al. 1960). In 1958, Emil Frei, Emil Freireich, and James Holland at the NCI performed combination chemotherapy trials for children with leukemia testing 6-mercaptopurine plus methotrexate. The ALCCSGA also initiated phase I clinical trials in children to test a number of drugs, including mitomycin C, 5-fluroro-2′-deoxyuridine, and actinomycin D. The development of the Acute Leukemia Group B followed shortly thereafter and later became the Cancer and Leukemia Group B (CALGB).

By 1959, the ALCCSGA had grown to 12 member institutions. The ALCCSGA would eventually become the Children's Cancer Study Group (CCSG), subsequently renamed the Children's Cancer Group (CCG). In 1956, the Southwest Cancer Chemotherapy Study Group (SWCCSG) was founded to study leukemia in children and adults. The SWCCSG was later renamed the Southwest Oncology Group (SWOG), and its pediatric division merged with that of the CALGB to become the Pediatric Oncology Group (POG). Together, the CCG and POG conducted 693 treatment studies in children with cancer. In 2000, the CCG and POG, along with the NCI's smaller disease-specific pediatric oncology cooperative groups, the International Rhabdomyosarcoma Study Group (IRSG) and the National Wilms Tumor Study Group (NWTS) merged to become the Children's Oncology Group (COG). Currently, the COG is the world's largest organization devoted to clinical, translational, and epidemiological research in childhood cancer, having conducted 270 treatment studies and 551 nontreatment studies (i.e., supportive care, screening, biology, specimen acquisition, and data analysis studies) since its inception.

1.4 Impact of Regulation to Improve Safety and Efficacy Federal Laws Providing a Regulatory Framework for Drug Development in Children

Unfortunately, catastrophic events and deaths in children from unsafe medicinal products led to the need for a series of laws and a system of regulations to ensure the safety and efficacy of drugs approved for use in children. These US laws, and the regulations that emerged in other parts of the world, and their impact on pediatric cancer drug development are detailed in Chap. 10.

The first of these addressed the adulteration of medicinal products. The Drug Importation Act of 1848 was passed after the blistering agent, Spanish flies (cantharides), was found to be adulterated with other insects and beads (Fig. 1.3). Early legislation addressing the safety of medicinal drug products included the Biologics Control Act of 1902 that was passed after the death in 1901 of a child from tetanus after treatment with a diphtheria antitoxin preparation. The Pure Food and Drugs Act of 1906 was passed after the deaths of a number of infants who were given Mrs. Winslow's Soothing Syrup that was intended to treat teething pain and colic. This product did not divulge its ingredients that included morphine (Fig. 1.4). In 1937, there was another tragedy involving a product known as elixir of sulfanilamide, manufactured by the S.E. Massengill Company in Bristol, Tennessee (Fig. 1.5). It was marketed as a "treatment of all conditions in which the hemolytic streptococci appear." It was marketed, in part, directly to children since the very insoluble sulfanilamide was dissolved to generate a liquid formulation thought to be appropriate for pediatric use. More than 100 people died, the majority being children, due to the highly toxic chemical diethylene glycol that was used as the solvent. Public outcry helped to facilitate the Roosevelt administration in its passage of the Food, Drug, and Cosmetic (FDC) Act of 1938 that gave the Food and Drug Administration (FDA) the authority to approve drugs that were proven safe. However, 1962 saw another devastating tragedy, again involving children, who were born with phocomelia, a severe

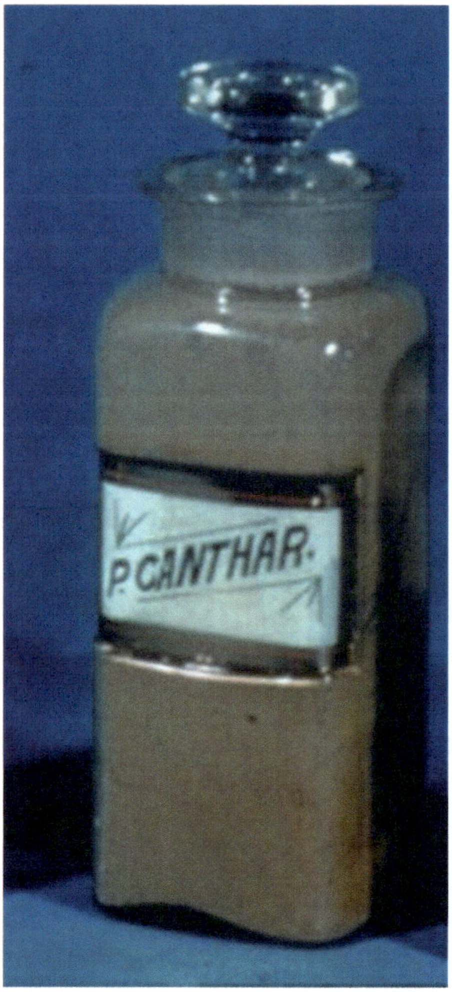

Fig. 1.3 Cantharides (Spanish flies)

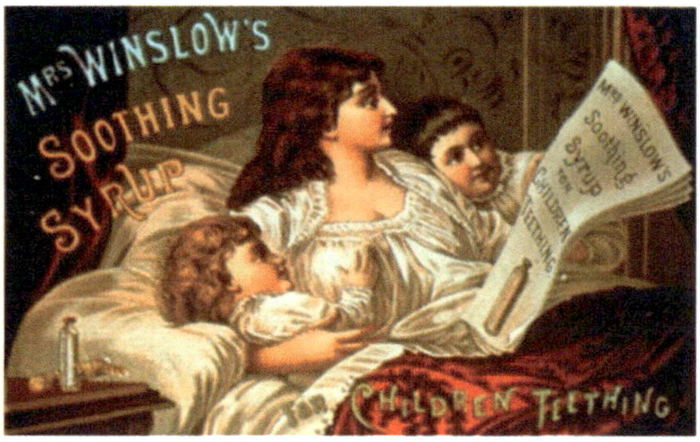

Fig. 1.4 Mrs. Winslow's Soothing Syrup

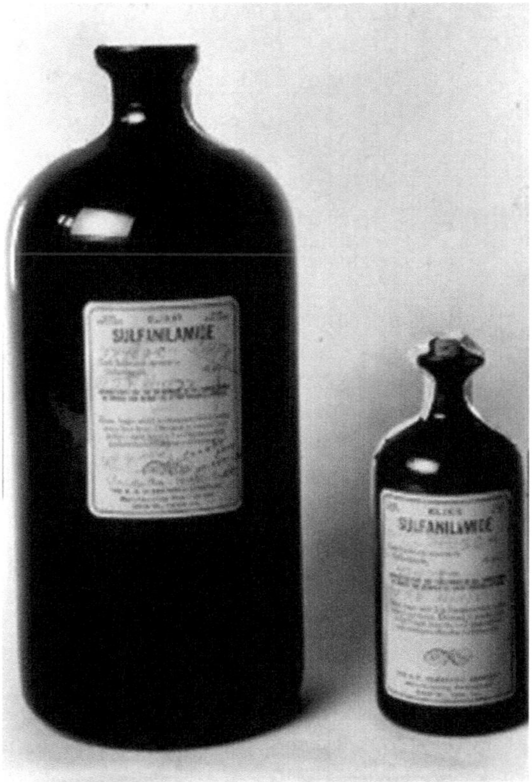

Fig. 1.5 Elixir sulfanilamide

congenital condition of upper and/or lower limb deformities resulting from their pregnant mother's use of the sedative, thalidomide, to treat morning sickness. In response, the Kefauver-Harris Amendment of 1962 was passed that provided a framework for drug manufacturers to prove that their products were not only safe but also effective.

In 1997, the Food, Drug, and Cosmetic Act was amended as the Food and Drug Administration Modernization Act (FDAMA) which provided 6 months of marketing exclusivity as an incentive to manufacturers who voluntarily conducted studies of drugs in children. In 2003, the Pediatric Research Equity Act was passed, following the rescinding of the Pediatric Rule to require pediatric assessments of new drugs when the clinical indications for which the drugs were developed existed in children and the drugs were likely to be used in the pediatric population. In 2002, the exclusivity provision released as part of FDAMA was reauthorized as the Best Pharmaceuticals for Children Act (BPCA). For various reasons, it is perhaps useful to view the FDA's approval of drugs that include a pediatric indication before, and after, passage of the FDAMA (Tables 1.1 and 1.2).

Table 1.1 Drugs with an indication for children with cancer, approved by the FDA prior to FDAMA

Drug	Initial pediatric approval	Currently approved indications
Mercaptopurine	1953	ALL
Methotrexate	1959	ALL, meningeal leukemia, OS, NHL
Cyclophosphamide	1959	Leukemia, lymphoma, NBL, retinoblastoma
Vincristine	1963	ALL, lymphomas, WT, RMS, NBL
Dactinomycin	1964	ES, sarcoma botryoides
Vinblastine	1965	HL, histiocytosis, testicular germ cell carcinoma
Thioguanine	1966	AML
Cytarabine	1969	AML
Procarbazine	1969	HL
Doxorubicin	1974	WT, NBL, STS, HL, other lymphoma, ALL, AML
Lomustine	1976	Brain tumors, HL
L-Asparaginase	1978	Leukemia
Daunorubicin	1979	ALL
PEG-asparaginase	1994	ALL
Tretinoin	1995	APML
Teniposide	2002	Refractory ALL

ALL acute lymphoblastic leukemia, *OS* osteosarcoma, *NHL* non-Hodgkin's lymphoma, *NBL* neuroblastoma, *WT* Wilms' tumor, *RMS* rhabdomyosarcoma, *ES* Ewing sarcoma, *HL* Hodgkin's lymphoma, *AML* acute myeloid leukemia, *STS* soft tissue sarcoma, *APML* acute promyelocytic leukemia

Table 1.2 Drugs with an indication for children with cancer, approved by the FDA after FDAMA

Drug	Initial pediatric approval	Currently approved indications
Arsenic trioxide	2000	APML
Clofarabine	2004	Refractory ALL
Nelarabine	2005	T-cell ALL
Erwinia asparaginase	2011	ALL
Everolimus	2012	SEGA
Denosumab	2013	Giant cell tumor of the bone
6-Mercaptopurine oral solution	2014	ALL
Dinutuximab	2015	High-risk NBL
Pembrolizumab	2017	Refractory classical HL
	2017	MSI-H- or MM repair-deficient solid tumor
	2018	Refractory primary MLBCL
	2018	Metastatic Merkel cell carcinoma
	2020	Refractory classical HL
	2020	Mutational burden-high solid tumors
Avelumab	2017	Metastatic Merkel cell carcinoma
Gemtuzumab	2017	R/R CD33+ AML
	2020	Newly diagnosed CD33+ AML
Tisagenlecleucel	2017	R/R ALL
Dasatinib	2017	Ph + AML in chronic phase, Ph + ALL
Imatinib	2017	Ph + ALL, Ph + CML
Ipilimumab	2017	Unresectable or metastatic melanoma
Nilotinib	2018	Ph + CML in chronic phase
Emapalumab	2018	R/R primary HLH
Larotrectinib	2018	Solid tumors with NTRK gene fusion
Tagraxofusp	2018	BPDCN
Calaspargase	2018	ALL
Entrectinib	2019	Solid tumors with NTRK gene fusion
Naxitamab	2020	R/R NBL
Tazemetostat	2020	Metastatic or locally advanced epithelioid sarcoma
Pralsetinib	2020	RET-mutated medullary thyroid cancer
Selpercatinib	2020	RET fusion-positive thyroid cancer
Selumetinib	2020	NF1, inoperable plexiform neurofibromas
Crizotinib	2021	R/R ALCL
Asparaginase erwinia chrysanthemi	2021	ALL, lymphoblastic lymphoma

APML acute promyelocytic leukemia, *ALL* acute lymphoblastic leukemia, *SEGA* subependymal giant cell astrocytoma, *NBL* neuroblastoma, *HL* Hodgkin's lymphoma, *MSI-H* microsatellite instability-high, *MM* mismatch, *MLBCL* mediastinal large B-cell lymphoma, *AML* acute myeloid leukemia, *CML* chronic myeloid leukemia, *HLH* hemophagocytic lymphohistiocytosis, *BPDCN* blastic plasmacytoid dendritic cell neoplasm, *ALCL* anaplastic large cell lymphoma

Although PREA and BPCA resulted in the addition of pediatric use language in product labeling of more than 800 drug products since the passage of these respective pieces of legislation, the contribution of these laws to cancer drug development was due solely to BPCA; no cancer drug has been subject to a PREA-mandated study since the requirement is indication-based and most cancers seen in adults rarely, if ever, occur in children. In those rare situations where diseases span the adult and pediatric populations, the orphan disease designation exempts the sponsor from the PREA requirement. This unintended oversight has been finally and recently addressed by the RACE (Research Acceleration for Cure and Equity) for Children Act, incorporated as part of the Food and Drug Administration Reauthorization Act (FDARA) passed in 2017. Section 504 of FDARA amends Section 505B of the FD&C Act to authorize

FDA to require early pediatric assessment of new cancer drugs developed for cancers in adults when the molecular target to which that drug is directed is substantially relevant to the growth or progression of a cancer that occurs in children. The impact of this new law on the regulatory environment for pediatric cancer drug development nationally and global is discussed in Chap. 10.

1.5 Indications

The historical paradigm resulted in the approval of 16 cancer drugs prior to 1997 for children with a cancer indication (Table 1.1), with 28 drugs approved since 1997 (Table 1.2). The first cancer drug approved by the FDA for children with cancer was 6-mercaptopurine, approved in 1953 for children with ALL. Looking at all 44 drugs that are approved by the FDA for various pediatric cancer indications, the vast majority are for children with hematologic malignancies (n = 37 indications) with fewer drugs approved for solid tumor indications (n = 24 indications). Sixteen FDA-approved therapies have ALL as an indication, with four for acute myeloid leukemia (AML), two for acute promyelocytic leukemia (APML), two for chronic myeloid leukemia (CML), seven for various forms of non-Hodgkin's lymphoma (NHL), five drugs for Hodgkin's lymphoma, and one for blastic plasmacytoid dendritic cell neoplasm (BPDCN).

Despite significant effort and numerous clinical trials, there are fewer approved drugs for children with solid tumors, with the largest number (n = 4) for children with neuroblastoma. For other solid tumors, there are only small numbers of approved drugs. Disappointingly, most of these drugs are quite old. For example, only one drug, vincristine, is approved for the treatment of children with rhabdomyosarcoma, with this approval in 1963. Similarly, there is only one drug, dactinomycin, approved for the treatment of children with Ewing sarcoma, with this approval in 1964. However, dactinomycin is no longer a component of standard of care for children with Ewing sarcoma.

Interestingly, and consistent with the great advances in the biology of cancer in children and adults, six drugs have recently been approved based on a biologic target that is largely "agnostic" of the organ of origin. These drugs are directed at several interesting biologic targets, including RET, NTRK, microsatellite instability, mismatch repair deficiency, and tumor mutational burden. In addition, the development of more novel agents like the chimeric antigen receptor T-cell (CAR-T) product tisagenlecleucel received its initial approval for a pediatric oncology indication (i.e., relapsed or refractory ALL).

1.6 Summary

Since its inception, the FDA has approved only 44 drugs for children with cancer, in striking contrast to more than 600 drugs for adults with cancer. Despite this difference, it is clear that the development of new therapies for children with cancer has, in large part, driven the process of investigating the safety and effectiveness of all cancer drugs. Notably, the development of chemotherapy approaches was pioneered by Farber's work in children with ALL along with that of Frei, Holland, and Freireich; the first cooperative cancer group was focused on children with ALL; and most significant laws at ensuring the safety and efficacy of new drugs were in response to injury and deaths in children exposed to unsafe and ineffective products. It can also be argued that the first "targeted" therapy (L-asparaginase) was developed and approved for children with ALL. L-Asparaginase targets a specific molecular target, the amino acid asparagine, which is essential for the survival of acute lymphoblastic leukemia cells.

With the remarkable advances in science and insights into the biology of these cancers, it is anticipated that an increasing number of innovative drug products and biologics will be developed and approved in the future. But unique to the assessment of success in the treatment of children with cancer is not only cure of their cancer but more accurate assessments of excess risk of death that is the result of increased lifetime morbidity and mortality.

It is known that survivors of childhood cancer have an increased risk of death due to cardiac disease, pulmonary disease, new cancers, and a number of chronic health conditions (Begg and Schrag 2002; Mertens et al. 2008, 2015; Williams et al. 2021). The future of pediatric cancer therapy development will therefore require not only more effective cancer treatments but, critically, less toxic therapy.

References

Begg CB, Schrag D (2002) Attribution of death following cancer treatment. J Natl Cancer Inst 94:1044–1045

Heyn RM, Brubaler CA, Burchenal JH et al (1960) The comparison of 6-mercaptopurine with the combination of 6-mercaptopurine and azaserine in the treatment of acute leukemia in children: results of a cooperative study. Blood 15:350–259

Howlander NNA, Krapcho M, Miller D et al (1975–2017) SEER cancer statistics review. National Cancer Institute, Bethesda, MD. http://seer.cancer.gov/csr/1975_2017, based on Nov 2019 SEER data submission, posted to the SEER website, Apr 2020

Hunger SP, Mulligan CG (2015) Acute lymphoblastic leukemia in children. N Engl J Med 373:1541–1552

Mertens AC, Liu Q, Neglia JP et al (2008) Cause-specific late mortality among 5-year survivors of childhood cancer: the childhood cancer survivor study. J Natl Cancer Inst 100:1368–1379

Mertens AC, Yong J, Dietz AC et al (2015) Conditional survival in pediatric malignancies: analysis of data from the childhood cancer survivor study and the surveillance, epidemiology, and end results program. Cancer 121:1108–1117

Mukherjee S (2010) The emperor of all maladies. Scribner, New York

O'Leary M, Krailo M, Anderson JR et al (2008) Progress in childhood cancer: 50 years of research collaboration. A report from the Children's Oncology Group. Semin Oncol 35:484–493

Smith MA, Altefruse SF, Adamson PD et al (2014) Declining childhood and adolescent cancer mortality. Cancer 120:2497–2506

Williams AM, Liu Q, Bhakta N et al (2021) Rethinking success in pediatric oncology: beyond 5-year survival. J Clin Oncol 39:2227–2231

Targeted Small Molecule Drug Discovery

2

Jorge DiMartino

Contents

2.1 Introduction

Until relatively recently, the discovery of substances to treat human diseases, including cancer, has relied largely on serendipity and observation. Much of the pharmacologic armamentarium at the disposal of oncologists today, antimetabolites, DNA-damaging agents, and antimitotics were, much like the original antibiotics, derived from natural sources and first tested in humans based on extrapolation of their effects in other diseases or accidental exposures. Perhaps most famously, some of the early alkylating agents began as weapons of war before their usefulness in prolonging life was discovered (Conant 2020). Even as these drugs remain the cornerstone of therapy in many malignancies, our increasingly sophisticated understanding of the molecular drivers of cancer, combined with the advent of technologies that enable massively parallel evaluation of chemical space, has ushered in an era of molecularly targeted therapies. In this chapter, we will consider the various steps in the process of discovering novel chemical matter directed at a prospectively defined target. Starting with what makes for a compelling therapeutic target, we will cover the methods whereby small molecule

J. DiMartino (✉)
Clinical Development, Kronos Bio Inc.,
San Mateo, CA, USA
e-mail: Jorge.dimartino@kronosbio.com

J. DiMartino et al. (eds.), *Pediatric Cancer Therapeutics Development*, Pediatric Oncology,
https://doi.org/10.1007/978-3-031-06357-2_2

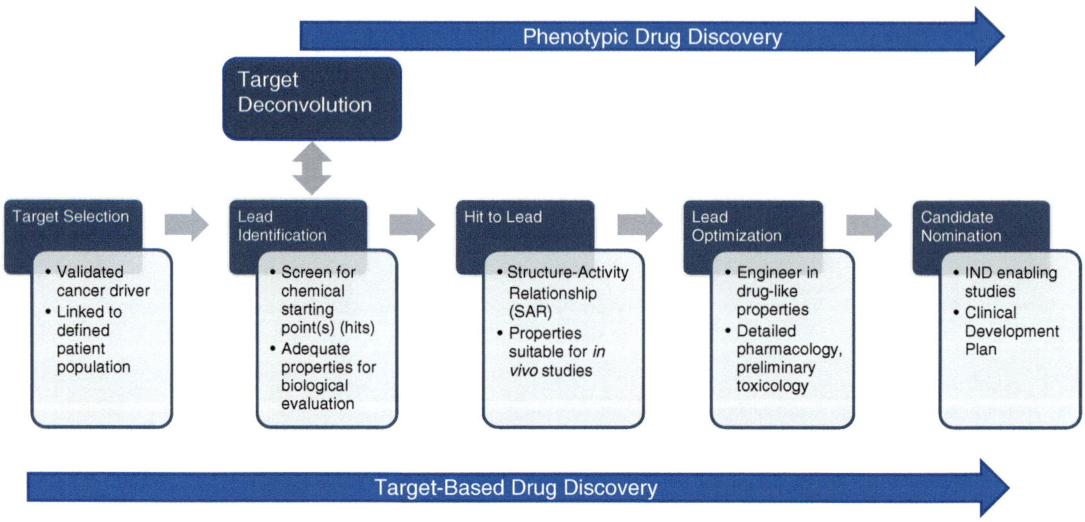

Fig. 2.1 Stages in the drug discovery process. Target-based drug discovery starts with selection of a target on which to base a screening effort to identify leads. Phenotypic drug discovery starts with identification of leads from a compound library in a target-agnostic manner but may require identification of the molecular target to drive molecule evolution. Both proceed from lead identification through subsequent steps to engineer drug-like properties into early chemical hits

starting points are identified and how these "hits" are elaborated to improve their potency and selectivity for the intended target as well as their pharmacologic properties to arrive at a development candidate (DC). Because the focus is on a molecular target, rather than a specific disease or tumor type, the principles described herein apply equally to adult and pediatric cancer.

2.2 Stage Gating

Targeted drug discovery requires a team of experts across multiple disciplines including molecular and cell biologists, biochemists, medicinal chemists, and others, working together over several years to arrive at a drug candidate for clinical development. To maximize the overall probability of success for this endeavor, the use of these resources should be carefully orchestrated to ensure adequate representation of scientists with the expertise needed for a given point the discovery process. For example, it would be wasteful to deploy a team of medicinal chemists for a project in which the biological validity of the target is still being assessed or where screening efforts have just begun. A system of stages with gates or requirements to progress from one stage to the next is commonly used to provide a common frame of reference for allocating resources in biotechnology or pharmaceutical companies (Fig. 2.1). The names and numbers of individual stages and requirements for advancement vary at different companies, but the sequence, from identifying a target to naming a clinical candidate, is universal. A simple schema, as depicted in Fig. 2.1, provides a convenient framework to discuss key aspects of targeted cancer drug discovery.

2.3 Phenotypic Drug Discovery

Drug discovery approaches can be broadly classified as phenotypic or target-based as shown in Fig. 2.2. Before the knowledge and methods to explicitly pursue molecular targets in cancer were widely available, drug discovery was driven by identifying compounds that affected phenotypes associated with cancer such as cell division (DeVita and DeVita-Raeburn 2015; Mukherjee 2010). Many of the mainstays of modern cancer therapy were identified based on phenotypic effects in animals or on cultured cancer cells with-

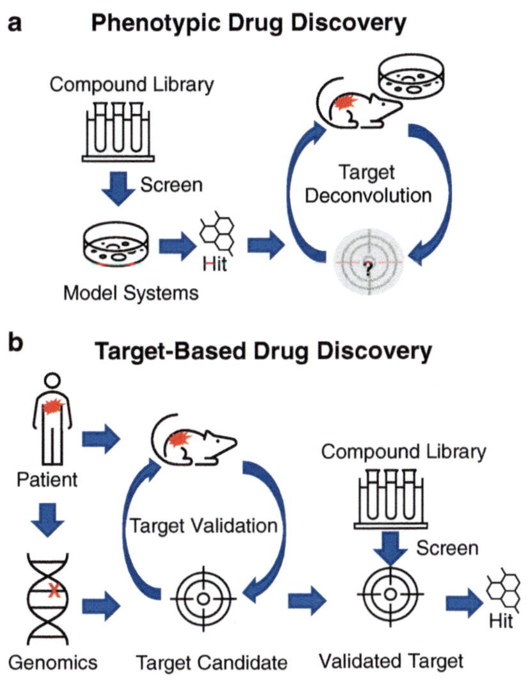

Fig. 2.2 Phenotypic vs target-based drug discovery. Phenotypic approaches screen a compound library on live cells to identify compounds that have the desired effect on cell properties. Because the mechanism whereby the compound achieves the desired phenotypic effect is unknown, efforts to identify the target may be required to facilitate subsequent development. Target-based discovery starts with the nomination of a candidate target implicated as a driver of the disease. Depending on the level of confidence about the target's role in the disease, extensive validation efforts may be required before committing to a screen. Biochemical screening of a compound library against the target yields chemical starting points for subsequent progression to a drug-like molecule

out any a priori knowledge of their respective targets or mechanisms. The astute observation that nitrogen mustards, derived from phosgene gas, a chemical weapon, depleted rapidly dividing cells in the bone marrow and lymph nodes of rabbits set the stage for their experimental use in lymphoma patients (Conant 2020). As cell culture methods became widely available in the 1950s, unbiased screening of compounds against cells in vitro became a productive approach to identify new agents or anticancer applications of agents that were being developed for other diseases. The phenotypic effect that served as the endpoint for these screens was inhibition of cell growth or induction of cell death which, at that time, was assessed using vital stains and counting. A relative handful of cell lines were established at that time, including the murine L1210 leukemia cell line which served as a workhorse model for many screens as well as an allograft model for in vivo testing of antileukemic compounds (Research Paradigm 1955–1975). The screens were laborious, and throughput of compounds was limited, but tens of thousands of potential chemotherapeutic agents were screened in this manner.

The introduction of robotic pipetting and miniaturization of cell culture conditions in the latter half of the twentieth century and beginning of the twenty-first enabled a massive increase in the throughput of phenotypic screens. The recognition that drugs may exert anticancer effects, in part, by modulating nonmalignant cells in the tumor microenvironment also led to screening for phenotypic endpoints other than growth inhibition. Lenalidomide, a cornerstone of therapy for multiple myeloma, was identified through screens of compounds that were structurally related to thalidomide and that modulated cytokine production in cultured lymphocytes as well as having antiproliferative activity against multiple myeloma cell lines (Zeldis et al. 2011). Recent advancements, such as high-content imaging of live cells, aided by sophisticated computational analysis algorithms, provide the opportunity to further expand phenotypic effects beyond simple viability readouts (Scheeder et al. 2018; Horvath et al. 2016). Live imaging can detect effects of a compound on cell morphology, granularity, and migration individually or as an integrated multidimensional readout in a fully automated manner depending on the programming. In addition to screening with libraries of synthetic chemicals with defined structures, phenotypic screens have been valuable for the interrogation of libraries of naturally occurring compounds from various sources. Lurbinectedin, recently approved for the treatment of small cell lung cancer, was discovered by screening a library of compounds derived from marine organisms for antiproliferative effects against cancer cell lines (Pereira et al. 2019). Based on the historical success with this approach, phenotypic screening is being employed in some settings to identify novel cancer therapeutics.

The major advantage of compounds that are identified on the basis of concentration-dependent biological activity is that they start off with some of the physicochemical properties, such as aqueous solubility and cell permeability, which are essential for an oral or parenterally administered drug. In contrast to hits from a biochemical binding or enzymatic inhibition screen (described below) which often require extensive efforts to address problems with solubility or cell-based potency, phenotypic screening hits can often transition quickly from cell-based to in vivo studies in tumor xenograft models and are potentially more readily elaborated into pharmacologic preparations suitable for human dosing. The disadvantages of the phenotypic approach become evident when planning for the clinical evaluation of the agent in patients. These challenges are discussed in greater detail in Chap. 5.

Because of these limitations, modern phenotypic screens are often combined with efforts to deconvolute or reverse engineer the identity of the molecular target that is engaged by the hit. The explosion in knowledge of the molecular profiles of the many available cancer cell lines that is now publicly available through resources like the Cancer Cell Line Encyclopedia makes it possible to correlate patterns of sensitivity or resistance to a compound with the presence or absence of specific mutations or gene expression profiles in the sensitive or resistant cell lines (CCLE 2012). Alternatively, functional genomic approaches ranging from random mutagenesis to genome-wide knockout screens using Clustered Regularly Interspaced Short Palindromic Repeats (CRISPR) can be applied to identify genes that confer sensitivity or resistance to the agent in vitro (Shalem et al. 2015; Nijman 2015). For example, a sensitive cell line can be exposed to a mutagenic agent, such as *N*-ethyl-*N*-nitrosourea (ENU) followed by selection for survival in lethal concentrations of the phenotypic hit of interest. Exome sequencing of emerging resistant clones can point to genes whose mutation mediates resistance to the hit and help to identify the target or pathway involved. Genome-wide CRISPR-based approaches can be used in much the same way with the exception that the guide RNAs (sgRNA) introduced to direct the Cas-9 endonuclease to specific genes can be more readily identified than point mutations induced by ENU mutagenesis. In addition to identifying genes whose excision confers resistance to the antiproliferative effects of a compound, CRISPR knockouts can be used in a synthetic lethality screen to identify genes that cooperate with the compound to make a resistant cell line sensitive. This type of drop-out screen uses next-generation sequencing (NGS) to quantify the abundance of specific sgRNAs before and after a period of treatment with the compound of interest or with a sham treatment. Guides that knock out genes that confer sensitivity to the compound will be preferentially depleted in the compound-treated cultures as compared to the sham-treated cultures. It should be noted that these approaches do not always identify the target that the compound interacts with directly. Often, several genes are identified that may confer sensitivity or resistance as a result of adjacent dependencies or interacting pathways, and additional experiments are required to clarify the relationship between the genetic hit and the phenotypic hit.

A more direct approach to target deconvolution uses biophysical detection of target compound interaction. A commonly used method involves conjugating the compound of interest to a solid support, such as a microbead, exposing the conjugate to a cell lysate for binding to occur and then isolating the interacting protein(s) by centrifugation (pull-down) or elution from a column. Peptide sequencing can then be used to identify the protein(s) enriched in this way. This was the approach used by Handa and collaborators to identify cereblon as the molecular target of thalidomide, decades after its tragic introduction into humans and the discovery of its utility in the treatment of multiple myeloma (Ito et al. 2010). Despite the apparent elegance of this approach, its technical complexity presents numerous challenges to its successful execution. The conjugation of the compound to the solid substrate must be achieved in an orientation that does not hide the molecule's target binding moiety. This is constrained by the available reactive moieties used for the conjugation chemistry and the lack of knowledge of what part(s) of the molecule interacts with the target. Beyond that challenge, nonspecific binding to the molecule-bead complex in a complex mixture of proteins extracted from lysed cells can yield artifactual results. Deep expertise in chemistry and protein biochemistry and a willingness to try out multiple conditions for generating the lysate, incubation for binding, and pull-down or elution are required to even have a chance at a successful target identification effort. Whether through functional genetic or physicochemical approaches, target identification for a phenotypic hit is not a trivial exercise. Moreover, even identification of a target with great confidence does not always inform the development plan. It has been known for decades that dihydrofolate reductase (DHFR) is the molecular target of methotrexate and that beta tubulin is the target of the taxanes. This knowledge does not explain why one compound is useful for leukemia and the other for breast cancer. Even the identification of cereblon as the target of thalidomide and lenalidomide did not explain the mechanism of action of these drugs until it was shown that engagement of this E3 ligase subunit by these and structurally similar drugs induced the proteomic degradation of the transcription factors aiolos and ikaros, transcription factors that are critical for the pathogenesis of malignant plasma cells (Licht et al. 2015). Despite these limitations, phenotypic screening remains an important tool in drug discovery (Moffat et al. 2017). The remainder of the chapter will focus on target-based drug discovery.

2.4 Target-Based Drug Discovery: Considerations for Target Selection/Identification

The dominant approach to cancer drug discovery today leverages the explosion of knowledge of the molecular genetics and biochemistry of cancer to identify and explicitly pursue targets for pharmacologic intervention. Molecular targets include a wide range of intracellular enzymes, cell surface receptors, or ion channels and even structural components of large macromolecular complexes such as the proteasome. Although a complete survey of cancer target classes is beyond the scope of this chapter, there are many excellent reviews (Hahn et al. 2021; Hoelder et al. 2012; Yap and Workman 2012). Suffice it to say that a target can be any molecule that has been implicated, through genetic or other observations, in the pathogenesis of cancer. The paradigm shift to developing drugs based on molecular targets rather than tissue of origin or histology of the tumor will ultimately benefit pediatric oncology drug development. Even though the tissue of origin of cancers is different between children and adults, many of the molecular drivers of those cancers are shared. Cancer drugs developed initially for adult tumors are being tested in pediatric indications that share the same target.

Assembling a package of data implicating the intended target as a key driver of a particular type of cancer is critical, not only to justify the enormous commitment of resources that will be required to identify and advance chemical matter toward human testing but also to help guide the process. As with most difficult journeys, in drug discovery, it helps to begin with the end in mind. A good thought experiment at this step is to imagine that the perfect modulator of the intended target already exists and is ready for human testing. An ideal target enables a hypothesis-driven clinical development plan. This will be covered in greater detail in Chap. 5.

Most targets do not come with a built-in therapeutic hypothesis, and the process of selecting a target requires assembling a package of data that provides confidence that the target is a driver of a particular type of cancer. The academic cancer research literature has long been a rich source of potential molecular targets. Years of work in multiple laboratories have provided ample validation for the idea that pharmacologically neutralizing the mutated form of the RAS protein, for example, would have potent anti-tumor effects (Ryan and Corcoran 2018). Because many of the more obvious tumor driver targets have resisted efforts to develop pharmacologic inhibitors, there is a continual search for new potential targets. The explosion of knowledge about cancer genomics has led to the identification of target opportunities such as $BRAF^{V600E}$, a recurring mutation in melanoma, which has been successfully pursued (Kim et al. 2014). Similarly, recurring mutations in the isocitrate dehydrogenase (IDH) genes in AML led to the development of inhibitors that are currently approved for clinical use (Kim 2017; Norsworthy et al. 2019). In both cases, the commitment to pursue drug discovery efforts relied on molecular genetic data that suggested these were, in fact, drivers of the disease phenotype. This included the presence of the mutation across the malignant clone, suggesting that it was an early or foundational event in malignant transformation. Moreover, retention of the mutant allele in the face of the significant genomic instability associated with cancer speaks to a role for the mutation not only in the initiation of malignant transformation but also in the maintenance of this phenotype.

Such genetic "smoking gun" evidence implicating a molecular target as a disease driver is not always available or clear-cut, and validation efforts include experiments aimed at addressing the causal role of a target in establishing and maintaining tumor viability. For example, a suspected oncogenic driver mutation can be evaluated for its ability to confer neoplastic properties to normal cells in culture by enforced expression of a cDNA in transfected cells. Alternatively, the mutated gene can be used to generate a transgenic mouse to evaluate its causal relationship to tumor formation. In addition to interrogating the role of the mutated gene in tumor initiation, functional genomic tools can be used to evaluate the impact of eliminating the gene product on the growth and survival of a tumor expressing the mutant (Shalem et al. 2015; Nijman 2015). Methods for this type of genetic manipulation have evolved significantly in recent years and include the use of siRNA/shRNA to knock down the target mRNA, either transiently or inducibly, as well as CRISPR/Cas-9 systems in which the gene encoding the potential target is knocked out of the genome. In some cases, there are available chemical probes or tool compounds that modulate the target in question. These chemicals generally lack properties that could make them useful as drugs but can be used to evaluate the impact of target engagement in preclinical models (Arrowsmith et al. 2015). Each of these approaches has its limitations. For example, the complete ablation of a target by CRISPR far exceeds the degree of target inhibition that could be achieved pharmacologically and may overestimate the functional impact of drugging that target. Moreover, small molecule drugs typically inhibit a specific function of the target such as a catalytic domain, whereas knockdown and knockout approaches remove both the catalytic function and any structural or scaffolding role the target may play in the assembly or stability of multi-protein complexes (Shi et al. 2015). The use of chemical probes or tool compounds can be a useful adjunct to functional genomic approaches in target validation with the caveat that many of these compounds exhibit poor selectivity, engaging not only the target of interest but also close paralogs or even unrelated molecules (Arrowsmith et al. 2015). Because of these limitations, a robust target validation campaign relies on multiple cross-validating approaches. Discordant results between, for example, CRISPR and a tool inhibitor compound, if not well-understood, should give pause to pursuing a discovery program.

In addition to establishing a causal role for the target in driving the malignant phenotype, generating a testable hypothesis about which patients are likely to respond is an important component of target selection. In cases such as BRAF or ALK fusions, this is fairly straightforward in that the mutation defines both the target of the drug and the patient subset most likely to benefit from treatment with the drug. In the decades since the publication of the human genome, extensive cancer genomics efforts have unearthed a number of potentially druggable targets. These have predominantly been putative activating mutations in signaling kinases and have yielded important advances benefiting cancer patients. As a consequence of these advances and the ever-decreasing cost of DNA sequencing, genomic analysis of patient's tumors is becoming a more routine part of clinical oncology practice (Cancer Target Discovery and Development Network 2016). A sobering lesson from this exercise is that the vast majority of patients lack what has been termed an actionable mutation in their tumors (Ng et al. 2018; McGranahan et al. 2015). This is not only because suitable inhibitors have not yet been developed for all potential targets but because the mutations themselves do not suggest immediate targets. For example, it is estimated that 20% of human tumors have mutations in components of nucleosome remodeling complexes that play a key role in regulating access of transcription factors to enhancers and promoters (Kadoch and Crabtree 2015). These are almost exclusively loss of function rather than activating mutations and, therefore, do not suggest an immediate pharmacologic approach. To move beyond the current era of genomics-driven target identification will require novel approaches to link cancer mutations to corresponding therapeutic targets. Such approaches include synthetic lethality, where a loss of function in one gene leads to a critical dependence on another gene that can serve as a drug target. This was the approach that led to the development of the EZH2 inhibitor tazemetostat in rare sarcomas with loss of function mutations in the SWI/SNF nucleosome remodeling complex (Kim et al. 2015). Tremendous public data resources, such as the Cancer Dependency Map from the Broad Institute, have recently become available to enable both industry and academic drug discovery efforts (Tsherniak et al. 2017).

In summary, validation of a potential cancer target follows a weight-of-evidence approach, using orthogonal experimental approaches to build and reinforce confidence that a particular target merits the substantial effort that will be required to identify suitable chemical matter against it and to advance that chemical matter toward a drug-like molecule for human testing. Whether the intended target is an intracellular enzyme or a cell surface antigen, the experimental approach to its validation should be carefully planned and take into account the available tools and knowledge of the biology. Invalidating a target can be just as valuable as validating it by preventing the expenditure of resources to discover a drug without a clear path forward to clinical validation.

2.5 Target-Based Drug Discovery: Identifying Chemical Starting Points

Having established that a particular target merits the effort of a discovery campaign, the next step in target-based drug discovery is the identification of chemical or biologic starting points that can be evolved into a drug candidate. These starting points are merely the first steps in a long and iterative path from target concept to a Phase 1-ready compound. In the terminology of drug discovery, a hit is a compound that emerges from a screen, while leads are selected from among a number of hits based on more selective criteria. Because the path is filled with false starts and blind alleys, multiple potential leads are generated, of which only one or a few may be suitable for subsequent medicinal chemistry efforts. Which of the many hit discovery approaches to employ in a discovery campaign depends on the nature of the target as well as the capabilities of the team undertaking the effort.

An early consideration in small molecule drug discovery, prior to initiating screening efforts, is evaluating the available knowledge about the structure of the target. Small molecules can engage protein targets through a variety of three-dimensional interactions in aqueous media including hydrophobic or electrostatic interactions (Anderson 2003). Those interactions can modulate the function of the target protein, for example, by competing with a substrate or cofactor for the same binding site or by inducing a conformational change. Structural information for potential target proteins can be obtained through X-ray crystallography, nuclear magnetic resonance (NMR), or homology modeling approaches (Petros and Fesik 1994; Bordoli et al. 2009). An immense body of data on protein structures is available through the RCSB Protein Data Bank (n.d.). 3-D structures can provide valuable information about potential binding pockets, grooves, or other features that a small molecule of defined structure could bind in a specific manner (Shuker et al. 1996). Combined with knowledge of the amino acid sequence of the protein and its functional domains, this information can be used to refine the physical screening approach or even to perform a virtual screen. Using immensely powerful computer algorithms, it is possible to test thousands of small molecules in silico by docking or fitting their structures into features of protein crystal structures, taking into account electrostatic charges, presence or absence of water molecules, and other physical and thermodynamic variables. Predicted hits can then be followed up with "wet lab" experiments in which binding of the actual chemical to the target can be measured (McInnes 2007). This can greatly speed the discovery process if promising hits can be identified without having to set up and optimize a physical screen. Even if the primary screening approach is in vitro rather than in silico, structural data can be used to evaluate and prioritize screening hits based on how their structure is predicted to interact with key features of the target protein or even to start to optimize the hit by adding or removing chemical moieties to enhance binding potency or selectivity (Cui et al. 2011; Raman et al. 2019).

Although computational methods have become an important part of the hit identification process, biochemical screening is indispensable. A successful screening campaign requires access to a compound library of the appropriate composition and the ability to design and execute an assay to measure interaction between the compound and the target. Compound libraries can be enormous collections of chemical entities encompassing a wide range of structures or more focused collections with variations around a common feature. The former type of library, known as a diversity library, can have as few as tens of thousands of compounds in academic settings to as many as hundreds of thousands or even millions of compounds in the case of large pharmaceutical companies. Diversity libraries are curated to contain representation of multiple diverse families of structures or chemotypes and are useful for an unbiased approach to finding target interacting compounds or when there are no known structures that interact with the feature of interest in the target (Fox et al. 2006). In other cases, for example, when the target is a protein kinase, a focused library of a few thousand compounds that is enriched for structures that are likely to interact with known features of kinases can be used (Jacoby et al. 2018). This can reduce the number of false positive or nonspecific hits that are often identified in screens of larger unbiased screens. The compounds in these libraries are typically commercially available (i.e., not patented) although companies often supplement their compound libraries with chemical entities discovered in the course of other medicinal chemistry efforts.

The development of a biochemical assay to detect interaction between a compound in the library and the target of interest is a critical step in a screening campaign. It starts with identifying a source of the target protein to screen against. Generally, this requires isolating highly purified protein from cell or tissue extracts or, more commonly, recombinantly expressing the target in a prokaryotic or eukaryotic system (Hunt 2005). An advantage to the recombinant expression approach is that an epitope tag can be added to the target to aid in its purification and to attach it to a solid substrate for screening purposes. It is essential that the target protein retains its native structure and, in some cases, its enzymatic activity when purified to homogeneity or expressed as a recombinant protein. Certain classes of proteins, such as transcription factors, have intrinsically disordered domains that can only adopt their native structure when complexed with other proteins in large multi-subunit complexes (Tarczewska and Greb-Markiewicz 2019). Screening for binding to a largely unfolded protein like this cannot yield any specific or useful interactions. The reaction that is measured in a screening assay depends primarily on the nature of the target and the throughput of compounds required (i.e., the size of the library and available equipment). Enzymatic assays may be appropriate for targets with catalytic activity, while measuring binding of compounds is more suitable for targets like receptors that do not have enzymatic activity. As a rule, the simpler the assay format, the better. Enzymatic assays may require the addition of substrates, quenchers, often with washing steps in between and other reagents, to measure the products of the reaction, usually with colorimetric or luminescent readouts. Minimizing the steps involved and standardizing reagents is critical to ensure reliability of an assay that may be conducted in parallel in hundreds or thousands of 384 or 1536 well microtiter plates. The reliability or reproducibility of a screen is commonly expressed as a *Z* score that reflects the variability around the high and low end of the range of assay signals (Zhang et al. 1999). *Z* scores range from 0 to 1, and a score of 0.6 or more is considered a reliable assay in an industry screen.

An alternative approach to the use of diversity or focused libraries, which contain organic compounds of molecular weight around 500, is the use of fragment libraries. As the name implies, fragment libraries contain small or lower molecular weight structures that can be simple but highly diverse and interact with features of the target more freely but with lower affinity than the larger structures contained in diversity or focused sets (Jhoti 2007; Feyfant et al. 2011). Because these interactions are low affinity and incapable of inhibiting enzymatic or other protein function, detecting binding requires incubating high concentration of compounds with protein crystals and methods such as NMR spectroscopy to detect binding. A particularly interesting form of fragment libraries are so-called DNA-encoded libraries (DELs) in which a unique oligonucleotide code is attached to each fragment. After incubating the library with the target and washing steps, the identity of fragments enriched in the bound fraction is achieved by sequencing and counting the reads associated with each fragment (Brenner and Lerner 1992; Goodnow et al. 2017). Fragments can then be combined with other fragments directly or via linker fragments to create molecules that interact more stably and with higher affinity to the target. This relies on structure-guided design as described above.

2.6 Hit-to-Lead

Screening hits are only the first step in a long path to a clinical candidate that includes selecting which hits to advance to lead compounds for hit-to-lead (H2L) efforts, which lead or leads to take into lead optimization (LO) and, if all goes well, the nomination of a development candidate (DC) for IND-enabling studies. In the pharmaceutical industry, this process is guided by the target candidate profile (TCP), a list of specifications describing the ideal properties the candidate should have for the intended clinical application of the drug. If the drug's ultimate use will be for chronic, daily administration, an orally bioavailable form is critical. If, on the other hand, the drug is to be dosed a few days a month, an intravenous route of administration could be adequate. A threshold level of potency against the target, usually expressed as the concentration that reduces the response (binding or enzymatic activity) by half (IC_{50}) or that results in half of the maximal response (EC_{50}) is used as a standardized way to compare across hits. Additional requirements may include selectivity for the intended target over closely related paralogs of the target to minimize off-target toxicity. The importance of achieving a particular potency threshold depends on the anticipated pharmacokinetic properties of the drug and on the risk of off-target toxicity. A drug that can achieve limited plasma exposure, e.g., due to poor oral bioavailability, needs to be more potent than a highly bioavailable drug. High exposures, on the other hand, may magnify the risks of off-target toxicity if the drug is not sufficiently selective. Crafting a realistic TCP, with input from experienced drug developers, early in the discovery process is critical, but it should also be mentioned that the TCP is not set in stone. It can evolve over the span of a discovery effort to accommodate changes in the treatment landscape or technical innovations.

Medicinal chemists are responsible for driving the evolution of compounds toward DCs based on the specifications starting with the selection of hits to advance into leads. Essentially, this means selecting from among hits that have already undergone extensive validation through orthogonal screens and counter-screens to ensure that they truly engage with the target in a structure-driven manner. Hits at this stage typically have low (micromolar) potency and a host of potential physicochemical liabilities that need to be addressed and other key attributes that need to be preserved or enhanced. It is a common practice to select several leads representing different structural classes of compounds to increase the likelihood of generating at least one successful lead. The number selected depends on the output from the screen and the availability of chemists to synthesize and evaluate multiple analogues. The process of evolving leads through synthetic organic chemistry is iterative and driven by a growing body of knowledge about which chemical groups can affect solubility, metabolic stability, mutagenic potential, and many other factors that can affect drug-like properties. A classic example of the acquired knowledge that informs medicinal chemistry efforts is captured in Lipinski's rule of 5 (Lipinski et al. 2001). Based on empirical analysis of factors that impact cell permeability and oral absorption, Lipinski and others observed that the majority of existing oral drugs share many common features. These include molecular weights of less than 500, *C*log*P* (a measure of hydrophobicity) less than 5, fewer than 5 hydrogen bond donors or acceptors, etc. Keeping these and other design principles in mind, along with a helping of what can best be described as chemical intuition, medicinal chemists can take a hit with poor physicochemical properties and drive it toward a more drug-like molecule.

It is at this hit-to-lead stage that a reliable cell-based assay for target engagement also becomes important. While biochemical assays continue to play an important role in establishing the structure-activity relationship (SAR), this process in oncology drug discovery often relies on growth inhibition or cytotoxicity assays in cancer cell lines. The cell line(s) chosen to drive the cycles of SAR should have a clear dependence on the target in question to avoid driving the chemistry toward optimizing an off-target or nonspecific toxic effect. A cancer cell line that is not dependent on the target can serve as an important control to avoid this common pitfall. Many other types of cell-based assays have been developed including assays to measure changes in cell state such as differentiation, or to evaluate effects on reporter genes engineered into the cell line (Rozanov et al. 2019). This is where having a sound therapeutic hypothesis about the role of the target in the biology of the malignancy can be very helpful. As new molecules are synthesized, they undergo testing not only for the physical properties that the modification was intended to address but also in relevant cell line models to ensure that the desired activity and potency are retained or improved. This testing is carried out in a hierarchical cascade of assays that is tailored to the needs and challenges of a specific program.

An important part of any H2L cascade is addressing the compound's distribution, metabolism, and pharmacokinetic (DMPK) properties, also referred to as absorption, distribution, metabolism, and excretion (ADME). The best biochemical or cell-based performance of a molecule is of no use if it cannot achieve adequate plasma and tissue exposure in a patient. A drug, as opposed to a chemical compound, needs to enter the circulation either directly through intravenous administration or through absorption from the gut. It also needs to remain in circulation for some period of time and to partition into tissues such as tumor. This requires physicochemical properties that allow permeation into and across gut epithelium or vascular endothelial cells. Structures that are substrates for drug efflux pumps, present in many tissues, can also limit penetration. Metabolic enzymes can also rapidly attack and inactivate compounds in the liver. DMPK assessment of compound liabilities encompasses a range of standard assay formats that interrogate these properties in vitro. The colon carcinoma cell line Caco-2, for example, is commonly used to predict potential for permeability across the gut epithelium (Hubatsch et al. 2007). The compound is added to media above a monolayer of cells grown on a permeable membrane support. A coefficient of permeability is calculated by measuring the rate of compound flux from the media over to a chamber below the membrane. This can help predict gut permeability. In vitro assays are also used to evaluate a compound's susceptibility to drug efflux pumps and to metabolism by cytochrome enzymes (Gameiro et al. 2017). Incubating compounds in preparations of hepatocytes or liver microsomes is used to determine whether and in what way chemical structures are broken down and what the metabolic byproducts of this metabolism are. Finally, pharmacokinetic assessment of a compound in a pharmacology species, usually the mouse, is a critical step to advance a compound from H2L into the next stage of discovery.

2.7 Lead Optimization

If the hit-to-lead phase of discovery has been successful, there should be at least one molecule to advance into lead optimization (LO). As its name suggests, the objective of this stage is to optimize the drug-like properties of the compound to realize, as much as possible, the specifications in the TCP. This includes delivering proof of in vivo target-driven anti-tumor activity and an understanding of the relationship between exposure, target engagement, and efficacy in preclinical models. Any lead compounds that do not achieve adequate systemic exposure in animal models, either with oral or parenteral administration, typically do not advance from H2L to LO, despite how attractive their potency or selectivity might look in biochemical or cell-based assays (Waring et al. 2015). Even though the pool of potential candidates decreases with each successive stage gate transition in the discovery process, the resources required to clear the next gate go up. In LO, this increased cost is driven by more intensive medicinal chemistry efforts to refine the drug-like properties of the molecule more closely with the TCP and by the extensive in vivo pharmacology studies. Because of this, resource-constrained developers may require the lead candidate to demonstrate proof of anti-tumor activity in at least one animal model prior to advancing into investing in a LO program.

Animal models selected for in vivo pharmacology should, as much as possible, read out target-dependent anti-tumor effects of the compound rather than nonspecific or poorly understood cytotoxicity. In some cases, the same cell lines that have been used for in vitro experiments can be grown as subcutaneous xenografts in immunocompromised mice (Kerbel 2003). Not all cell lines grow robustly as xenografts, however, and it is also helpful to test the therapeutic hypothesis in multiple orthogonal models. These can include patient-derived xenografts (PDX), syngeneic allografts, and genetically engineered mouse models (GEMMs) (Okada et al. 2019; Webster et al. 2020). PDX models use fragments of resected tumor tissue from cancer patients that can be grown as subcutaneous implants in immunocompromised mouse strains. These models can be extensively characterized for mutation status, gene expression, and other molecular features and can be passaged serially in mice to generate a reliable experimental reagent. Growth inhibition of a PDX bearing the same mutation or gene expression profile that defines target dependence can provide robust proof-of-principle for the therapeutic hypothesis. One limitation of both cell line xenograft and PDX models is that both require an immunocompromised host and are, therefore, inappropriate to study anti-tumor effects mediated by the host immune system. Syngeneic allograft models and GEMMs enable the study of a murine tumor in the correct histocompatibility background in an immunocompetent host (Schaffer et al. 2010).

Consistent data from multiple models can provide robust validation of the target hypothesis and even an idea of the range of responses and sensitivity and resistance in various target-driven models. For working out the relationship between exposure, target engagement, and anti-tumor activity, however, it is best to focus efforts on a single "work-horse" model. The objective of these experiments is to gain a better understanding of the plasma and tissue exposure and target engagement parameters associated with response (Garralda et al. 2017). These experiments can inform the design of the 28-day GLP toxicology studies as well as human dose-finding studies. By varying dose and schedule of administration, it can be determined whether tumor response is most sensitive to the maximum plasma concentration (C_{max}), area under the concentration/time curve (AUC), or time above trough concentrations of the compound. Because the pharmacokinetic parameters of the compound in humans will be different from the mouse, it is critical to associate these PK parameters with target engagement or PD parameters such as the magnitude and duration of target modulation associated with response (Parchment and Doroshow 2016). These data can define the criteria for selecting a dose and schedule at the end of dose-finding studies in humans and provide context for toxicity.

In addition to proof-of-principle for the target, observing anti-tumor activity in a mouse xenograft model without overt toxicity (significant weight loss or even death) can provide some confidence that a therapeutic index exists for the compound. To more thoroughly de-risk the potential for significant toxicity, however, requires more formal toxicology studies as outlined in the ICH-S9 regulatory guidance (2010). At this stage, these types of studies can be conducted without invoking the rigid regulatory standards defined as Good Laboratory Practice (GLP). These will be described in greater detail in the next chapter. Dose-ranging toxicity studies typically administer high single doses and lower repeated doses up to 7 days to one rodent and in some cases to a non-rodent species. These dose-ranging toxicology studies to look for exaggerated pharmacologic effects of the compound and for the relationship of dose, exposure, and toxicity. In addition to informing the design of the IND-enabling toxicology studies, comparing the plasma concentrations of compound associated with severe toxicity or lethality to the concentrations required for anti-tumor activity can give an idea of how wide the therapeutic margin might be in the clinic.

2.8 Candidate Nomination

Lead compounds that meet or exceed the specifications of the TCP are considered development candidates (DCs). Nominating a DC is a major milestone in a discovery effort and a major decision for a drug development organization. In nominating a DC, the organization is committing to enter human testing within a year to 18 months which comes with a significant price tag. The process of selecting a target, conducting a screen to identify hits, and progressing those hits through H2L and LO take, on average, 3–5 years and $430 million (DiMasi et al. 2016). These costs, however, pale in comparison with the spend that will be required to drive the candidate to the next major milestone at the end of a first-in-humans clinical trial. These costs include scaling up manufacturing of the compound itself to provide sufficient material for formal toxicology studies conducted under GLP as well as for human testing (Garralda et al. 2017). The GLP toxicology studies themselves, which require one rodent and one non-rodent species dosed over a 28-day period with the compound at various doses as well as a matched group of animals dosed with a vehicle control, can cost millions of dollars. The data from these studies is used to select a starting dose with an ample safety margin for human trials and identifies potential target toxicities for the basis for the clinical safety monitoring plan in these trials. It is very unusual in oncology drug discovery to identify a "show-stopper" toxicity at this point. Cancer is a life-threatening condition, and toxicities that would be considered unacceptable in other therapeutic areas are unfortunately commonplace for cancer drugs. Nevertheless, a toxicity that is essentially catastrophic (i.e., potentially life-threatening, unmonitorable, and/or unreversible) can preclude a candidate from entering human studies. Such a toxicity should have revealed itself during the non-GLP dose-ranging toxicology studies but sometimes only become evident with more extended dosing in the GLP studies.

Manufacturing the active pharmaceutical ingredient (API) at a scale to supply the GLP toxicology studies and at a minimum, the Phase 1 program, is a significant at-risk investment that needs to be made well ahead of the start of these programs. Making compounds during H2L or LO is typically on small scales, on the order of a few grams to, perhaps, a few hundred grams to supply preclinical studies. At some point, as the lead that will become the DC starts to become evident, production needs to be scaled up to produce kilograms of compound in compliance with good manufacturing practice (GMP) regulations in the Food, Drug and Cosmetics Act Chapter V Part A (2018). This requires securing a stable supply of starting materials and, in most cases, establishing a contractual agreement with a Contract Drug Manufacturing Organization (CDMO). Although many large pharmaceutical companies have some GMP manufacturing capacity internally, they are often functioning at capacity to make marketed products and not available for products in research and development. The synthetic routes that were adequate to supply non-GMP-compliant compound during earlier stages of discovery are often inadequate for large-scale production of clinical material. The process chemistry that explores various ways of improving the reproducibility, yield, and purity of a compound is usually done internally. Although Phase 1 studies typically use simple preparations, such as API powder in a capsule, in some cases, formulation of the API with various excipients may be required to improve its stability or dissolution properties. The API is sometimes referred to as the drug substance, whereas the final form that will be dosed is called the drug product. Candidates that will be administered parenterally generally require some formulation work to address solubility issues. In addition to process chemistry, analytical methods to assess the purity of the drug product must be developed and validated. These synthetic, formulation and analytical methods are transferred to a CDMO.

Obtaining permission to initiate human trials from competent health authorities (HAs) such as the US Food and Drug Administration (FDA) and the European Medicines Agency (EMA) constitutes another resource-intensive workstream tied to candidate nomination (FDA 2021; EMA 2022). Preparing an Investigational New Drug (IND) application for FDA or a Clinical Trial Authorization (CTA) for EMA and other ex-US HAs can take many months and the coordinated activity of a large cross-functional team. At its core, an IND or CTA is a document that provides HA reviewers with information to evaluate whether human testing is warranted and does not expose human subjects to undue risks of toxicity or death. The pharmacology section provides in vitro and in vivo data to support the potential benefit of the drug in cancer, but most of the focus is on the nonclinical safety and manufacturing information and the planned clinical development of the drug to evaluate the risks. The safety testing to identify potential toxic effects of the drug will be described in great detail in the next chapter. Specialist reviewers at HAs pay particular attention to the chemistry, manufacturing, and controls (CMC) section of the application. This is where the sponsor lays out how the drug is made and characterizes the drug substance in terms of degree of purity and any residual contaminants in the final product either from solvents or other reagents in the manufacturing process or byproducts of synthesis. The analytical methods for this characterization and their validation are also described here. Finally, the IND or CTA includes an overall clinical plan, and a detailed clinical protocol for the first-in-humans trial is included as well as an investigator brochure that summarizes all of the information in the IND for trial site staff. The clinical protocol will be described in greater detail in Chap. 5 but, in essence, is where all of the information in the IND or CTA is integrated to describe an experiment to understand the safety, PK, PD, and, hopefully, a glimpse of clinical activity while mitigating any potential risks to patients.

In summary, the drug discovery process is a lengthy, costly, iterative process with many challenges and no guarantee of success but, nevertheless, one that is critical for improving and extending the lives of both adults and children with cancer. The considerable up-front investment required just to get from a target concept to a drug candidate and the drug development challenges and limited market opportunity associated with pediatric cancer explain why most companies do not explicitly pursue pediatric cancer targets. Fortunately, many of the targets that are being pursued for adult malignancies also play a role in childhood cancers, and every effort needs to be made to ensure that children have access to these drug candidates as early as is feasible in their development.

References

Anderson AC (2003) The process of structure-based drug design. Chem Biol 10:787–797. https://doi.org/10.1016/j.chembiol.2003.09.002

Arrowsmith CH, Audia JE, Austin C, Baell J, Bennett J, Blagg J, Bountra C, Brennan PE, Brown PJ, Bunnage ME, Buser-Doepner C, Campbell RM, Carter AJ, Cohen P, Copeland RA, Cravatt B, Dahlin JL, Dhanak D, Edwards AM, Frederiksen M, Frye SV, Gray N, Grimshaw CE, Hepworth D, Howe T, Huber KV, Jin J, Knapp S, Kotz JD, Kruger RG, Lowe D, Mader MM, Marsden B, Mueller-Fahrnow A, Müller S, O'Hagan RC, Overington JP, Owen

DR, Rosenberg SH, Roth B, Ross R, Schapira M, Schreiber SL, Shoichet B, Sundström M, Superti-Furga G, Taunton J, Toledo-Sherman L, Walpole C, Walters MA, Willson TM, Workman P, Young RN, Zuercher WJ (2015) The promise and peril of chemical probes. Nat Chem Biol 11(8):536–541. https://doi.org/10.1038/nchembio.1867. Erratum in: Nat Chem Biol. 2015;11(8):541. Roth, Brian [Corrected to Roth, Bryan] and Frederiksen, Mathias [Added]. Erratum in: Nat Chem Biol. 2015;11(11):887

Bordoli L, Kiefer F, Arnold K, Benkert P, Battey J, Schwede T (2009) Protein structure homology modeling using SWISS-MODEL workspace. Nat Protoc 4(1):1–13. https://doi.org/10.1038/nprot.2008.197

Brenner S, Lerner RA (1992) Encoded combinatorial chemistry. Proc Natl Acad Sci U S A 89:5381–5383

Cancer Target Discovery and Development Network (2016) Transforming big data into cancer-relevant insight: an initial, multi-tier approach to assess reproducibility and relevance. Mol Cancer Res 14(8):675–682. https://doi.org/10.1158/1541-7786.MCR-16-0090. Epub 2016 Jul 11

The Cancer Cell Line Encyclopedia enables predictive modelling of anticancer drug sensitivity. Nature 2012;483(7391):603–7. https://doi.org/10.1038/nature11003. https://sites.broadinstitute.org/ccle/

Conant J (2020) The Great Secret: the classified world war II disaster that launched the war on cancer. W.W. Norton & Co., New York

Cui JJ, Tran-Dubé M, Shen H, Nambu M, Kung PP, Pairish M, Jia L, Meng J, Funk L, Botrous I, McTigue M, Grodsky N, Ryan K, Padrique E, Alton G, Timofeevski S, Yamazaki S, Li Q, Zou H, Christensen J, Mroczkowski B, Bender S, Kania RS, Edwards MP (2011) Structure based drug design of crizotinib (PF-02341066), a potent and selective dual inhibitor of mesenchymal-epithelial transition factor (c-MET) kinase and anaplastic lymphoma kinase (ALK). J Med Chem 54:6342–6363. https://doi.org/10.1021/jm2007613. Epub 2011 Aug 18

DeVita V Jr, DeVita-Raeburn E (2015) The death of cancer. Macmillan, New York

DiMasi JA, Grabowski HG, Hansen RW (2016) Innovation in the pharmaceutical industry: new estimates of R&D costs. J Health Econ 47:20–33. https://doi.org/10.1016/j.jhealeco.2016.01.012. Epub 2016 Feb 12

EMA (2022) EMA CTA process. http://data.europa.eu/eli/reg/2014/536/oj

FDA (2021) FDA IND process. https://www.fda.gov/drugs/types-applications/investigational-new-drug-ind-application

Feyfant E, Cross JB, Paris K, Tsao DH (2011) Fragment-based drug design. Methods Mol Biol 685:241–252. https://doi.org/10.1007/978-1-60761-931-4_12

Fox S, Farr-Jones S, Sopchak L, Boggs A, Nicely HW, Khoury R, Biros M (2006) High-throughput screening: update on practices and success. J Biomol Screen 11(7):864–869. https://doi.org/10.1177/1087057106292473. Epub 2006 Sept 14

Gameiro M, Silva R, Rocha-Pereira C, Carmo H, Carvalho F, Bastos ML, Remião F (2017) Cellular models and in vitro assays for the screening of modulators of P-gp, MRP1 and BCRP. Molecules 22:600. https://doi.org/10.3390/molecules22040600

Garralda E, Dienstmann R, Tabernero J (2017) Pharmacokinetic/pharmacodynamic modeling for drug development in oncology. Am Soc Clin Oncol Educ Book 3(7):210–215. https://doi.org/10.1200/EDBK_180460

GMP (2018) GMP Guidance document. https://www.fda.gov/regulatory-information/search-fda-guidance-documents/guidance-industry-q7a-good-manufacturing-practice-guidance-active-pharmaceutical-ingredients

Goodnow RA, Dumelin CE, Keefe AD (2017) DNA-encoded chemistry: enabling the deeper sampling of chemical space. Nat Rev Drug Discov 16:131–147

Hahn WC, Bader JS, Braun TP, Califano A, Clemons PA, Druker BJ, Ewald AJ, Fu H, Jagu S, Kemp CJ, Kim W, Kuo CJ, McManus M, Mills GB, Mo X, Sahni N, Schreiber SL, Talamas JA, Tamayo P, Tyner JW, Wagner BK, Weiss WA, Gerhard DS, Cancer Target Discovery and Development Network (2021) An expanded universe of cancer targets. Cell 184:1142–1155. https://doi.org/10.1016/j.cell.2021.02.020

Hoelder S, Clarke PA, Workman P (2012) Discovery of small molecule cancer drugs: successes, challenges and opportunities. Mol Oncol 6:155–176

Horvath P, Aulner N, Bickle M, Davies AM, Nery ED, Ebner D, Montoya MC, Östling P, Pietiäinen V, Price LS, Shorte SL, Turcatti G, von Schantz C, Carragher NO (2016) Screening out irrelevant cell-based models of disease. Nat Rev Drug Discov 15(11):751–769. https://doi.org/10.1038/nrd.2016.175. Epub 2016 Sept 12

Hubatsch I, Ragnarsson EG, Artursson P (2007) Determination of drug permeability and prediction of drug absorption in Caco-2 monolayers. Nat Protoc 2:2111–2119. https://doi.org/10.1038/nprot.2007.303

Hunt I (2005) From gene to protein: a review of new and enabling technologies for multi-parallel protein expression. Protein Expr Purif 40:1–22. https://doi.org/10.1016/j.pep.2004.10.018

ICH-S9 (2010) ICH-S9 Guidance document. https://www.fda.gov/regulatory-information/search-fda-guidance-documents/s9-nonclinical-evaluation-anticancer-pharmaceuticals

Ito T, Ando H, Suzuki T, Ogura T, Hotta K, Imamura Y, Yamaguchi Y, Handa H (2010) Identification of a primary target of thalidomide teratogenicity. Science 327:1345–1350

Jacoby E, Wroblowski B, Buyck C, Neefs JM, Meyer C, Cummings MD, van Vlijmen H (2018) Protocols for the design of kinase-focused compound libraries. Mol Inform 37:e1700119. https://doi.org/10.1002/minf.201700119. Epub 2017 Nov 8

Jhoti H (2007) Fragment-based drug discovery using rational design. Ernst Schering Found Symp Proc 3:169–185. https://doi.org/10.1007/2789_2007_064

Kadoch C, Crabtree GR (2015) Mammalian SWI/SNF chromatin remodeling complexes and cancer: Mechanistic insights gained from human genomics. Sci Adv 1(5):e1500447. https://doi.org/10.1126/sciadv.1500447

Kerbel RS (2003) Human tumor xenografts as predictive preclinical models for anticancer drug activity in humans: better than commonly perceived-but they can be improved. Cancer Biol Ther 2(4 Suppl 1):S134–S139

Kim ES (2017) Enasidenib: first global approval. Drugs: 1705–1711. https://doi.org/10.1007/s40265-017-0813-2

Kim G, McKee AE, Ning YM, Hazarika M, Theoret M, Johnson JR, Xu QC, Tang S, Sridhara R, Jiang X, He K, Roscoe D, McGuinn WD, Helms WS, Russell AM, Miksinski SP, Zirkelbach JF, Earp J, Liu Q, Ibrahim A, Justice R, Pazdur R (2014) FDA approval summary: vemurafenib for treatment of unresectable or metastatic melanoma with the BRAFV600E mutation. Clin Cancer Res 20:4994–5000. https://doi.org/10.1158/1078-0432.CCR-14-0776. Epub 2014 Aug 5

Kim KH, Kim W, Howard TP, Vazquez F, Tsherniak A, Wu JN, Wang W, Haswell JR, Walensky LD, Hahn WC, Orkin SH, Roberts CW (2015) SWI/SNF-mutant cancers depend on catalytic and non-catalytic activity of EZH2. Nat Med 21:1491–1496. https://doi.org/10.1038/nm.3968. Epub 2015 Nov 9

Licht JD, Shortt J, Johnstone R (2015) From anecdote to targeted therapy: the curious case of thalidomide in multiple myeloma. Cancer Cell 25:9–11

Lipinski CA, Lombardo F, Dominy BW, Feeney PJ (2001) Experimental and computational approaches to estimate solubility and permeability in drug discovery and development settings. Adv Drug Deliv Rev 46:3–26

McGranahan N, Favero F, de Bruin EC, Birkbak NJ, Szallasi Z, Swanton C (2015) Clonal status of actionable driver events and the timing of mutational processes in cancer evolution. Sci Transl Med 7:283ra54. https://doi.org/10.1126/scitranslmed.aaa1408

McInnes C (2007) Virtual screening strategies in drug discovery. Curr Opin Chem Biol 11(5):494–502. https://doi.org/10.1016/j.cbpa.2007.08.033

Moffat JG, Vincent F, Lee JA, Eder J, Prunotto M (2017) Opportunities and challenges in phenotypic drug discovery: an industry perspective. Nat Rev Drug Discov 16(8):531–543. https://doi.org/10.1038/nrd.2017.111. Epub 2017 Jul 7

Mukherjee S (2010) The emperor of all maladies. Scribner, New York

Ng PK, Li J, Jeong KJ, Shao S, Chen H, Tsang YH, Sengupta S, Wang Z, Bhavana VH, Tran R, Soewito S, Minussi DC, Moreno D, Kong K, Dogruluk T, Lu H, Gao J, Tokheim C, Zhou DC, Johnson AM, Zeng J, Ip CKM, Ju Z, Wester M, Yu S, Li Y, Vellano CP, Schultz N, Karchin R, Ding L, Lu Y, Cheung LWT, Chen K, Shaw KR, Meric-Bernstam F, Scott KL, Yi S, Sahni N, Liang H, Mills GB (2018) Systematic functional annotation of somatic mutations in cancer. Cancer Cell 33:450–462.e10. https://doi.org/10.1016/j.ccell.2018.01.021

Nijman SMB (2015) Functional genomics to uncover drug mechanism of action. Nat Chem Biol 11:942–948

Norsworthy KJ, Luo L, Hsu V, Gudi R, Dorff SE, Przepiorka D, Deisseroth A, Shen YL, Sheth CM, Charlab R, Williams GM, Goldberg KB, Farrell AT, Pazdur R (2019) FDA approval summary: ivosidenib for relapsed or refractory acute myeloid leukemia with an isocitrate dehydrogenase-1 mutation. Clin Cancer Res 25:3205–3209. https://doi.org/10.1158/1078-0432.CCR-18-3749. Epub 2019 Jan 28

Okada S, Vaeteewoottacharn K, Kariya R (2019) Application of highly immunocompromised mice for the establishment of patient-derived xenograft (PDX) models. Cell 8(8):889. https://doi.org/10.3390/cells8080889

Parchment RE, Doroshow JH (2016) Pharmacodynamic endpoints as clinical trial objectives to answer important questions in oncology drug development. Semin Oncol 43:514–525. https://doi.org/10.1053/j.seminoncol.2016.07.002. Epub 2016 Jul 26

Pereira RB, Evdokimov NM, Lefranc F, Valentão P, Kornienko A, Pereira DM, Andrade PB, Gomes NGM (2019) Marine-derived anticancer agents: clinical benefits, innovative mechanisms, and new targets. Mar Drugs 17:329. https://doi.org/10.3390/md17060329

Petros AM, Fesik SW (1994) Nuclear magnetic resonance methods for studying protein-ligand complexes. Methods Enzymol 239:717–739. https://doi.org/10.1016/s0076-6879(94)39027-4

Raman S, Beilschmidt M, To M, Lin K, Lui F, Jmeian Y, Ng M, Fernandez M, Fu Y, Mascall K, Duque A, Wang X, Pan G, Angers S, Moffat J, Sidhu SS, Magram J, Sinclair AM, Fransson J, Julien JP (2019) Structure-guided design fine-tunes pharmacokinetics, tolerability, and antitumor profile of multispecific frizzled antibodies. Proc Natl Acad Sci U S A 116:6812–6817. https://doi.org/10.1073/pnas.1817246116. Epub 2019 Mar 20

RCSB Protein Data Bank (n.d.). https://www.rcsb.org/

Research Paradigm (1955–1975) Mouse L1210 leukemia model. https://dtp.cancer.gov/timeline/flash/milestones/M9_L1210.htm

Rozanov D, Cheltsov A, Nilsen A, Boniface C, Forquer I, Korkola J, Gray J, Tyner J, Tognon CE, Mills GB, Spellman P (2019) Targeting mitochondria in cancer therapy could provide a basis for the selective anticancer activity. PLoS One 14:e0205623. https://doi.org/10.1371/journal.pone.0205623

Ryan MB, Corcoran RB (2018) Therapeutic strategies to target RAS-mutant cancers. Nat Rev Clin Oncol 15:709–720. https://doi.org/10.1038/s41571-018-0105-0

Schaffer BS, Grayson MH, Wortham JM, Kubicek CB, McCleish AT, Prajapati SI, Nelon LD, Brady MM, Jung I, Hosoyama T, Sarro LM, Hanes MA, Rubin BP, Michalek JE, Clifford CB, Infante AJ, Keller C (2010) Immune competency of a hairless mouse strain for

improved preclinical studies in genetically engineered mice. Mol Cancer Ther 9(8):2354–2364. https://doi.org/10.1158/1535-7163.MCT-10-0207. Epub 2010 Jul 27
Scheeder C, Heigwer F, Boutros M (2018) Machine learning and image-based profiling in drug discovery. Curr Opin Syst Biol 10:43–52. https://doi.org/10.1016/j.coisb.2018.05.004
Shalem O, Sanjana NE, Zhang F (2015) High-throughput functional genomics using CRISPR-Cas9. Nat Rev Genet 16:299–311
Shi J, Wang E, Milazzo JP, Wang Z, Kinney JB, Vakoc CR (2015) Discovery of cancer drug targets by CRISPR-Cas9 screening of protein domains. Nat Biotechnol 33:661–667. https://doi.org/10.1038/nbt.3235. Epub 2015 May 11
Shuker SB, Hajduk PJ, Meadows RP, Fesik SW (1996) Discovering high-affinity ligands for proteins: SAR by NMR. Science 274:1531–1534. https://doi.org/10.1126/science.274.5292.1531
Tarczewska A, Greb-Markiewicz B (2019) The significance of the intrinsically disordered regions for the functions of the bHLH transcription factors. Int J Mol Sci 20:5306. https://doi.org/10.3390/ijms20215306
Tsherniak A, Vazquez F, Montgomery PG, Weir BA, Kryukov G, Cowley GS, Gill S, Harrington WF, Pantel S, Krill-Burger JM, Meyers RM, Ali L, Goodale A, Lee Y, Jiang G, Hsiao J, Gerath WFJ, Howell S, Merkel E, Ghandi M, Garraway LA, Root DE, Golub TR, Boehm JS, Hahn WC (2017) Defining a cancer dependency map. Cell 170:564–576.e16. https://doi.org/10.1016/j.cell.2017.06.010. https://depmap.org/portal/depmap/
Waring MJ, Arrowsmith J, Leach AR, Leeson PD, Mandrell S, Owen RM, Pairaudeau G, Pennie WD, Pickett SD, Wang J, Wallace O, Weir A (2015) An analysis of the attrition of drug candidates from four major pharmaceutical companies. Nat Rev Drug Discov 14:475–486. https://doi.org/10.1038/nrd4609. Epub 2015 Jun 19
Webster JD, Santagostino SF, Foreman O (2020) Applications and considerations for the use of genetically engineered mouse models in drug development. Cell Tissue Res 380(2):325–340. https://doi.org/10.1007/s00441-019-03101-y. Epub 2019 Sept 5
Yap TA, Workman P (2012) Exploiting the cancer genome: strategies for the discovery and clinical development of targeted molecular therapeutics. Annu Rev Pharmacol Toxicol 52:549–573. https://doi.org/10.1146/annurev-pharmtox-010611-134532
Zeldis JB, Knight R, Hussein M, Chopra R, Muller G (2011) A review of the history, properties, and use of the immunomodulatory compound lenalidomide. Ann N Y Acad Sci. https://doi.org/10.1111/j.1749-6632.2011.05974.x
Zhang JH, Chung TD, Oldenburg KR (1999) A simple statistical parameter for use in evaluation and validation of high throughput screening assays. J Biomol Screen 4:67–73. https://doi.org/10.1177/108705719900400206

3 An FDA Oncology Perspective of Juvenile Toxicity Studies to Support Pediatric Drug Development

John K. Leighton and Whitney Helms

Contents

3.1 Introduction

In 2016, the FDA Office of Oncologic Diseases (formerly the Office of Hematology and Oncology Products) published their view of the utility of juvenile animal studies (JAS) to support clinical development in pediatric patients for the treatment of cancer (Leighton et al. 2016). After reviewing the available data in our files and considering how clinical trials are conducted in pediatric populations, FDA Oncology concluded that JAS were generally not warranted, consistent with the position described in the ICH S9 Guidance for Industry: Nonclinical Evaluation for Anticancer Pharmaceuticals (FDA 2010). The reasons for both the Office's conclusion and the original basis for the statement in the guidance were that available clinical data in adult patients could be used to inform on monitoring and to set a start dose; that the life expectancy of pediatric patients in phase 1 or 2 trials was relatively short; that there was adequate monitoring for potential adverse events in this patient population; and that there were benefits to not delaying the clinical development of potentially promising drugs for pediatric patients with advanced cancer. They concluded that a JAS initiated or completed after a clinical trial in pediatric patients was ongoing or complete was of little

J. K. Leighton (✉) · W. Helms
Division of Hematology Oncology Toxicology, Office of Oncologic Diseases, Center for Drug Evaluation and Research, U.S. Food and Drug Administration, Silver Spring, MD, USA
e-mail: john.leighton@fda.hhs.gov

J. DiMartino et al. (eds.), *Pediatric Cancer Therapeutics Development*, Pediatric Oncology,
https://doi.org/10.1007/978-3-031-06357-2_3

to no value unless there was a specific question to be asked and the data to answer this question could not be obtained through clinical studies. It is usually the scenario in the oncology setting that clinical trials in adults are ongoing or complete prior to the initiation of clinical trials in pediatric patients, with the rare exception of the monoclonal antibodies to treat patients with neuroblastoma (dinutuximab and naxitamab). These drugs are discussed in more detail below. Also discussed in more detail below are the NTRK inhibitors; one of the drugs, larotrectinib, is approved for pediatric patients 28 days and older. Both drugs in this class are also approved for use in adults.

Since 2016 two new comprehensive reviews were published expressing contrasting opinions. In November 2017 EMA (2017) published a final document titled "Results of juvenile animal studies (JAS) and the impact on anti-cancer medicine development and use in children." Included among the benefits of JAS articulated in this paper were the need for more information, deferring inclusion of the youngest pediatric patients, waiver of additional pediatric studies in children less than 2 years of age, and recommendations on clinical trial design. Contrarily, Visalli et al. (2018) published a review titled "Lack of value of juvenile animal toxicity studies for supporting the safety of pediatric oncology phase 1 studies" looking at a dataset similar to that in the EMA paper that included 25 molecularly targeted drugs and 4 biologics. These authors concluded that the first pediatric dose was safe for all 29 drugs, that no life-threatening adverse events occurred in the first cohort, that the maximum tolerated dose (MTD) in pediatrics compared to the MTD in adults was close to 1, and that standard JAS would not have predicted the serious adverse events that did occur but were not picked up in standard clinical monitoring plans. The differing conclusions may be partly due to differences in the analysis: the EMA focused on differences in juvenile vs. adult animals, whereas Visalli et al. focused on dose setting and clinical monitoring when considering the value of JAS. A search of the PubMed database did not reveal any more recent reviews of JAS from 2016.

Now is perhaps an opportune time to reexamine the utility of JAS in oncology drug development. Have we learned anything in the studies that have been conducted? Since the 2016 publication by Leighton et al., ICH published a Question and Answers document for ICH S9 (FDA 2018b) that does not address JAS, and the ICH S11 (FDA 2021). This paper will briefly summarize the positions described in the S9 Q&A and S11 Guidance documents regarding JAS and oncology drugs as well as FDA Oncology's analysis of JAS conducted over the last few years, with particular focus on the approved anti-GD2 antibodies and the NTRK inhibitors due to the available data and the roles of both of these targets in the CNS. JAS conducted for other products will not be discussed in this paper as FDA Oncology has not routinely requested JAS to support pediatric drug development. Note that presence of JAS data in a product label should not be taken as an indication that the study was specifically requested or of the added benefit of the study, as labeling practices call for the inclusion of information from a JAS in Section 8.4 of a product label regardless of the impact of the nonclinical study on the clinical trial.

This paper will not discuss the role of pharmacology studies in assessing whether a clinical trial in pediatric patients is appropriate. Arguably, these proof-of-concept and mechanistic studies are more important than juvenile toxicity studies in that they lay the foundation for the initial Pediatric Study Plan and the study; without an adequate mechanistic understanding of the drug in the context of the disease, patients may be enrolling in a study which will be of little value, if any, for their treatment. For example, in vitro or in vivo nonclinical data (including in silico data, mechanism-based in vitro data, and appropriate tumor models) can inform the potential response to a treatment, and thus provide support for the inclusion of children from 2 to under 12 (see the final FDA Guidance on Cancer Clinical Trial Eligibility, March 2020a).

3.2 Should a JAS Be Considered?

A juvenile animal study (JAS) to support an oncology indication in a pediatric population is often not needed. But on rare occasions, a JAS may be considered, such as when there are no data in adults (product to be developed in children only) and a long life expectancy is anticipated for the study participants. While ICH S11 is mainly for non-oncology indications, the weight of evidence (WoE) approach described in this guidance may be consulted when considering a JAS. Given the nature of the disease and the monitoring usually in place for clinical trials for oncology drugs, the available clinical data and nonclinical studies in adult animals are usually considered sufficient to initiate a pediatric trial, and, thus, a JAS is not usually warranted. This principle was outlined in ICH S9. The rationale for FDA Oncology's position that JAS are generally not warranted was further articulated by Leighton et al. (2016) and need not be repeated here. If there are age-dependent safety concerns regarding the conduct of a clinical trial in pediatric population, then a staggered age enrollment may be considered.

3.2.1 ICH S11: Nonclinical Safety Testing in Support of Development of Pediatric Medicines

The ICH S11 Guidance, finalized in 2020, does not replace the recommendations in ICH S9 but can be consulted as needed, e.g., for JAS design when a study is warranted. The objective of the S11 Guidance, like most ICH guidances, is to promote harmonization and to apply the principles of the 3Rs; reduce, refine, and replace the use of animals where appropriate. Consistent with ICH S9, the S11 Guidance states that nonclinical studies should be undertaken only when available nonclinical and clinical data are judged to be inadequate to support the safety of a clinical trial in pediatric patients. The S11 Guidance provides key factors to consider in a weight of evidence determination to assess whether additional nonclinical studies are needed, and information on the design of nonclinical studies to support a pediatric development program. The guidance also discusses that for severely debilitating and life-threatening diseases, the information obtained should be weighed against the potential delay in clinical development, a consideration that would generally encompass anticancer drugs proposed for use in pediatric patients.

3.2.2 ICH S9: Nonclinical Evaluation for Anticancer Pharmaceuticals Questions and Answers

The main ICH S9 Guidance on nonclinical development for anticancer pharmaceuticals was published in 2010 and stated that in general JAS were not warranted to support the development of drugs intended for the treatment of patients with cancer; however, even after publication of the guidance, the Agency noted that developers were still often conducting JAS and submitting these studies to INDs or to marketing applications. The reason for the continued frequency of JAS conducted to support the safety of oncology drugs was not obvious; it could have been a timing issue with studies initiated prior to finalizing the guidance, or perhaps regulatory agencies in other regions were requesting these studies. To provide additional clarity around this and other topics discussed in ICH S9, a Concept Paper (CP; available at ich.org) was proposed to the ICH Steering Committee and endorsed on 23 October 2014. The CP did not specifically mention juvenile toxicity studies. Nevertheless, in response to feedback received from various stakeholders in developing the Q&A, the S9 Implementation Working Group (IWG) formed after adoption of the CP received questions for clarification on this topic. A draft Q&A was published on 8 June 2016 at Regulations.gov (docket # FDA 2016-D-2569) that included the following juvenile animal discussion:

Q: The guideline states that juvenile animal studies should be considered only when human safety data and previous animal data are insufficient. Under what situations would a juvenile animal study be warranted? What should be the goal of a juvenile animal study to support development in paediatric patients with cancer?

Draft response: Juvenile toxicity studies should only be performed when available animal models are believed to generate data relevant for paediatric safety, and there is a clear value for such data for supporting clinical paediatric development. This is normally not the case for paediatric clinical trials in children with limited available therapeutic options and short life expectancy. Clinical data from adults is typically available prior to initiation of these paediatric trials; this data is used to set a starting dose and inform monitoring plans. In addition, these trials are usually done in a controlled setting with substantial safety monitoring. Pharmacology data and toxicology data from adult animals can also inform on safety.

When clinical development is pursued in children with longer life expectancy, the need for juvenile toxicity testing should be a case by case decision based on the available knowledge on pharmacology, nonclinical and clinical safety and the presence of safety concerns where a juvenile toxicity study could add important information. When studies are needed, ICH S11 should be consulted to address the design of the juvenile animal study. A dialogue with the regulatory agency is also encouraged.

To support the clinical development in a paediatric-only indication, the age of animals in the repeat-dose toxicity studies should be chosen to cover the age of the patient population in the initial clinical trials.

The FDA did not receive any comments to the docket regarding this question during the public comment period, but objections were raised in the deliberations of the IWG subsequent to the publication of the draft Step 2 guidance. The IWG explored various wordings to achieve harmonization, but could not reach consensus and, thus, decided that removing the reference to JAS entirely would allow sponsors more freedom to have discussions with regional regulators. For this reason, the Step 2 draft language was removed, and there is no reference to JAS in the final S9 Q&A guidance published in 2018.

3.3 Dinutuximab and Naxitamab

The anti-GD2 antibodies Unituxin (dinutuximab) (FDA 2015) and Danyelza (naxitamab-GQGK) (FDA 2020b) were approved in 2015 and 2020, respectively. Both products were follow-ons to murine antibodies against human GD2 originally developed in academic settings in the 1980s. As expected of a murine antibody, development of human anti-murine antibodies limited clinical utility leading developers to develop chimeric or fully humanized versions of the products as clinical development proceeded. The biology, chemistry, and nonclinical and clinical development of the anti-GD2 antibodies have been reviewed by Sait and Modak (2017). A major side effect noted in these trials is neuropathic pain, which was moderated in those patients developing an immunogenic response.

Dinutuximab (ch14.18), a chimeric IgG1 antibody produced in the murine SP2/0 cell line, is now a standard therapy for treatment of pediatric patients with high-risk neuroblastoma. It was also studied in adults at Memorial Sloan Kettering between 1979 and 2015 for the same indication (Suzuki et al. 2018). The major side effect of dinutuximab is neuropathic pain, probably related to the pharmacologic activity of the drug. There were no long-term toxicology studies conducted with dinutuximab, and the majority of the clinical experience was in combination with other therapies (IL-2 and/or GM-CSF). There was limited chronic toxicity data in either human adults or in animals, and questions related to recovery of neurotoxicity remained, particularly in still developing brains. For these reasons a post-marketing requirement (PMR) to conduct a JAS in cynomolgus monkeys of 5-month duration was requested for dinutuximab to further understand the potential neurotoxicity and potential for recovery. The PMR requested a detailed evaluation of the central and peripheral nervous systems, with 7–8 slices of the brain for histopathological assessment and long-term evaluation for potential effects on nociception and pain threshold at the end of an appropriate recovery period. Section 8.4 of the original label has since been updated to reflect the results of this JAS. The main findings of the study were degeneration in the dorsal root ganglia that persisted 6 months after cessation of dosing, although with lesser severity, and decreased nerve conduction velocity that also showed signs of slow reversibility after 6 months.

Naxitamab (hu3F8-IgG1) is a humanized version of m3F8 (a murine version of the antibody).

It is reported to be associated with much less immunogenicity than its murine precursor, and higher doses are tolerated (Sait and Modak 2017). Due to concerns regarding the relevance of the model chosen to assess the toxicity of this product (the nude rat) and the age of the only indicated patient population, a JAS in a relevant species similar in design to that requested for dinutuximab was also requested as a PMR for naxitamab. According to the PMR timelines, a final report is expected in July 2023.

3.4 TRK Inhibitors

Trk proteins have an established role in neuronal development (Smeyne et al. 1994; Tucker et al. 2001). Published reports of congenital somatic mutations in TRK proteins or their ligands suggest a relationship between deficient Trk signaling and development of schizophrenia, mood disorders, obesity, and peripheral sensory and motor disorders (Indo et al. 1996; Knable 1999; Kranz et al. 2015; Lewis et al. 2005; Otnaess et al. 2009; Yeo et al. 2004). An awareness of the link between deficiencies in these pathways and CNS effects in humans might raise the value JAS for drugs targeting these pathways, particularly as other studies typically conducted to support clinical development of oncology drugs may not fully capture these endpoints. For example, while embryo-fetal development studies can detect malformations in brain structure, they are not designed to assess motor development or psychiatric function, and while a pre- and postnatal development study may be capable of evaluating some endpoints of concern, these studies are not typically recommended for a drug intended to treat patients with advanced cancer.

Vitrakvi (larotrectinib sulfate) (FDA 2018a) was approved in 2018 for used in adult and pediatric patients with solid tumors that have the neurotrophic tyrosine receptor kinase (NTRK) gene fusion. The results of a JAS submitted with the original application are described in Section 8.4 of the label and in more detail in the nonclinical review. As part of the administrative record for NDA 210861, the Applicant, Loxo, described the design of a JAS that was requested by the European Medicines Agency and the Pediatric Subcommittee of the Oncology Drugs Advisory Committee. In two separate studies, juvenile animals were dosed from day 7 to 27, and from day 28 to 70; the main findings were transient central nervous system-related signs, including head flick, tremor, and circling in both sexes. These studies also demonstrated potential effects on learning and memory, consistent with known effects of TrkA signaling deficiencies in humans associated with the rare recessive disorder, congenital insensitivity to pain, and anhidrosis (CIPA; Indo et al. 1996).

Rozlytrek (entrectinib) (FDA 2019) was approved in 2019 with a similar indication regarding the NTRK gene fusion. JAS data are described in Section 8.4 of the product label. In a 13-week JAS where animals were dosed from the neonatal stage to adulthood (day 7–97), the main findings were decreased body weight gain and delayed sexual maturation, neurobehavioral deficits, and decreased femur length. Both JAS did show evidence of neurobehavioral changes compared to untreated controls; nevertheless, toxicity to the central nervous system is an expected finding based on expression of TRKs and their known roles on neural development and behavior, and there were similar signs in adult animals. While the JAS did suggest a potential for increased effects or effects at lower doses in pediatric patient populations compared to adults, findings of increased severity are not uncommon in JAS for other targets either and do not represent new toxicities compared to those identified in adult studies.

3.5 Conclusion

FDA Oncology's general approach to use of JAS to support pediatric oncology indications has been well articulated by ICH S9 and by Leighton et al. (2016). There has been no significant new data to suggest that the current approach needs to be reconsidered at this time. FDA Oncology has requested JAS on a rare basis, to address specific questions and concerns. This approach is consistent with the principles outlined by the FDA Roadmap regarding reducing, refining, and replacing the use of animals for nonclinical studies when warranted. Not routinely requesting JAS to support the development of drugs to treat pediatric patients with cancer clearly reduces animal use, especially use of nonhuman primates, often the only pharmacologically relevant model for biotherapeutics including immune-oncology drugs and antibody-drug conjugates.

References

EMA (2017) Results of juvenile animal studies (JAS) and impact on anti-cancer medicine development and use in children: project report. https://www.ema.europa.eu/en/documents/scientific-guideline/results-juvenile-animal-studies-jas-impact-anti-cancer-medicine-development-use-children_en.pdf. Accessed 19 Feb 2021

FDA (2010) Guidance for industry: nonclinical evaluation for anticancer pharmaceuticals. https://www.fda.gov/regulatory-information/search-fda-guidance-documents/s9-nonclinical-evaluation-anticancer-pharmaceuticals. Accessed 24 Feb 2021

FDA (2015) FDA summary review for Unituxin (dinutuximab, BLA 125516). Dated 10 Mar 2015. Available at: drugs@fda, https://www.accessdata.fda.gov/scripts/cder/daf/

FDA (2018a) FDA summary review for Vitrakvi (larotrectinib, NDA 210861). Dated 26 Nov 2018. Available at: drugs@fda, https://www.accessdata.fda.gov/scripts/cder/daf/

FDA (2018b) Guidance for industry: nonclinical evaluation for anticancer pharmaceuticals: questions and answers. https://www.fda.gov/regulatory-information/search-fda-guidance-documents/s9-nonclinical-evaluation-anticancer-pharmaceuticals-questions-and-answers. Accessed 24 Feb 2021

FDA (2019) FDA summary review for Rozlytrek (entrectinib, NDA 212275). Dated 15 Aug 2019. Available at: drugs@fda, https://www.accessdata.fda.gov/scripts/cder/daf/

FDA (2020a) Guidance for industry and IRBs: cancer clinical trial eligibility criteria: minimum age considerations for inclusion of pediatric patients

FDA (2020b) FDA summary review for Danyelza (naxitamab-GQGK, BLA 761171). Dated 22 Nov 2020. Available at: drugs@fda, https://www.accessdata.fda.gov/scripts/cder/daf/

FDA (2021) S11 guidance for industry: nonclinical safety testing in support of development of pediatric pharmaceuticals. Available at https://www.fda.gov/media/148478/download. Accessed July 13 2022

Indo Y, Tsuruta M, Hayashida Y, Karim MA, Ohta K, Kawano T, Mitsubuchi H, Tonoki H, Awaya Y, Matsuda I (1996) Mutations in the TRKA/NGF receptor gene in patients with congenital insensitivity to pain with anhidrosis. Nat Genet 13:485–488

Knable MB (1999) Schizophrenia and bipolar disorder: findings from studies of the Stanley Foundation brain collection. Schizophr Res 32:149–152

Kranz TM, Goetz RR, Walsh-Messinger J, Goetz D, Antonius D, Dolgalev I, Heguy A, Seandel M, Malaspina D, Chao MV (2015) Rare variants in the neurotrophin signaling pathway implicated in schizophrenia risk. Schizophr Res 168:421–428

Leighton JK, Saber H, Reaman G, Pazdur R (2016) An FDA oncology view of juvenile animal studies in support of initial pediatric studies for anticancer drugs. Reg Toxicol Pharmacol 79:142–143

Lewis DA, Hashimoto T, Volk DW (2005) Cortical inhibitory neurons and schizophrenia. Nat Rev Neurosci 4:321–324

Otnaess MK, Djurovic S, Rimol LM, Kulle B, Kähler AK, Jönsson EG, Agartz I, Sundet K, Hall H, Timm S, Hansen T, Callicott JH, Melle I, Werge T, Andreassen OA (2009) Evidence for a possible association of neurotrophin receptor (NTRK-3) gene polymorphisms with hippocampal function and schizophrenia. Neurobiol Dis 200:518–524

Sait S, Modak S (2017) Anti-GD2 immunotherapy for neuroblastoma. Expert Rev Anticaner Ther 17:889–904

Smeyne RJ, Klein R, Schnapp A, Long LK, Bryant S, Lewin A, Lira SA, Barbacid M (1994) Severe sensory and sympathetic neuropathies in mice carrying a disrupted Trk/NGF receptor gene. Nature 368:246–249

Suzuki M, Kushner BH, Kramer K, Basu EM, Roberts SS, Hammond WJ, LaQuaglia MP, Wolden SL, Cheung NKV, Modak S (2018) Treatment and outcome of adult-onset neuroblastoma. Int J Cancer 143:1249–1258

Tucker KL, Meyer M, Barde YA (2001) Neurotrophins are required for nerve growth during development. Nat Neurosci 4:29–37

Visalli T, Bower N, Kokate T, Andrews PA (2018) Lack of value of juvenile animal toxicity studies for supporting the safety of pediatric oncology phase I trials. Reg Toxicol Pharmacol 96:167–177

Yeo GSH, Hung C-CC, Rochford J, Keogh J, Gray J, Sivaramakrishnan S, O'Rahilly S, Farooqi IS (2004) A de novo mutation affecting human TrkB associated with severe obesity and developmental delay. Nat Neurosci 7:1187–1189

Design and Statistical Considerations for Early Phase Clinical Trials in Pediatric Oncology

4

Jirui Wang and Xiaofang Yan

Contents

4.1 Introduction

Development of a scientifically rigorous study design that addresses the study questions is a key component of clinical trials in oncology. The development of the study design is a collaborative effort between clinical investigators and biostatisticians. An appropriate study design is critical to the success of a clinical trial as it will facilitate the ability of the trial to answer the study questions; will define the number of patients required for enrollment to answer these questions and the duration of the study; and, in early phase studies, will enable the identification of the desired dose to move into subsequent studies (e.g., maximum tolerated dose (MTD); recommended Phase II dose (RP2D)). In early stage pediatric oncology studies, the identification of a safe dose is critically important, as this dose may vary from adult

J. Wang (✉) · X. Yan
Biostatistician, Medpace, Inc., Cincinnati, OH, USA
e-mail: j.wang7@medpace.com

J. DiMartino et al. (eds.), *Pediatric Cancer Therapeutics Development*, Pediatric Oncology,
https://doi.org/10.1007/978-3-031-06357-2_4

Table 4.1 Summary of study designs

Category of study designs	Description
Rule-based design (algorithm-based design)	All the rules for dose escalation, de-escalation, or staying at the current dose are defined in the protocol and prior to conduct of the clinical trial: • Traditional 3 + 3 design • Accelerated titration design • Rolling six design
Model-based design	Some assumptions of a parametric statistical model for the dose-toxicity curve are presented in the protocol. Then, the estimate of the dose-toxicity curve is continuously updated to guide the dose assignment and MTD selection based on accumulating trial data, on a real-time basis: • Continual reassessment method (CRM) • Escalation with overdose control (EWOC) • Time-to-event continual reassessment method (TITE-CRM) • Bayesian logistic regression model (BLRM) • Time-to-event escalation with overdose control (TITE-EWOC)
Model-assisted design	Combines the ideas of both rule-based and model-based designs. The rules for dose escalation, de-escalation, or staying at the current dose are determined before the start of patient enrollment but based on a parametric statistical model: • Modified toxicity probability interval (mTPI) design • Keyboard design • mTPI-2 design • Bayesian optimal interval (BOIN) design

doses. In this chapter, we introduce Phase I clinical trial designs from three categories based on statistical assumptions (Table 4.1): rule-based/algorithm-based designs; model-based designs; and model-assisted design (Wei et al. 2019). This chapter will also discuss the advantages and disadvantages of these study designs in pediatric oncology studies.

The starting dose in adult oncology studies is calculated based on nonclinical safety data in animal models (Shen et al. 2019). However, most pediatric clinical trials are conducted after the completion of adult Phase I clinical trials that can provide historical data for the determination of the starting dose (Smith et al. 1998). Typically, pediatric oncology studies start at approximately 80% of the adult MTD/RP2D (Marsoni et al. 1985; Lee et al. 2005). This prevents the trial from starting with doses that are too low and potentially ineffective doses, unnecessarily exposing children to toxicity without likelihood of benefit and accelerates the dose escalation period. However, for drugs where there is no MTD in adults, there can be consideration to starting at the adult RP2D, as determined in adult, single-agent studies. Pediatric oncology studies starting at the adult RP2D would be designed with plans for dose de-escalation, if necessary.

4.2 Rule-Based Designs

4.2.1 Traditional 3 + 3 Design

The most traditional and straightforward design in clinical trials is the 3 + 3 study design (Storer 1989). The detailed procedure is described in the FDA Guidance for Industry Clinical Considerations for Therapeutic Cancer Vaccines (FDA 2011) which is summarized as follows:

1. Three patients are enrolled into a pre-defined starting dose level:
   (a) If there is no DLT observed in these three patients, then escalate the dose level, and enroll three additional patients into the new dose level. Move to Step 2.
   (b) If there is only one DLT observed in these three patients, then stay on the same dose level, and enroll three additional patients in the current dose level:
      - If there is no DLT observed in these three patients (i.e., one DLT in six patients), then escalate the dose level, and enroll three additional patients into the new dose level. Move to Step 2.
      - If there is one DLT or more observed in these three additional patients (i.e., ≥2 DLTs in six patients), then stop the trial and choose the previous dose level as MTD.

(c) If there are more than one DLT observed in these three patients, then stop the trial and choose the previous dose level as MTD.

2. Repeat Step 1 for each new dose level.

This study design has all the advantages of rule-based designs. It is simple to understand the design structure and is convenient for clinical operational teams to implement since the parameters for dose escalation are clearly defined. However, this commonly used study design has significant disadvantages and constraints. Statistically, it can only estimate the MTD when the target probability of DLT is between 20% and 33% (Le Tourneau et al. 2009). The 3 + 3 design is "memory-less" since it is based on only the last, most recently enrolled three (or six) patients. This design also requires many escalation steps with doses that may be too low to be effective, leading to suboptimal treatment (if the drug is, in fact, effective) for a large number of patients. It is also difficult to predict the final sample size since all that is known is the cohort size (three or six patients) at each dose level. Another concern of 3 + 3 study design in pediatric oncology studies is that this design has significant operational limitations since most of these studies are multicenter clinical trials (Doussau et al. 2016).

However, in both adult and pediatric oncology studies, the conservative 3 + 3 design is still one of the most popular and commonly used study designs despite criticism of its inefficiency and underestimation of MTD.

4.2.2 Accelerated Titration Design

The accelerated titration design was proposed by Simon et al. (1997). This study design extends the traditional 3 + 3 design to reduce the number of patients enrolled at lower dose levels by adding an initial accelerated phase before the start of a 3 + 3 study design phase.

During the initial accelerated phase, there is only one patient per dose level cohort enrolled at lower dose levels until the pre-defined stopping rules for DLTs or toxicities are met. After the initial accelerated phase, a traditional 3 + 3 design is implemented with cohorts of three to six patients at the higher dose levels.

Simon et al. performed simulations based on four Phase I designs (Simon et al. 1997): Design 1 was a traditional 3 + 3 design, while Designs 2, 3, and 4 were accelerated titration designs with different assumptions (Table 4.2). The simulation results showed that the average number of required patients in a Phase I trial was reduced from 39.9 for Design 1 to 24.4, 20.7, and 21.2 for Designs 2, 3, and 4, respectively.

Therefore, the accelerated titration design has an advantage to have fewer required patients, especially when there are many dose levels planned. Some accelerated titration designs also allow for intra-patient dose escalation during the initial accelerated phase to further reduce the number of patients and provide some patients the opportunity to receive the investigation agent at higher dose levels (Ivy et al. 2010). This has the potential to make the accelerated

Table 4.2 Summary of phase I simulations by Simon et al. (1997)

Design	Initial accelerated phase	3 + 3 phase	Condition to 3 + 3 phase	Average # of patients
1	Not applicable	40% dose increments	Not applicable	39.9
2	Single-patient cohorts 40% dose escalation	40% dose increments	At least one first-course DLT, *or* one second first-course intermediate toxicity	24.4
3	Single-patient cohorts 100% dose escalation	40% dose increments	At least one first-course DLT, *or* one second first-course intermediate toxicity	20.7
4	Single-patient cohorts 100% dose escalation	40% dose increments	At least one any course DLT, *or* one any course intermediate toxicity	21.2

titration design more attractive to adult patients enrolled in FIH Phase I trials. However, in pediatric oncology clinical trials, the accelerated titration design is not compelling since most starting doses are based on the MTD in adult trials and can be too low when compared to the true MTD.

4.2.3 Rolling Six Design

In order to shorten the timeline of pediatric oncology Phase I trials, the rolling six design was proposed by Skolnik et al. (2008). It is another rule-based design that also extends the 3 + 3 study design (Skolnik et al. 2008).

In the rolling six design, two to six patients can be enrolled continuously on the same dose level. The escalation and de-escalation rules can be summarized as follows:

1. If 0/3, 0/4, 0/5, 0/6, or 1/6 patients are observed with DLTs, then escalate to the dose level.
2. If 0/2, 1/2, 1/3, 1/4, or 1/5 patients are observed with DLTs, then stay on the same level, and enroll more patients up to a total of 6.
3. If there are more than two DLTs observed, then de-escalate the dose level.
4. If six patients have been enrolled on the current dose level, escalation/de-escalation decision will not be made until at least five of those six patients have completed the DLT period.

The dose level assigned to a new patient is based on the following three components:

1. The number of patients currently enrolled and evaluable
2. The number of patients experiencing a DLT
3. The number of patients at risk of experiencing a DLT

In 1000 study simulations performed by Skolnik et al. (2008), the average (±standard deviation) time of study duration was 294 (±75 days) for the rolling 6 design versus 350 (±84) days for the traditional 3 + 3 design. This design successfully shortens the study duration for pediatric oncology studies in situations where there is prior information about the adult starting dose (Le Tourneau et al. 2009). Since this study design was specifically developed for pediatric oncology clinical trials, it has been increasingly implemented over the last decade (Doussau et al. 2016).

4.3 Model-Based Designs

4.3.1 Continual Reassessment Method (CRM)

One of the earliest model based-designs using Bayesian statistics, the continual reassessment method (CRM), was proposed by O'Quigley et al. (1990). This predated the accelerated titration and rolling six designs. In 2003, it was applied in a simulation study on pediatric Phase I oncology clinical trials by Onar-Thomas and Xiong (2010).

As an example of an adaptive design, a Bayesian statistical model is used to fit a dose-toxicity curve to find the dose (e.g., MTD) with the toxicity rate closest to the target rate. The target DLT rate is fixed at the beginning of the study, and only one patient is required for each dose level or cohort. The assumptions of the prior distributions for the parameters of the dose-toxicity curve are made based on historical data. Dose escalation decisions can then be made by investigators and biostatisticians based on the whole updated posterior distribution of toxicity at each dose, based on accumulating DLT information. The dose level recommended for the next patient is the one minimizing the difference between its probability of toxicity and the target toxicity rate.

There are three essential steps in a CRM study (Zhou et al. 2018):

1. Assume a parametric model for dose-toxicity curve, like a power model:

$$p_j = \alpha_j^{\exp(\alpha)},$$

while p_j denotes the true DLT probability of dose level j, α is the unknown parameter, and

$0 < \alpha_1 < \cdots < \alpha_J < 1$ are prior guesses for the DLT probability at each dose.

2. Update the estimate of the dose-toxicity curve based on the accumulating DLT data across all dose levels, and assign the next cohort of patients to the "optimal" dose, defined as the dose whose posterior mean estimate of the DLT probability is closest to the target DLT probability.
3. Rules to forbid skipping doses and safety stopping rules.

For the Bayesian CRM, advantages include the assumption that the target DLT level is more flexible compared to the traditional 3 + 3 design. This design allows for a more precise estimate of the MTD. Therefore, more patients can be treated at a potentially therapeutic dose level. In a comparison of simulations among study designs for pediatric oncology Phase I clinical trials, CRM was also been found to be more efficient than two algorithm-based methods (3 + 3 and rolling six) and reduce the number of skipped children (Doussau et al. 2012).

However, like all Bayesian models, justification of prior distributions considered in the CRM design analysis is always critical. Incorrect assumptions will expose patients to overtreatment risk. With respect to operational considerations, it is more complicated to constantly update the posterior distribution based on accrued DLT information after each cohort. This requires timely collaboration between statisticians, investigators, and clinical operational team throughout the dose escalation period.

The CRM design is still not been widely utilized in clinical trials, but various modifications have been made to improve the performance of the CRM design, including the escalation with overdose control (EWOC) design in 1998 (Babb et al. 1998), the time-to-event continual reassessment method (TITE-CRM) in 2000 (Cheung and Chappell 2000), an adaptive CRM design called TriCRM in 2006 (Zhang et al. 2006), a Bayesian-based extension of TriCRM in 2007 (Mandrekar et al. 2007), the Bayesian logistic regression model (BLRM) in 2008 (Neuenschwander et al. 2008), and time-to-event escalation with overdose control (TITE-EWOC) in 2011 (Mauguen et al. 2011). In the following sections, we will introduce the EWOC, BLRM, TITE-CRM, and TITE-EWOC study designs.

4.3.2 EWOC and BLRM

EWOC and BLRM are similar when compared to the CRM. They both assume a Bayesian two-parameter logistic regression model for dose-toxicity curves that actively control for the risk of overdosing. But these two designs use two different definitions to estimate the optimal dose.

The EWOC selects the optimal dose by selecting the highest dose whose posterior probability of being higher than the MTD is equal to or less than a pre-specified threshold, such as 25% or 30%. The EWOC was applied in a Phase I dose escalation study of oral gefitinib and irinotecan in children with refractory solid tumors that was published in 2014. In this study, the pre-specified threshold to control the overdosing risk was set at 30% (Brennan et al. 2014).

The BLRM defines the optimal dose that has the highest posterior probability of being within a pre-specified dosing interval (δ_1, δ_2). Another feature of the BLRM is that the dose skipping is not allowed.

In conclusion, in order to find the optimal dose with lower risk of overdose, the EWOC puts a constraint on the probability, while the BLRM puts a constraint on the dose directly.

4.3.3 TITE-CRM and TITE-EWOC

In the model-based designs discussed above, the dose-toxicity curve has to be updated by statisticians after all previous patients have completed their safety and toxicity evaluations. Enrollment of additional patients is delayed in studies with long DLT assessment periods (e.g., DLT assessment periods greater than 28 days). Time-to-event approaches combine existing model-based designs to estimate the next dose level from all previous patients with some data from patients still in the DLT assessment period, or in patients in whom follow-up is pending (Doussau et al. 2016).

The TITE-CRM was proposed in 2000 to estimate of the cumulative probability of late-onset toxicity over several cycles when some patients have not yet completed the DLT assessment period (Cheung and Chappell 2000). In 2006, Normolle and Lawrence (2006)) used Monte Carlo simulations of 60,000 Phase I studies to demonstrate that TITE-CRM trials are considerably shorter compared with traditional 3 + 3 and CRM study designs when toxicity observation times are long. However, Le Tourneau et al. (2009) pointed out that in two pancreatic cancer trials (Muler et al. 2004; Desai et al. 2007), the TITE-CRM design had accrual of more patients to dose levels below the RP2D as compared to those using a traditional 3 + 3 design.

Similar to the TITE-CRM, when statisticians update the estimates based on the Bayesian model in the TITE-EWOC design, the observations of patients who have not completed the follow-up period are likely to be down-weighted. Mauguen et al. (2011) showed that compared with the EWOC design, trial duration can be significantly decreased with the TITE-EWOC, without a major impact on the probability of overdose risk or the number of DLTs. This design also avoids waiting time in pediatric cancer chemoradiation trials (Doussau et al. 2016).

4.4 Model-Assisted Designs

4.4.1 Modified Toxicity Probability Interval (mTPI) Design

In 2007, Ji et al. (2007) proposed a Phase I dose-finding approach with simple escalation and de-escalation rules based on toxicity probability intervals (TPI). In 2010, Ji et al. (2010) presented a modified TPI (mTPI) design to improve efficiency while maintaining the simplicity of the original TPI design.

In the mTPI design, three intervals are specified to denote the proper dosing interval (δ_1, δ_2), the underdosing interval (0, δ_1), and the overdosing interval (δ_2, 1). The mTPI makes the decision about dose escalation and de-escalation based on the unit probability mass (UPM) of the three intervals (Fig. 4.1). Let p_{cur} denote the DLT probability of the current dose. The UPM is defined as the posterior probability that p_{cur} is within the interval, divided by the length of the interval.

By assuming the target toxicity rate, dose levels, and potential toxicity rate at each dose level, a Monte Carlo experiment can be performed to identify the operating characteristics, including estimated number of patients and the observed number of toxicities. Given the simulation results, dose escalation and de-escalation can be determined before the onset of the trial, which makes the mTPI design easy to use for investigators. This creates an advantage for the mTPI design, namely, the ease of implementation of studies with this design.

Two further modifications of the mTPI were proposed in 2017: the mTPI-2 design (Guo et al. 2017) and the keyboard design (Yan et al. 2017). These two study designs are very similar and have almost the same operating characteristics in simulations, but the keyboard design is conceptually easier to understand.

4.4.2 Keyboard Design

The keyboard design was proposed to improve the performance of the mTPI design (Yan et al. 2017), since the original mTPI has a higher risk of overdosing patients due to the use of the UPM to guide dose escalation. The

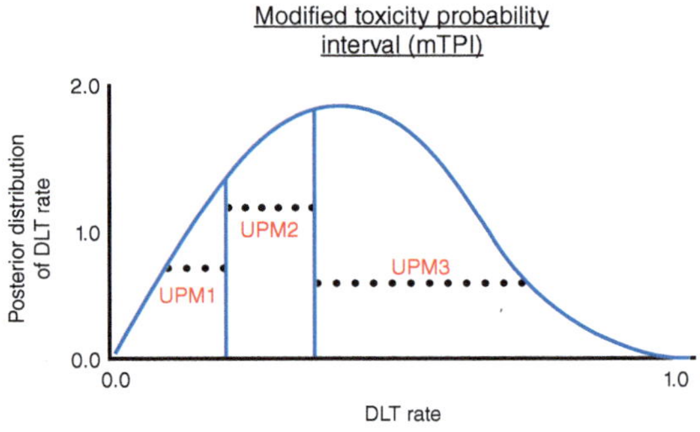

Fig. 4.1 mTPI calculates and compares the UPMs of the underdosing, proper dosing, and overdosing intervals

keyboard design constructs a series of equal-width dosing intervals, referred to as "keys," to guide dose escalation and de-escalation (Fig. 4.2).

The keyboard design starts by eliciting the proper dosing interval (referred to as the target key) from clinicians, and then forms a series of equal-width keys on both sides of the target key. The keyboard design makes the decision of dose escalation and de-escalation based on the location of the "strongest" key, defined as the key that has the largest area under the posterior distribution curve of p_{cur}. The rule of dose escalation and de-escalation is intuitive by comparing the location of target key and strongest key.

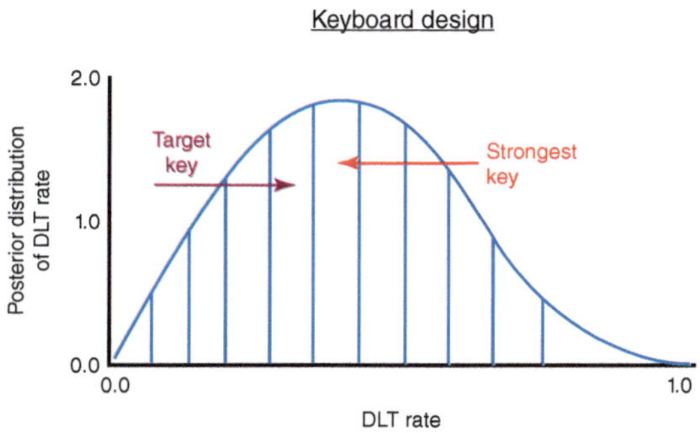

Fig. 4.2 The keyboard design forms a series of equal-width keys and bases the decision on the position of the strongest key with respect to the target key

4.4.3 Bayesian Optimal Interval (BOIN) Design

The BOIN design is another model-assisted design that has overdose toxicity controls (Liu and Yuan 2015; Yuan et al. 2016). Unlike the mTPI and keyboard designs, the BOIN design makes the decision of dose escalation and de-escalation simply by comparing the observed DLT rate with a pair of fixed, predetermined dose escalation and de-escalation boundaries (Fig. 4.3).

The respective dose escalation and de-escalation boundaries are derived from a pair of pre-specified toxicity probability thresholds: the highest DLT probability that is predicted to be underdosing such that dose escalation is needed and the lowest DLT probability that is predicted to be overdosing such that dose de-escalation is needed.

The BOIN design can target any pre-specified DLT rate without limitations. During the escalation phase, the process is very transparent and assessable for non-statisticians.

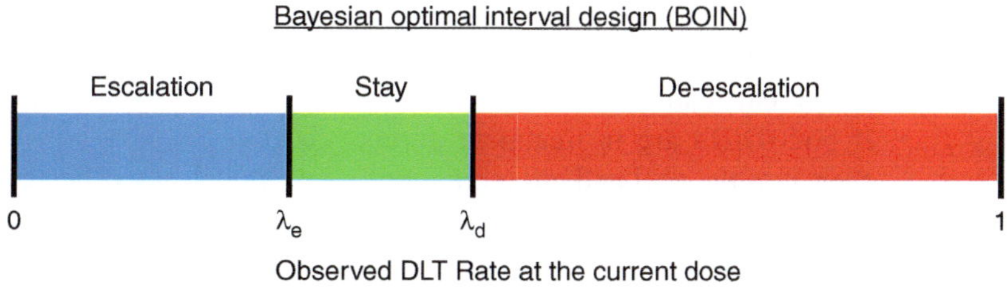

Fig. 4.3 BOIN compares the observed DLT rate at the current dose with the pre-specified dose escalation and de-escalation boundaries

4.5 New Designs

Because the practical demands of recent advances in oncology treatments, many new study designs are under development or being tested prospectively in upcoming clinical trials (George et al. 2016). Some of these new designs have been incorporated into clinical trials, but have not yet been published and validated statistically.

4.5.1 Modified 4 + 4 Design

As the name suggests, the 4 + 4 design is a modification of the traditional 3 + 3 design. In addition to the three patients treated by study drug in each cohort, it adds one more patient on placebo. The 4 + 4 design is blinded and needs the safety review committee (SRC) involvement for the evaluation for each cohort.

The following guidelines are provided for each dose level:

1. If 0/4 patients are observed with DLTs, then escalate the dose level.
2. If 1/4 patients are observed with DLTs, then stay on the same level and enroll 4 more patients:
   (a) If 1/8 patients are observed with DLTs, then escalate the dose level.
   (b) If 2/8 patients are observed with DLTs, then SRC is unblinded to treatment:
      - If there are ≥1 DLTs in placebo group, then escalate the dose level.
      - If both DLTs are in treatment group, then stop the trial and choose the previous dose level as MTD.
3. If 2/4 patients are observed with DLTs, then SRC is unblinded to treatment:
   (a) If there is 1 DLT in treatment group, then stay on the same level and enroll 4 more patients:
      - If 1/8 patients are observed with DLTs, then escalate the dose level.
      - If 2/8 patients are observed with DLTs, then SRC unblinded to treatment:
         – If there is 1 DLT in placebo group, then escalate the dose level.
         – If both DLTs are in treatment group, then stop the trial and choose the previous dose level as MTD.
   (b) If there are two DLTs in treatment group, then stop the trial and choose the previous dose level as MTD.
4. If 3/4 patients are observed with DLTs, then the trial stops and the previous dose level is defined as the MTD.

This design is perhaps applicable to the studies where it is difficult to ascertain the difference between adverse events related to the investigational agent and adverse events that are expected due to the underlying disease. In this scenario, the placebo group can help increase the probability to escalate the dose level. This idea can also be borrowed into oncology studies by replacing the placebo group with a control group of the other lines of therapy if efficacy is a secondary objective in Phase I.

4.6 Conclusions

While there is great interest and enthusiasm about model-based study designs, over the past decade, the rule-based designs, like the traditional 3 + 3 design and newer rolling six study design, are still the most commonly used in pediatric oncology trials. As noted above, these study designs are easy to execute since the rules about dose escalation and de-escalation are a priori defined in the protocol based on observed DLTs.

Model-based designs have significant advantages on reducing numbers of study patients and shortening study durations. However, they require significant involvement of statisticians for the development of the study design, for monitoring of the study, and in dose escalation/de-escalation decisions. Model-based designs are also operationally complicated, due to a requirement for repeated model fitting, conceptual and computational complexity, and nontransparent approach to decision-making.

The model-assisted designs combine the superior performance of model-based designs with the simplicity of algorithm-based designs. They offer more flexible approaches to patient enrollment while retaining clear escalation and de-escalation rules. Because of their good performance and simplicity, model-assisted designs have been increasingly used in practice. In addition, many software and online tools are now available to support the simulation of operating characteristics for both model-based and model-assisted designs. But since model-assisted designs are relatively new, they are not commonly utilized in pediatric oncology trials. In the future, we believe more model-assisted designs will be developed by investigators and biostatisticians and applied to pediatric oncology studies.

References

Babb J, Rogatko A, Zacks S (1998) Cancer phase I clinical trials: efficient dose escalation with overdose control. Stat Med 17(10):1103–1120. https://doi.org/10.1002/(sici)1097-0258(19980530)17:10<1103::aid-sim793>3.0.co;2-9

Brennan RC, Furman W, Mao S, Wu J, Turner DC, Stewart CF, Santana V, McGregor LM (2014) Phase I dose escalation and pharmacokinetic study of oral gefitinib and irinotecan in children with refractory solid tumors. Cancer Chemother Pharmacol 74(6):1191–1198. https://doi.org/10.1007/s00280-014-2593-7. Epub 2014 Sept 26

Cheung YK, Chappell R (2000) Sequential designs for phase I clinical trials with late-onset toxicities. Biometrics 56(4):1177–1182. https://doi.org/10.1111/j.0006-341x.2000.01177.x

Desai SP, Ben-Josef E, Normolle DP, Francis IR, Greenson JK, Simeone DM, Chang AE, Colletti LM, Lawrence TS, Zalupski MM (2007) Phase I study of oxaliplatin, full-dose gemcitabine, and concurrent radiation therapy in pancreatic cancer. J Clin Oncol 25(29):4587–4592. https://doi.org/10.1200/JCO.2007.12.0592

Doussau A, Asselain B, Le Deley MC, Geoerger B, Doz F, Vassal G, Paoletti X (2012) Dose-finding designs in pediatric phase I clinical trials: comparison by simulations in a realistic timeline framework. Contemp Clin Trials 33(4):657–665. https://doi.org/10.1016/j.cct.2011.11.015. Epub 2012 Apr 13

Doussau A, Geoerger B, Jiménez I, Paoletti X (2016) Innovations for phase I dose-finding designs in pediatric oncology clinical trials. Contemp Clin Trials 47:217–227. https://doi.org/10.1016/j.cct.2016.01.009

FDA (2011) Guidance for industry: clinical considerations for therapeutic cancer vaccines, Oct 2011. Available from: https://www.fda.gov/regulatory-information/search-fda-guidance-documents/clinical-considerations-therapeutic-cancer-vaccines

George SL, Wang X, Pang H (2016) Cancer clinical trials: current and controversial issues in design and analysis. CRC Press, Boca Raton

Guo W, Wang SJ, Yang S, Lynn H, Ji Y (2017) A Bayesian interval dose-finding design addressing Ockham's razor: mTPI-2. Contemp Clin Trials 58:23–33

Ivy SP, Siu LL, Garrett-Mayer E, Rubinstein L (2010) Approaches to phase 1 clinical trial design focused on safety, efficiency, and selected patient populations: a report from the clinical trial design task force of the national cancer institute investigational drug steering committee. Clin Cancer Res 16(6):1726–1736. https://doi.org/10.1158/1078-0432.CCR-09-1961. Epub 2010 Mar 9

Ji Y, Li Y, Bekele BN (2007) Dose-finding in phase I clinical trials based on toxicity probability intervals. Clin Trials 4(3):235–244

Ji Y, Liu P, Li Y, Bekele BN (2010) A modified toxicity probability interval method for dose-finding trials. Clin Trials 7(6):653–663. https://doi.org/10.1177/1740774510382799. Epub 2010 Oct 8

Le Tourneau C, Lee JJ, Siu LL (2009) Dose escalation methods in phase I cancer clinical trials. J Natl Cancer Inst 101(10):708–720. https://doi.org/10.1093/jnci/djp079

Lee DP, Skolnik JM, Adamson PC (2005) Pediatric phase I trials in oncology: an analysis of study conduct efficiency. J Clin Oncol 23(33):8431–8441. https://doi.org/10.1200/JCO.2005.02.1568

Liu S, Yuan Y (2015) Bayesian optimal interval designs for phase I clinical trials. J R Stat Soc Ser C Appl Stat 64:507–523

Mandrekar SJ, Cui Y, Sargent DJ (2007) An adaptive phase I design for identifying a biologically optimal dose for dual agent drug combinations. Stat Med 26(11):2317–2330. https://doi.org/10.1002/sim.2707

Marsoni S, Ungerleider RS, Hurson SB et al (1985) Tolerance to antineoplastic agents in children and adults. Cancer Treat Rep 69:1263–1269

Mauguen A, Le Deley MC, Zohar S (2011) Dose-finding approach for dose escalation with overdose control considering incomplete observations. Stat Med 30(13):1584–1594. https://doi.org/10.1002/sim.4128. Epub 2011 Feb 24

Muler JH, McGinn CJ, Normolle D, Lawrence T, Brown D, Hejna G, Zalupski MM (2004) Phase I trial using a time-to-event continual reassessment strategy for dose escalation of cisplatin combined with gemcitabine and radiation therapy in pancreatic cancer. J Clin Oncol 22(2):238–243. https://doi.org/10.1200/JCO.2004.03.129. Epub 2003 Dec 9

Neuenschwander B, Branson M, Gsponer T (2008) Critical aspects of the Bayesian approach to phase I cancer trials. Stat Med 27(13):2420–2439. https://doi.org/10.1002/sim.3230

Normolle D, Lawrence T (2006) Designing dose-escalation trials with late-onset toxicities using the time-to-event con-

tinual reassessment method. J Clin Oncol 24(27):4426–4433. https://doi.org/10.1200/JCO.2005.04.3844
O'Quigley J, Pepe M, Fisher L (1990) Continual reassessment method: a practical design for phase 1 clinical trials in cancer. Biometrics 46(1):33–48
Onar-Thomas A, Xiong Z (2010) A simulation-based comparison of the traditional method, Rolling-6 design and a frequentist version of the continual reassessment method with special attention to trial duration in pediatric phase I oncology trials. Contemp Clin Trials 31(3):259–270. https://doi.org/10.1016/j.cct.2010.03.006. Epub 2010 Mar 15
Shen J, Swift B, Mamelok R, Pine S, Sinclair J, Attar M (2019) Design and conduct considerations for first-in-human trials. Clin Transl Sci 12(1):6–19. https://doi.org/10.1111/cts.12582
Simon R, Freidlin B, Rubinstein L, Arbuck SG, Collins J, Christian MC (1997) Accelerated titration designs for phase I clinical trials in oncology. J Natl Cancer Inst 89(15):1138–1147. https://doi.org/10.1093/jnci/89.15.1138
Skolnik JM, Barrett JS, Jayaraman B, Patel D, Adamson PC (2008) Shortening the timeline of pediatric phase I trials: the rolling six design. J Clin Oncol 26(2):190–195. https://doi.org/10.1200/JCO.2007.12.7712
Smith M, Bernstein M, Bleyer WA et al (1998) Conduct of phase I trials in children with cancer. J Clin Oncol 16:966–978
Storer BE (1989 Sep) Design and analysis of phase I clinical trials. Biometrics 45(3):925–937
Wei L, Pan X, Fernandez S (2019) Practical considerations for the implementation of adaptive designs for oncology phase I dose-finding trials. Future Drug Discov 1(2):FDD18. https://doi.org/10.4155/fdd-2019-0021. Published 2019 Oct 11
Yan F, Mandrekar SJ, Yuan Y (2017) Keyboard: a novel Bayesian toxicity probability interval design for phase I clinical trials. Clin Cancer Res 23(15):3994–4003. https://doi.org/10.1158/1078-0432.CCR-17-0220
Yuan Y, Hess KR, Hilsenbeck SG, Gilbert MR (2016) Bayesian optimal interval design: a simple and well-performing design for phase I oncology trials. Clin Cancer Res 22(17):4291–4301
Zhang W, Sargent DJ, Mandrekar S (2006) An adaptive dose-finding design incorporating both toxicity and efficacy. Stat Med 25(14):2365–2383. https://doi.org/10.1002/sim.2325
Zhou H, Yuan Y, Nie L (2018) Accuracy, safety, and reliability of novel phase I trial designs. Clin Cancer Res 24(18):4357–4364

Exploratory Clinical Development: From First in Humans to Phase 3 Ready

5

Jorge DiMartino

Contents

5.1 Introduction

In the traditional drug development paradigm, clinical development starting with Phase 1 trials has been viewed as separate from the discovery research that produced the drug candidate. Getting from the first human dosed to a Phase 3-ready asset followed an empirical approach, literally clinical trial and error, to define dose and schedule of administration and to select indications for development. The advent of target-driven drug discovery as well as the sheer volume of drugs in development and economic pressures has made this traditional model for drug development unsustainable. Although the Phases, 1, 2, and 3 are still used in the naming of studies, oncology drug development, at least in the industry setting, is now thought of in terms of two major phases: the exploratory phase, which encompasses dose and schedule selection up through clinical proof of concept (PoC), and the confirmatory phase which is aimed at obtaining regulatory approval. During the exploratory phase, there continue to be many touchpoints with the discovery research stage of a molecule's life cycle, and an ongoing dialogue between the clinical/translational team and the discovery team is essential. As much as developers understand about a molecule and its target before it enters the clinic, human testing often yields new insights and potential pitfalls that need to be addressed through the virtuous cycle of bedside to bench

J. DiMartino (✉)
Clinical Development, Kronos Bio Inc., San Mateo, CA, USA
e-mail: Jorge.dimartino@kronosbio.com

J. DiMartino et al. (eds.), *Pediatric Cancer Therapeutics Development*, Pediatric Oncology,
https://doi.org/10.1007/978-3-031-06357-2_5

and back to bedside. The confirmatory phase of clinical development is subject to extensive regulatory oversight. Although this stage has also evolved in response to the explosion in knowledge behind targeted drug development, describing recent regulatory changes as they relate to registrational studies is beyond the scope of this chapter. Here we will focus on how drug developers get from first-in-humans (FIH) Phase 1 trials to PoC, defined functionally as the point when a drug is ready to enter registrational trials. In principle, this should be the same process for adult and pediatric cancers. In practice, however, FIH trials are typically done in adults, and pediatric development begins with at least some knowledge of the dose, schedule, and safety profile of a new agent. A potential leading role for pediatric cancer will be discussed in this context.

5.2 The Therapeutic Hypothesis

Implicit in the modern approach to oncology drug development is the dependence on a well-defined therapeutic hypothesis about how the drug delivers clinical benefit for patients. A robust therapeutic hypothesis incorporates five elements:

- The identity of the molecular target that is engaged by the drug candidate, its role in the initiation, and/or maintenance of the cancer phenotype.
- The downstream consequences, biochemical and phenotypic, of target engagement by the drug candidate that lead to the desired anticancer effect.
- The target engagement parameters required to achieve the desired anticancer effect, i.e., magnitude and duration of target inhibition or agonism.
- The molecular context (e.g., mutational background) of dependence on the target, i.e., the clinical setting within which target engagement of the appropriate magnitude and duration leads to the desired anticancer effect.
- The anticipated clinical outcome associated with the desired anticancer effect, e.g., tumor regression vs differentiation or stasis.

A well-defined hypothesis can provide a basis for expecting to find a window between a dose and schedule that is efficacious and one that is unacceptably toxic (i.e., a therapeutic index). It can help to set goal posts for a dose escalation study and to identify a patient population whose tumors are expected to respond to the drug at a reasonably high rate. In short, it enables a hypothesis-driven early clinical development program that can deliver clinical PoC data, or, just as importantly, invalidate a target hypothesis or drug candidate efficiently and informatively. Efficiency at this stage of the drug development process means not only avoiding ongoing financial expenditures with multiple protracted clinical trials but, more importantly, not exposing more patients than is absolutely necessary to an experimental drug candidate with an uncertain future. Moreover, a therapeutic hypothesis means that even failure can be informative, for example, by invalidating aspects of the hypothesis or determining that a drug candidate's pharmacologic properties preclude attainment of PK or PD objectives.

5.3 Dose and Schedule Determination

One thing that has not changed in the modern oncology drug development paradigm is that first-in-humans (FIH) trials are, first and foremost, about safety (FDA 2005). An important qualifier here is that these trials seek to understand the safety profile of a drug candidate at a dose and schedule that are expected to have at least the potential for anti-tumor activity. At one extreme, a homeopathic dose of an agent could be found to be safe but would not necessarily merit taking the agent forward into a signal-seeking Phase 2 study based simply on the absence of adverse effects. At the other extreme, a maximal tolerated dose (MTD) can be defined on a particular schedule of administration. Depending on the therapeutic hypothesis, the MTD may well be the desired dose to explore further for clinical activity, but this is not always the case. The classical concept of MTD applies well to broadly cytotoxic agents that target cell processes that are common to both cancer cells and rapidly dividing normal tissues, such as DNA replication and the mitotic spindle apparatus. The unifying hypothesis for these agents is that toxicity to normal tissues is "on target" and inseparable from the mechanism of efficacy. Based on this model, the goal is to deliver a dose of the drug that achieves substantial killing of both tumor cells and normal hematopoietic or epithelial progenitor cells over a brief period of 1 or a few days and then to provide a holiday during which the normal tissue is allowed to recover.

While this approach has been useful historically, it cannot be applied universally to molecularly targeted agents. This is because, although many of these agents have significant toxicity to normal tissue, these toxic effects are not always related to engagement of the intended target and their relationship to the mechanism of efficacy is uncertain at best (Lin et al. 2019). The MTD may thus be an unnecessarily high dose of the drug relative to what is needed to achieve efficacy. Because MTD is based on acute toxicity (usually in the first 28 days of dosing) and many molecularly targeted agents are meant to be taken chronically, an unnecessarily high dose with even modest toxicity could lead to dose interruptions, reductions, or discontinuations that could limit a drug's efficacy (Bullock et al. 2016). Even worse, if the toxicity that defines MTD is driven by an off-target effect, the compound may not even be achieving the desired magnitude of target engagement, exposing patients to adverse effects without the potential for benefit. In other cases, it may not be possible to define an MTD, either because the target is not essential for normal tissue or because exposures that would lead to toxicity cannot be achieved due to limitations of bioavailability and pill burden or the prohibitive cost of producing the drug on that scale (Cook et al. 2015). For all these reasons, having a predefined objective for plasma exposure and target engagement parameters that are necessary (if not sufficient) for anti-tumor activity is essential for establishing the recommended Phase 2 dose (RP2D).

Naturally, the best marker of target engagement on which to base a dose and schedule selection would be anti-tumor activity itself. Unfortunately, this is not realistic for a number of reasons. Phase 1 oncology trials typically enroll a heterogeneous population of heavily pre-treated patients who are unlikely to respond to anything, especially monotherapy with a targeted agent (Horstmann et al. 2005). Moreover, depending on the genetic context of target dependence, achieving the desired PK and PD parameters may be necessary, but not sufficient for anti-tumor effects. The only practical way to establish PK and PD objectives for dose-finding studies is in the preclinical setting using in vitro and in vivo models. As described in Chap. 2, this work is usually initiated during the lead optimization (LO) stage of the drug discovery process or as soon as there are adequate tool compounds and models available. These experiments seek to define the relationship between plasma exposure, target engagement, and anti-tumor activity by exploring various doses and schedules of drug treatment. Target engagement markers are generally biochemical changes that occur as a direct result of target modulation such as phosphorylation of a kinase target or acetylation or methylation of a histone tail for an epigenetic modulator (Garralda et al. 2017). Ideally, these biochemical changes can be measured in both tumor tissue and in more easily accessible surrogate tissues such as blood cells or skin. This is because in the dose escalation phase of a FIH trial, it is challenging to obtain serial tumor biopsies (i.e., baseline and on treatment) to measure these changes. By collecting and analyzing both tumor and surrogate tissue in drug-treated xenograft models, these experiments can not only define the PK/PD/efficacy relationship, they can also define the relationship of tumor PD to surrogate tissue

PD. A threshold level and duration of PD effect in tumor and surrogate tissue from an informative preclinical model, together with an understanding of the PK parameters associated with efficacy, can be an important component of a dose selection strategy in a FIH trial (Parchment and Doroshow 2016).

From a practical perspective, real-time safety data is the most critical determinant of the progress of a FIH trial. Selection of the starting dose is based on the GLP toxicology studies that were conducted prior to the IND filing and chosen to provide an ample margin of safety (FDA 2005). Dose escalation decisions are undertaken by a Dose Escalation Committee (DEC) composed of the study physicians with representation from the industry sponsor of the drug as appropriate. As a rule, these studies seek to define an MTD, whether or not this ends up being the RP2D. Over the last 10–15 years, the traditional deterministic 3 + 3 design for these trials has been replaced by Bayesian dose escalation models that provide greater flexibility and accuracy in defining an MTD (Doussau et al. 2012; Jaki et al. 2013). Whether the approach is deterministic or Bayesian, the DEC evaluates all adverse events (AEs) that have occurred in a given dose cohort including protocol-defined dose-limiting toxicities (DLTs) to decide if a dose escalation step is warranted and the magnitude of the increment. PK and PD data typically lags behind the dose escalation decisions but is reviewed as it becomes available and could impact a dose escalation decision if, for example, it becomes clear that the last escalation step did not result in a significant increase in exposure or PD (i.e., approaching saturation, maximal inhibition, or futility). Selecting the RP2D requires an integration of all of the available data in the context of the prespecified goals for PK and PD as well as the safety profile that would support further development. If, for example, preclinical models suggest that more than 50% inhibition of the intended target is needed for efficacy and unacceptable toxicity (i.e., the MTD) is encountered at doses that only achieve 10–20% inhibition, it might be unwise to move forward into efficacy testing with that dose.

5.4 Clinical Proof of Concept (PoC)

Proof of concept (PoC) is one of those fraught terms in drug development that can mean many different things to different people. A useful definition of clinical PoC is that it comprises a package of data that supports investing in a costly and often lengthy Phase 3 trial for regulatory approval. This kind of investment requires a reasonable level of confidence that the Phase 3 study will be successful based on observing evidence of target-dependent activity on a clinically measurable endpoint in previous early phase studies (Chen and Beckman 2014). This is different from simply observing clinical activity in two important ways. For conventional cytotoxic chemotherapeutics, the observation of anti-tumor activity in one tumor type versus another has always been empirical. There is nothing about the mechanism of these agents that provides a rationale for their observed activity. DNA cross-linking agents, alkylating agents, and topoisomerase inhibitors all cause DNA damage, but each was found to be more active in some malignancies than in others. Identifying a promising indication for a new agent without a clear idea of what tumor type or subset thereof will be sensitive can require multiple studies, many of which will be negative or equivocal. Even when a promising activity signal is detected in a specific histologic tumor type in Phase 2, there is no guarantee that it will hold up in a larger Phase 3 study. This is because of the extensive heterogeneity within any given type of cancer. Heterogeneity applies not only to clinical variables, such as previous lines of therapy, which can be controlled for but also to molecular heterogeneity (Zolotovskaia et al. 2020). Phase 2 and Phase 3 populations may thus differ in terms of the representation of underlying factors that predispose a patient's tumor to be sensitive or resistant to the agent. A consequence of moving into Phase 3 studies on the basis of empirically observed, poorly understood signals of activity is a high failure rate for these large and costly studies (Jardim et al. 2017).

This is where having a strong therapeutic hypothesis becomes critical again by providing a basis for interpreting clinical activity in the context of target dependency. When a BRAF inhibitor shows activity in $BRAF^{V600E}$-mutated melanoma but not in $BRAF^{wt}$ melanoma, there should be a reasonable expectation that this will hold up in larger studies (Larkin et al. 2014). Similarly, the inhibitor of mutated IDH2, enasidenib, showed early evidence of clinical activity in AML patients with IDH2 mutations as expected. This allowed the program to move quickly to registration on the basis of an extended Phase 1 study. This type of activity is convincing not only to industry sponsors but to regulatory authorities as well. The enasidenib story also brings up another important aspect of defining PoC, the nature of the clinical activity resulting from successfully modulating the drug target. The traditional definition of activity, which is still the most common, is the killing of tumor cells as evidenced by radiographic regression of a lesion on a CT or MRI scan in solid tumors or the induction of a period of marrow aplasia followed by recovery without leukemic blasts (complete response) in the acute leukemias. A recent exception to this were responses to enasidenib in IDH2-mutated AML patients (Stein et al. 2019). These responses were characterized initially by a recovery of platelet and neutrophil counts with only gradual reductions in the proportion of blasts and essentially no marrow aplasia. This is entirely consistent with the role of IDH2 mutations in blocking the differentiation of myeloid progenitors and with the removal of that blockade by the action of enasidenib (Amatangelo et al. 2017). Restoration of hematologic function, even without immediate elimination of all blasts, provides clinical benefit to patients and, importantly, extends survival. The therapeutic hypothesis should, therefore, not only provide an idea of the clinical context within which there is a high likelihood of response but also an idea of how that response would manifest to support PoC.

The establishment of surrogate endpoints for PoC trials remains an ongoing challenge. The hematologic malignancies have benefitted from the ease of access to malignant cells with a blood draw. This allowed the immediate appreciation of reductions in white blood cell counts in CML patients treated with imatinib and the appearance of mature neutrophils in IDH2-mutated AML patients treated with enasidenib (Amatangelo et al. 2017; Capdeville et al. 2002). For lymphomas and solid tumors, however, objective responses based on RECIST criteria provide the only reliable way to assess activity within the single-arm, open-label study design that describe most Phase 2 trials. This is primarily because radiographic imaging of the primary mass or metastases is readily performed and quantitated objectively. We know that these responses do not always translate into the gold standard for clinical benefit which is survival (Grimaldi et al. 2018). Nevertheless, response rates remain important due to the difficulty of interpreting a time-to-event endpoint like survival in the context of an uncontrolled single-arm study. While uncontrolled growth is certainly one aspect of the cancer phenotype, there are many other hallmarks, as defined in the classic publication by Hanahan and Weinberg, which are critical to sustain a tumor (Hanahan and Weinberg 2011). These include things like deregulating tumor metabolism, activating invasion and metastasis, and genomic instability. Drugging targets that drive these behaviors could, conceivably, prolong survival without necessarily inducing cell death within the tumor on a scale that would result in a significant radiographic regression. For example, the androgen receptor antagonist, enzalutamide, clearly prolongs survival in men with castrate-resistant prostate cancer despite the fact that it does not produce a measurable objective response rate.

A randomized Phase 2 study can be conducted to establish PoC if the PoC will be based on a time-to-event endpoint like survival or if it is important to demonstrate an improvement in response rate over an existing treatment. An added benefit of this approach is that it can provide an estimate of the treatment effect to help size the Phase 3 study appropriately. The main disadvantage to a randomized Phase 2 study is the cost and impact to the development timeline. An adequately powered randomized Phase 2 can require upward of 100 subjects and begins to approach a small Phase 3 in terms of cost and duration. This brings us back to the original need for data to support this kind of investment of resources as well as patients. Novel approaches in development that could supplement or replace, in some cases at least, traditional RECIST-based response assessment are being evaluated. These include functional imaging, of which FDG-PET is the most well established (Wahl et al. 2009). Loss of glucose uptake by a tumor that was PET-avid prior to treatment is clearly indicative of a drug effect that is reasonably likely to result in a beneficial effect (Lei et al. 2016). Dynamic contrast-enhanced (DCE) MRI can be used to evaluate microvascularity in tumors, while diffusion-weighted MRI measures intracellular and extracellular water content to estimate the cellularity of tissue (Torigian et al. 2007). Imaging before and after treatment with an agent expected to impact these parameters could provide proof-of-mechanism to increase confidence to proceed with a subsequent trial. Non-imaging-based approaches to study tumor responses to a novel agent include circulating tumor cells (CTC) and circulating tumor DNA (ctDNA) (Cabel et al. 2017; Cristiano et al. 2019). CTC are well validated in some diseases such as prostate cancer and can be tracked over time, before and after drug treatment to measure anti-tumor activity. Quantitating tumor-specific mutations by sequencing ctDNA can also be used to evaluate tumor responses over time (Ma et al. 2020). All of these approaches will need to be validated in specific tumor types with specific drug candidates before they become firmly established endpoints to support decision-making by drug developers, to say nothing of regulatory agencies.

5.5 Putting It All Together: Combined Phase 1–2 Studies

The advent of hypothesis-driven studies in the exploratory phase of cancer drug development has resulted in the phenomenon, at least in adult oncology studies in the USA, of what has variously been referred to as a Phase 1–2 study or a Phase 1 study with expansion cohorts (Geoerger et al. 2020; Schafer et al. 2020; FDA 2022). In either case, the idea is to transition nearly seamlessly from a dose-finding stage, usually enrolling an unselected patient population, followed by a single-arm expansion at the RP2D in at least one patient population that is expected to be enriched for responders. The enrichment can be on the basis of a particular tumor histology, clinicopathologic or molecular biomarker-defined subset, depending on the target and therapeutic hypothesis. In some cases, multiple parallel cohorts are open, resulting in FIH trials that enroll 100 or more patients (Bang et al. 2020). Although this may seem inefficient, the idea is to get the drug, at the right dose and schedule, into the patients who, according to the therapeutic hypothesis, have the highest likelihood of responding. Ironically, by allowing a drug to fail early in its development, this approach can be very efficient. Failure can come during the dose-finding phase if the PK and PD objectives cannot be achieved due to toxicity or poor PK properties. If the PK and PD objectives are achieved but no activity is observed in the population with the greatest likelihood of response, there is little enthusiasm for testing the drug in other populations with even less of a rationale for sensitivity. If, on the other hand, the expected activity is seen in the expected patient population, the drug and target have been, to a significant extent, de-risked, and investing in further development, including other patient subsets and combinations, can proceed with confidence.

This is the theory. In practice, there is rarely a therapeutic hypothesis that is so focused around a particular population, leading to multiple parallel expansion cohorts, each with its own rationale, to increase the likelihood of observing activity. This has been the case for many of the drugs targeting the PI3K/AKT/mTOR signaling pathway (Yap et al. 2015; Polivka Jr and Janku 2014; Mayer and Arteaga 2016). These are targets that have been implicated in multiple cancer types though, often, without a mutational roadmap to select specific patients whose tumors are addicted. The expansion cohorts in these trials were often defined on the basis of histology, e.g., lung, breast, or colorectal cancer. While some patients experienced dramatic responses in some of these cohorts, they were mostly anecdotal, without a clear rhyme or reason for the lack of response in similar patients. Combined with the on- and off-target toxicities associated with these targets, including rashes and mucositis, this spotty activity was not sufficient to support registrational trials in many cases. The only exceptions to this were the isoform-selective PI3K inhibitors, alpelisib for PI3Kα and idelalisib for PI3Kδ (Narayan et al. 2020; Markham 2014). Alpelisib has been approved for breast cancer based on the presence of activating PIK3Ca mutations in a subset of HER-2-positive breast cancer patients. PI3Kδ is expressed selectively in lymphoid tissues and plays a key role in B-cell receptor signaling which is a driver in CLL. It showed activity in patients with relapsed CLL and is now FDA approved in that indication. These examples highlight the importance of having a well-defined therapeutic hypothesis to guide exploratory drug development.

Although clinical activity consistent with the therapeutic hypothesis is critical to supporting the decision to advance to registrational trials, it is by no means the only requirement. Meeting regulatory requirements ahead of a label-enabling trial means many more boxes will need to be checked. These boxes relate primarily to safety and dose and schedule justification. The US FDA and other health authorities need to make a comprehensive assessment of the risks and potential benefits of allowing a new drug onto the market. This requires a safety database of at least a few hundred patients treated across multiple studies in most cases. A package of studies addressing drug-drug interactions and PK in special populations, such as patients with hepatic impairment, may also be required. Finally, a justification for the dose and schedule selected has become an important component of negotiations with regulatory authorities. This can involve population PK modeling and other analyses of dose and exposure in relation to toxicity and efficacy across earlier studies. The intent of all this is to be able to provide adequate information in the label for physicians to prescribe the drug safely to their patients (FDA 2020). In situations where the intended approved patient population is exceedingly rare, it may not be possible to provide all of this information ahead of a planned registrational trial.

If the unmet need is sufficiently dire and the promise of the drug is based on a strong mechanistic rationale that supports the observed efficacy, it may be possible to negotiate acquisition of these data in parallel with the registrational trial or as a post-marketing commitment (FDA 2014). These options are summarized in the FDA guidance document on expedited programs for serious conditions and includes fast track or breakthrough designations, priority review, and accelerated approval pathway. With sufficiently compelling efficacy and safety data and a well-understood mechanism, the exploratory phase of development can essentially become confirmatory, giving patients in need access to new therapies in an expedient fashion.

5.6 A Role for Pediatric Cancer in Exploratory Drug Development

The importance of a sound, biologically plausible therapeutic hypothesis to guide exploratory drug development provides an important avenue for moving testing of new agents into children with cancer sooner than has been the case historically. Once a safe and potentially active dose has been established in adults, the indication with the clearest biological rationale may be a pediatric cancer. This has been the case with the EZH2 inhibitor tazemetostat. A synthetic lethal dependency on EZH2 occurs in tumors with mutations in components of the SWI/SNF nuclear remodeling complex (Kim et al. 2015). These mutations are found in almost all cases of malignant rhabdoid tumor (MRT), a rare tumor type but one which occurs in children (St Pierre and Kadoch 2017). A Phase 1 trial of tazemetostat in children with MRT and other SWI-/SNF-mutated tumors is currently enrolling (NCT02601937). Similarly, larotrectinib, an inhibitor of the neurotrophic receptor tyrosine kinase (NTRK), is active in tumors with NTRK gene fusions, including infantile fibrosarcomas (Cocco et al. 2018). This rare but biologically well-defined pediatric tumor contributed to the approval of larotrectinib in a basket trial design enrolling multiple tumor types, adult and pediatric, based on the presence to NTRK gene fusions (Scott 2019). When the adult MTD/RP2D has been established, a limited dose-ranging trial can determine an acceptable dose in pediatric patients, enabling efficacy testing in biomarker-defined populations to begin. As the understanding of pathogenic drivers of pediatric cancers increases, along with the availability of drugs targeting those drivers, there will be more opportunities to test those drugs early, benefiting both adult and pediatric patients by delivering clinical PoC.

References

Amatangelo MD, Quek L, Shih A, Stein EM, Roshal M, David MD, Marteyn B, Farnoud NR, de Botton S, Bernard OA, Wu B, Yen KE, Tallman MS, Papaemmanuil E, Penard-Lacronique V, Thakurta A, Vyas P, Levine RL (2017) Enasidenib induces acute myeloid leukemia cell differentiation to promote clinical response. Blood 130(6):732–741. https://doi.org/10.1182/blood-2017-04-779447. Epub 2017 Jun 6

Bang YJ, Su WC, Schuler M, Nam DH, Lim WT, Bauer TM, Azaro A, Poon RTP, Hong D, Lin CC, Akimov M, Ghebremariam S, Zhao S, Giovannini M, Ma B (2020) Phase 1 study of capmatinib in MET-positive solid tumor patients: dose escalation and expansion of selected cohorts. Cancer Sci 111(2):536–547. https://doi.org/10.1111/cas.14254. Epub 2019 Dec 30

Bullock JM, Rahman A, Liu Q (2016) Lessons learned: dose selection of small molecule-targeted oncology drugs. Clin Cancer Res 22(11):2630–2638. https://doi.org/10.1158/1078-0432.CCR-15-2646

Cabel L, Proudhon C, Gortais H, Loirat D, Coussy F, Pierga JY, Bidard FC (2017) Circulating tumor cells: clinical validity and utility. Int J Clin Oncol 22(3):421–430. https://doi.org/10.1007/s10147-017-1105-2. Epub 2017 Feb 25

Capdeville R, Buchdunger E, Zimmermann J, Matter A (2002) Glivec (STI571, imatinib), a rationally developed, targeted anticancer drug. Nat Rev Drug Discov 1(7):493–502. https://doi.org/10.1038/nrd839

Chen C, Beckman RA (2014) Maximizing return on socioeconomic investment in phase II proof-of-concept trials. Clin Cancer Res 20(7):1730–1734. https://doi.org/10.1158/1078-0432.CCR-13-2312. Epub 2014 Feb 13

Cocco E, Scaltriti M, Drilon A (2018) NTRK fusion-positive cancers and TRK inhibitor therapy. Nat Rev Clin Oncol 15(12):731–747. https://doi.org/10.1038/s41571-018-0113-0

Cook N, Hansen AR, Siu LL, Abdul Razak AR (2015) Early phase clinical trials to identify optimal dosing and safety. Mol Oncol 9(5):997–1007. https://doi.org/10.1016/j.molonc.2014.07.025. Epub 2014 Aug 14

Cristiano S, Leal A, Phallen J, Fiksel J, Adleff V, Bruhm DC, Jensen SØ, Medina JE, Hruban C, White JR, Palsgrove DN, Niknafs N, Anagnostou V, Forde P, Naidoo J, Marrone K, Brahmer J, Woodward BD, Husain H, van Rooijen KL, Ørntoft MW, Madsen AH, van de Velde CJH, Verheij M, Cats A, Punt CJA, Vink GR, van Grieken NCT, Koopman M, Fijneman RJA, Johansen JS, Nielsen HJ, Meijer GA, Andersen CL, Scharpf RB, Velculescu VE (2019) Genome-wide cell-free DNA fragmentation in patients with cancer. Nature 570(7761):385–389. https://doi.org/10.1038/s41586-019-1272-6. Epub 2019 May 29

Doussau A, Asselain B, Le Deley MC, Geoerger B, Doz F, Vassal G, Paoletti X (2012) Dose-finding designs in pediatric phase I clinical trials: comparison by simulations in a realistic timeline framework. Contemp Clin Trials 33(4):657–665. https://doi.org/10.1016/j.cct.2011.11.015. Epub 2012 Apr 13

FDA (2005). https://www.fda.gov/regulatory-information/search-fda-guidance-documents/estimating-maximum-safe-starting-dose-initial-clinical-trials-therapeutics-adult-healthy-volunteers

FDA (2014). https://www.fda.gov/regulatory-information/search-fda-guidance-documents/expedited-programs-serious-conditions-drugs-and-biologics

FDA (2020). https://www.fda.gov/about-fda/project-renewal/about-oncology-prescription-drug-labeling#

FDA (2022). https://www.fda.gov/regulatory-information/search-fda-guidance-documents/expansion-cohorts-use-first-human-clinical-trials-expedite-development-oncology-drugs-and-biologics

Garralda E, Dienstmann R, Tabernero J (2017) Pharmacokinetic/pharmacodynamic modeling for drug development in oncology. Am Soc Clin Oncol Educ Book 37:210–215. https://doi.org/10.1200/EDBK_180460

Geoerger B, Zwaan CM, Marshall LV, Michon J, Bourdeaut F, Casanova M, Corradini N, Rossato G, Farid-Kapadia M, Shemesh CS, Hutchinson KE, Donaldson F, Liao M, Caron H, Trippett T (2020) Atezolizumab for children and young adults with previously treated solid tumours, non-Hodgkin lymphoma, and Hodgkin lymphoma (iMATRIX): a multicentre phase 1-2 study. Lancet Oncol 21(1):134–144. https://doi.org/10.1016/S1470-2045(19)30693-X. Epub 2019 Nov 25

Grimaldi S, Terroir M, Caramella C (2018) Advances in oncological treatment: limitations of RECIST 1.1 criteria. Q J Nucl Med Mol Imaging 62(2):129–139. https://doi.org/10.23736/S1824-4785.17.03038-2. Epub 2017 Nov 22

Hanahan D, Weinberg RA (2011) Hallmarks of cancer: the next generation. Cell 144(5):646–674. https://doi.org/10.1016/j.cell.2011.02.013

Horstmann E, McCabe MS, Grochow L, Yamamoto S, Rubinstein L, Budd T, Shoemaker D, Emanuel EJ, Grady C (2005) Risks and benefits of phase 1 oncology trials, 1991 through 2002. N Engl J Med 352(9):895–904. https://doi.org/10.1056/NEJMsa042220

Jaki T, Clive S, Weir CJ (2013) Principles of dose finding studies in cancer: a comparison of trial designs. Cancer Chemother Pharmacol 71(5):1107–1114. https://doi.org/10.1007/s00280-012-2059-8. Epub 2013 Jan 9

Jardim DL, Groves ES, Breitfeld PP, Kurzrock R (2017) Factors associated with failure of oncology drugs in late-stage clinical development: a systematic review. Cancer Treat Rev 52:12–21. https://doi.org/10.1016/j.ctrv.2016.10.009. Epub 2016 Nov 4

Kim KH, Kim W, Howard TP, Vazquez F, Tsherniak A, Wu JN, Wang W, Haswell JR, Walensky LD, Hahn WC, Orkin SH, Roberts CW (2015) SWI/SNF-mutant cancers depend on catalytic and non-catalytic activity of EZH2. Nat Med 21(12):1491–1496. https://doi.org/10.1038/nm.3968. Epub 2015 Nov 9

Larkin J, Del Vecchio M, Ascierto PA, Krajsova I, Schachter J, Neyns B, Espinosa E, Garbe C, Sileni VC, Gogas H, Miller WH Jr, Mandalà M, Hospers GA, Arance A, Queirolo P, Hauschild A, Brown MP, Mitchell L, Veronese L, Blank CU (2014) Vemurafenib in patients with BRAF(V600) mutated metastatic melanoma: an open-label, multicentre, safety study. Lancet Oncol 15(4):436–444. https://doi.org/10.1016/S1470-2045(14)70051-8. Epub 2014 Feb 27

Lei L, Wang X, Chen Z (2016) PET/CT imaging for monitoring recurrence and evaluating response to treatment in breast cancer. Adv Clin Exp Med 25(2):377–382. https://doi.org/10.17219/acem/29853

Lin A, Giuliano CJ, Palladino A, John KM, Abramowicz C, Yuan ML, Sausville EL, Lukow DA, Liu L, Chait AR, Galluzzo ZC, Tucker C, Sheltzer JM (2019) Off-target toxicity is a common mechanism of action of cancer drugs undergoing clinical trials. Sci Transl Med 11(509):eaaw8412. https://doi.org/10.1126/scitranslmed.aaw8412

Ma F, Guan Y, Yi Z, Chang L, Li Q, Chen S, Zhu W, Guan X, Li C, Qian H, Xia X, Yang L, Zhang J, Husain H, Liao Z, Futreal A, Huang J, Yi X, Xu B (2020) Assessing tumor heterogeneity using ctDNA to predict and monitor therapeutic response in metastatic breast cancer. Int J Cancer 146(5):1359–1368. https://doi.org/10.1002/ijc.32536. Epub 2019 Jul 4. Erratum in: Int J Cancer. 2020;146(12):E8

Markham A (2014) Idelalisib: first global approval. Drugs 74(14):1701–1707. https://doi.org/10.1007/s40265-014-0285-6. Erratum in: Drugs. 2014;74(15):1839

Mayer IA, Arteaga CL (2016) The PI3K/AKT pathway as a target for cancer treatment. Annu Rev Med 67:11–28. https://doi.org/10.1146/annurev-med-062913-051343. Epub 2015 Oct 14

Narayan P, Prowell TM, Gao JJ, Fernandes LL, Li E, Jiang X, Qiu J, Fan J, Song P, Yu J, Zhang X, King-Kallimanis BL, Chen W, Ricks TK, Gong Y, Wang X, Windsor K, Rhieu SY, Geiser G, Banerjee A, Chen X, Reyes Turcu F, Chatterjee DK, Pathak A, Seidman J, Ghosh S, Philip R, Goldberg KB, Kluetz PG, Tang S, Amiri-Kordestani L, Theoret MR, Pazdur R, Beaver JA (2020) FDA approval summary: alpelisib plus fulvestrant for patients with HR-positive, HER2-negative, PIK3CA-mutated, advanced or metastatic breast cancer. Clin Cancer Res. https://doi.org/10.1158/1078-0432.CCR-20-3652. Epub ahead of print

Parchment RE, Doroshow JH (2016) Pharmacodynamic endpoints as clinical trial objectives to answer important questions in oncology drug development. Semin Oncol 43:514–525. https://doi.org/10.1053/j.seminoncol.2016.07.002. Epub 2016 Jul 26

Polivka J Jr, Janku F (2014) Molecular targets for cancer therapy in the PI3K/AKT/mTOR pathway. Pharmacol Ther 142(2):164–175. https://doi.org/10.1016/j.pharmthera.2013.12.004. Epub 2013 Dec 9

Schafer ES, Rau RE, Berg SL, Liu X, Minard CG, Bishop AJR, Romero JC, Hicks MJ, Nelson MD Jr, Voss S, Reid JM, Fox E, Weigel BJ, Blaney SM (2020) Phase 1/2 trial of talazoparib in combination with temozolomide in children and adolescents with refractory/recurrent solid tumors including Ewing sarcoma: a Children's Oncology Group Phase 1 Consortium study (ADVL1411). Pediatr Blood Cancer 67(2):e28073. https://doi.org/10.1002/pbc.28073. Epub 2019 Nov 14

Scott LJ (2019) Larotrectinib: first global approval. Drugs 79(2):201–206. https://doi.org/10.1007/s40265-018-1044-x

St Pierre R, Kadoch C (2017) Mammalian SWI/SNF complexes in cancer: emerging therapeutic opportunities. Curr Opin Genet Dev 42:56–67. https://doi.org/10.1016/j.gde.2017.02.004. Epub 2017 Apr 6

Stein EM, DiNardo CD, Fathi AT, Pollyea DA, Stone RM, Altman JK, Roboz GJ, Patel MR, Collins R, Flinn IW, Sekeres MA, Stein AS, Kantarjian HM, Levine RL, Vyas P, MacBeth KJ, Tosolini A, VanOostendorp J, Xu Q, Gupta I, Lila T, Risueno A, Yen KE, Wu B, Attar EC, Tallman MS, de Botton S (2019) Molecular remission and response patterns in patients with mutant-*IDH2* acute myeloid leukemia treated with enasidenib. Blood 133(7):676–687. https://doi.org/10.1182/blood-2018-08-869008. Epub 2018 Dec 3

Torigian DA, Huang SS, Houseni M, Alavi A (2007) Functional imaging of cancer with emphasis on molecular techniques. CA Cancer J Clin 57(4):206–224. https://doi.org/10.3322/canjclin.57.4.206. Erratum in: CA Cancer J Clin. 2007;57(6):380

Wahl RL, Jacene H, Kasamon Y, Lodge MA (2009) From RECIST to PERCIST: evolving considerations for PET response criteria in solid tumors. J Nucl Med 50(Suppl 1):122S–150S. https://doi.org/10.2967/jnumed.108.057307

Yap TA, Bjerke L, Clarke PA, Workman P (2015) Drugging PI3K in cancer: refining targets and therapeutic strategies. Curr Opin Pharmacol 23:98–107. https://doi.org/10.1016/j.coph.2015.05.016. Epub 2015 Jun 25

Zolotovskaia MA, Sorokin MI, Petrov IV, Poddubskaya EV, Moiseev AA, Sekacheva MI, Borisov NM, Tkachev VS, Garazha AV, Kaprin AD, Shegay PV, Giese A, Kim E, Roumiantsev SA, Buzdin AA (2020) Disparity between inter-patient molecular heterogeneity and repertoires of target drugs used for different types of cancer in clinical oncology. Int J Mol Sci 21(5):1580. https://doi.org/10.3390/ijms21051580

Gene and Cell Therapy: How to Build a BioDrug

6

Susanne Baumeister and Ann Woolfrey

Contents

S. Baumeister
Division of Pediatric Hematology-Oncology, Boston Children's Hospital, Boston, MA, USA

Department of Pediatric Oncology, Dana-Farber Cancer Institute, Boston, MA, USA

Harvard Medical School, Boston, MA, USA
e-mail: SUSANNE_BAUMEISTER@DFCI.HARVARD.EDU

A. Woolfrey (✉)
Clinical Research Division, Fred Hutchinson Cancer Research Center, Seattle, WA, USA

Medpace, Inc., Cincinnati, OH, USA
e-mail: a.woolfrey@medpace.com

J. DiMartino et al. (eds.), *Pediatric Cancer Therapeutics Development*, Pediatric Oncology,
https://doi.org/10.1007/978-3-031-06357-2_6

6.1 Introduction

BioDrugs, or advanced therapeutic medicinal products (ATMP), are novel medicines involving genes, tissues, or cells for use in the treatment of a variety of diseases. The European Medicines Agency (EMA) classifies ATMP into three general categories: (1) gene therapies, (2) somatic-cell therapies, and (3) tissue-engineered medicines (https://www.ema.europa.eu/en/human-regulatory/overview/advanced-therapy-medicinal-products-overview), although there is overlap in the types of technologies used to create BioDrugs in these categories. For example, techniques used to edit or insert genes may be used to create a BioDrug used for gene therapy or for somatic-cell therapy. Development of a successful BioDrug requires in-depth knowledge of cellular biology and molecular genetics, complex manufacturing procedures, and completion of rigorous clinical trials in patients with serious medical illness. This chapter provides a resource for pediatric hematologist/oncologists to learn about the fundamental technologies involved in BioDrug development and will focus on the development of BioDrugs in the first two categories: (1) *gene therapies*, defined as a BioDrug that contain genes for insertion into the human genome or that contain gene-editing machinery for intracellular correction of genetic diseases, and (2) *cell therapies*, defined as cell products or tissues that have been manipulated to change their biologic characteristics with the aim to cure human disease.

As ATMP become more available, it is important to understand the principles involved in their development and the components required to produce a BioDrug. The genes, gene-editing tools, delivery systems, tissues, and cells used to generate ATMP can be thought of as existing in a BioDrug ToolKit (Fig. 6.1), which contains various components or tools for use in development of a BioDrug. The main categories of "tools" used in production of a BioDrug include cells, genetic materials and editing systems, and delivery systems. A vast choice of tools exists within each category, which can be combined to generate novel therapeutic agents that can be applied ex vivo in laboratory-based cell cultures or in vivo by direct administration to a patient for treatment of life-threatening malignancies or hematologic disorders.

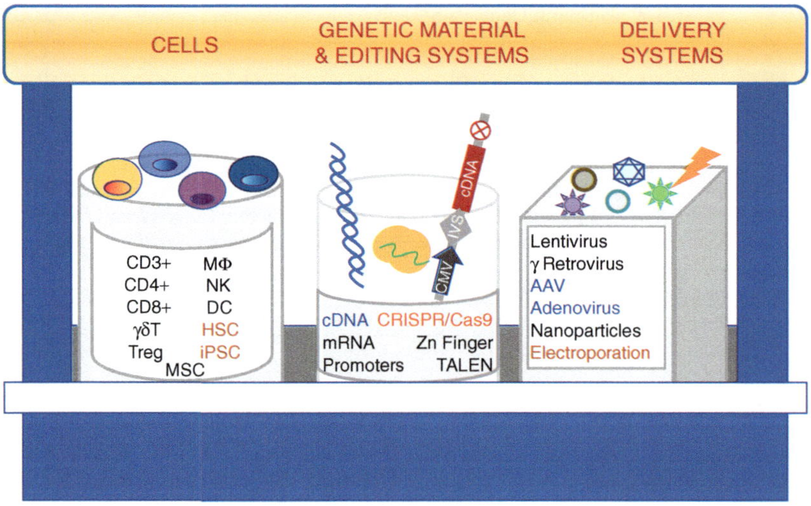

Fig. 6.1 The BioDrug ToolKit contains groups of tools and materials used to engineer cell and gene therapy. Combinations of cells, genetic material, and transgene delivery systems are used to engineer BioDrugs. Cells are selected for their biologic properties. The selection of the genetic material or editing systems is based on the desired genetic engineering approach. The selection of the delivery system is based on its carrying capacity and the efficiency of gene transduction

6.2 BioDrug ToolKit: Cells

The first important group of tools in developing a BioDrug are the cells or tissues that will be used either as targets of the BioDrug or as a component of the BioDrug itself. A cell may be used by itself as a BioDrug, or it may be genetically engineered to perform a specific function. BioDrug cells which are intended to be returned to the individual from which they were collected are termed "autologous" cells, whereas cells that are collected from one individual for administration to another individual are termed "allogeneic" cells. Allogeneic cells will differ genetically from the recipient and may express different major histocompatibility complex (MHC) antigens or minor histocompatibility antigens. The need to match the human leukocyte antigens (HLA) of the recipient with allogeneic cells depends upon the end use of the cells and whether long-term engraftment is desired. Depending on the type of immune cell, unmatched, unmanipulated allogeneic cells can mediate tissue damage in the recipient (i.e., graft-versus-host disease (GVHD)).

Cell products may be administered to the patient immediately after collection of the cells, such as in bone marrow transplantation procedures, or may also be cryopreserved for future use (Hornberger et al. 2019). Cryopreservation involves placing the cells in a solution with dimethyl sulfoxide (DMSO) which allows the cells to survive extremely low temperatures. The cell solution is cooled at a controlled rate until it can be stored in liquid nitrogen (approximately −195 °C). The shelf-life of cryopreserved cells depends on the cell type and cryopreservation methods.

The BioDrug ToolKit contains a variety of cells that can be developed for therapeutic use. The most commonly used cells are described here.

6.2.1 Hematopoietic Stem Cells (HSCs)

HSCs are capable of either self-renewal or differentiation into the various mature cells that comprise the hematopoietic system, including red cells, platelets, myeloid cells, and lymphocytes. HSCs reside in the bone marrow and can be obtained by direct aspiration of bone marrow or through mobilization of HSC into the bloodstream and removal via apheresis. HSCs are anchored in the marrow by adhesion to stromal cells; therefore, release of HSC into the peripheral blood requires interfering with these cellular bonds. The most efficient way to release HSC is through agents that disrupt adhesion bonds such as CXCR4-CXCL12. The most commonly used agents include granulocyte colony-stimulating factor (G-CSF) and more recently plerixafor (Giralt et al. 2014). While both bone marrow and mobilized peripheral blood stem cell (PBSC) products contain HSC, there are differences in composition that might affect the end use. Compared to mobilized PBSC, marrow products contain relatively more red cells and a lower proportion of T cells and may contain other bone marrow-derived cells, such as mesenchymal stromal cells. Bone marrow or mobilized PBSC may be administered to patients up to several days following collection, after which the viability is significantly reduced (Lazarus et al. 2009). When the intention is not for immediate use, both products may be cryopreserved and then thawed before administration to a patient or for use in generating an engineered cell product (Hornberger et al. 2019). HSCs also reside in the placenta and may be obtained by collection of postpartum umbilical cord blood and cryopreserved for future use.

In the setting of hematopoietic cell transplantation (HCT), HSCs can be viewed as a cell therapy product used to restore hematopoiesis after marrow-ablative therapy. HSCs also are used as the cellular component for the development of gene therapy products aimed at correcting genetic defects resulting in hematopoietic or immunologic diseases.

6.2.2 T Lymphocytes

T lymphocytes are the main effector cells of the adaptive immune system. Mature T cells recognize antigen via the T cell receptor (TCR), which is expressed early in T cell development (Davis and Bjorkman 1988). TCRs are heterodimers

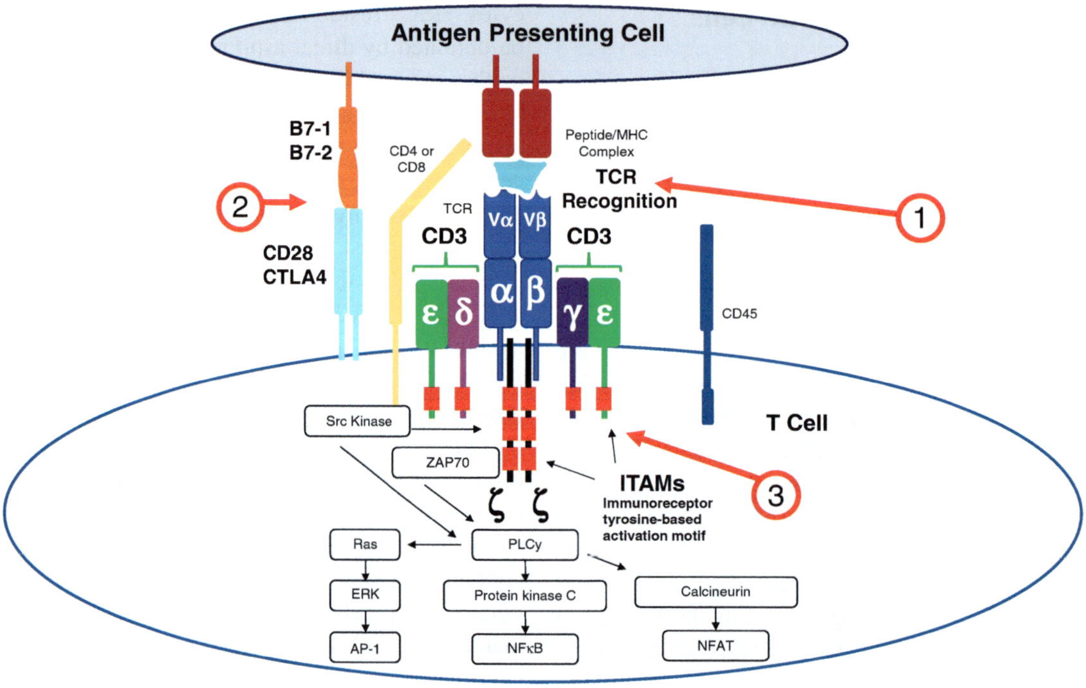

Fig. 6.2 The T cell recognition complex is comprised of (1) the T cell receptor (TCR); (2) the CD3 complex; and (3) the zeta (ζ) chain signaling molecules. The TCR is a heterodimer composed of alpha (α) and beta (β) chains. Each chain has a variable (V) and a constant region. When the TCR recognizes a peptide presented by a major histocompatibility antigen, signaling through the ζ chains results in phosphorylation of intracellular immunoreceptor tyrosine-based activation motifs (ITAMs). T cell activation involves three basic steps. Step 1: The T cell receptor recognizes the peptide in the context of the major histocompatibility complex (MHC) antigen of the antigen-presenting cell (APC). Step 2: A second signal or co-stimulatory signal is received by the T cell from the APC. Step 3: The TCR signal in concert with the co-stimulatory stimulates intracellular signaling leading to recruitment of ZAP-70 and Src kinase activation and subsequent generation of cytokines that promote T cell proliferation

comprised of α- and β-polypeptides linked by disulfide bonds. Each polypeptide has a variable region (Vα and Vβ, respectively) and a constant region (Fig. 6.2). The variable regions of the heterodimers are translated from a series of randomly juxtaposed sections of the V, D, and J genetic regions. When expressed on the cell surface, the TCR heterodimer associates with the CD3 heterodimeric complex externally, and internally associates with the ζ chain.

The entire complex, including the TCR, CD3, and ζ chain, is required for T cell antigen recognition and signaling (Alcover et al. 2018). In the simplest sense, activation and proliferation of antigen-specific T cells requires three main steps (Fig. 6.2): the first is TCR recognition of an antigen presented in the groove of a MHC molecule, which in humans are the human leukocyte antigens (HLA) (La Gruta et al. 2018; Smith-Garvin et al. 2009). Next a second signal or co-stimulatory signal must be received by the T cell from the antigen-presenting cell (APC). Importantly, if the second signal is not received, the T is rendered impotent or anergic (Sharpe and Freeman 2002; Azuma 2019). Co-signal receptors on the T cell include CD28, which interacts with B7-1 and B7-2 molecules, and the inducible T cell co-stimulator (ICOS), which interacts with the ICOS ligand. When stimulated, CD28 transmits a signal that in concert with the TCR signal results in the third step, phosphorylation of intracellular immunoreceptor tyrosine-based activation motifs (ITAMs) leading to recruitment of ZAP-70 and Src kinase activation and subsequent generation of cytokines such as IL-2 that promote clonal expansion.

To acquire sufficient numbers of T cells for cell therapy, large numbers of peripheral blood mononuclear cells (PBMC) are obtained by non-mobilized apheresis and then placed in culture conditions that support expansion of the desired T cell subset(s). Various T cell subsets have been used as a source for cell therapy products and can be selected from the apheresis product by their cell surface receptors. Most T cells within the product have heterodimeric TCRs composed of α- and β-polypeptides. αβT cells that express CD8 recognize peptides presented by class I HLA, whereas T cells that express CD4 recognize peptides presented by class II HLA. These subsets can be functionally defined further into naïve and memory subsets, which can be distinguished from each other by expression of other surface markers, e.g., CD62L, CCR7, and CD45RA expression on naïve T cells and CD45RO on memory T cell subsets (De Rosa et al. 2001). αβT cell subsets have been the predominant cell type used in the development of BioDrugs that target malignancies.

A small fraction of T cells have TCRs composed of γ- and δ-polypeptides, which play a role in both the adaptive and innate immune responses (Paul et al. 2014). γδT cells are found primarily in mucosal tissue and are capable of HLA-unrestricted cytotoxic activity, secrete cytokines that facilitate T and B cell activity, and are capable of antigen presentation. The development of BioDrugs using γδT cells is being explored as an alternative to αβT cells, based on their ability to infiltrate a wide variety of tumors and to recognize small phosphorylated non-peptide molecules emanated by tumor cells (Brandes et al. 2005; Gertner-Dardenne et al. 2012; Groh et al. 1999).

T regulatory (Treg) cells are another small population of CD4+ T cells that play a role in maintaining peripheral tolerance and preventing autoimmune disease. Tregs are characterized by surface expression of CD25 and intracellular FOXP3 (Owen et al. 2019). BioDrugs based on Treg cells currently are being explored for inducing tolerance in organ transplant recipients or mitigating GVHD after HCT and in patients with autoimmune diseases.

6.2.3 Natural Killer (NK) Cells

NK cells are large granular lymphocytes that play a pivotal role in the innate immune response to viral pathogens and tumors as well as have an adjunctive role in the adaptive immune response (Campbell and Hasegawa 2013; Caligiuri 2008; Sun et al. 2009). NK cells reside in lymphoid tissue as well as circulate in the blood and are characterized by surface expression of CD56 and lack of CD3 expression. NK cells interact with their environment through multiple inhibitory and activating receptors, including killer-cell immunoglobulin-like receptors (KIRs), CD16, or NKG2D, which engage MHC class I as well as non-MHC molecules. Activation of NK cells can occur either through engagement of a ligand with an activating receptor or by lack of engagement of an inhibitory KIR with its MHC class I ligand. Once activated, NK cells can directly kill target cells through perforin/granzyme production or through death receptor pathways (Smyth et al. 2001; Bryceson et al. 2006). Activated NK cells also produce gamma interferon (IFNγ), thus stimulating components of the adaptive immune response. NK are generated for cell therapy by apheresis and subsequent selection of CD56-positive cells, which are then placed in culture or cryopreserved (Kottaridis et al. 2015). NK cells currently are being developed as autologous or allogeneic cell therapies, either as unmanipulated cell products or as engineered tumor-directed cells.

6.2.4 Macrophages (MΦs)

MΦs reside in a variety of tissues and function to maintain homeostasis through cell-to-cell contact and elaboration of cytokines. Depending upon the microenvironment, MΦs become reversibly polarized toward a pro-inflammatory (M1) or an anti-inflammatory (M2) phenotype. M1 polarization occurs after stimulation of MΦs by pro-inflammatory agents such as IFNγ or lipopolysaccharide (LPS) which activate the NFκB pathway (Lee et al. 2016a; Mills et al. 2000). Pro-inflammatory MΦs play a role in the innate and adaptive immune systems through phagocytosis, antigen presentation, and cellular cytotoxicity. M2 polarization occurs in response to IL-4 signaling, as well as M-CSF, IL-10, IL-13, and TGF-β. These anti-inflammatory cytokines are prominent within the tumor microenvironment and result in polarization of tumor-associated MΦs (TAMs) (Italiani and Boraschi 2014). TAMs facilitate tumor persistence by contributing to the immunosuppressive environment and promoting angiogenesis and tumor invasion.

MΦs are obtained for cell therapy by apheresis or through lavage of alveolar or peritoneal tissues. Once collected, MΦs are placed into culture conditions that stimulate the M1 phenotype (Lee et al. 2016a). However, unlike T lymphocytes which can be expanded to large numbers in appropriate culture conditions, there is limited ability for MΦs to proliferate ex vivo. As an alternative approach, MΦs have been generated from conditional progenitor cell lines that allow differentiation to MΦs under specific culture conditions (Wang et al. 2006). M1 MΦs currently are currently being studied as the platform for solid tumor-directed engineered cell therapies (Klichinsky et al. 2020).

6.2.5 Dendritic Cells (DCs)

DCs are potent APCs involved in both the innate and adaptive immune responses. DCs arise from bone marrow CD34+ stem cells and reside in various tissues (Liu and Nussenzweig 2010). Mature DC subsets include myeloid/conventional DC1 (cDC1), myeloid/conventional DC2 (cDC2), and plasmacytoid DC (pDC) (Collin and Bigley 2018). DCs interact with their environment through multiple signaling receptors and produce various cytokines in response to stimulation. pDCs produce IFNα, TNF, IL-6, and granzyme B in response to receptor signaling by viral nucleic acids. cDC1 express MHC class I and present antigen to CD8+ T cells, as well as produce IFNα and IL-12. cDC2 also present antigen and secrete high levels of IL-12.

Dendritic cell therapy has been explored as a mechanism to increase anti-tumor immune responses through "vaccination" with cells that present tumor antigen to native CD8+ T cells (reviewed in depth in Sabado et al. 2017). DCs can be generated ex vivo from monocyte precursors or CD34+ HSC. Antigen loading of DCs is accomplished by incubation with proteins, RNA, or tumor cells along with GM-CSF to produce activated APCs. Sipuleucel-T is an example of an ex vivo cultured cell product that includes activated DCs, which is now approved for treatment of prostate cancer.

6.2.6 Mesenchymal Stem Cells (MSCs)

MSCs are defined by expression of CD73, CD90, and CD105, lack of HLA-DR expression, as well as the ability to adhere to plastic and to differentiate into mature mesenchymal tissues including adipocytes, chondrocytes, and osteoblasts (Wagner et al. 2005). MSCs can be derived from bone marrow, umbilical cord blood, as well as other adult and fetal tissues (Ullah et al. 2015). Tissue or blood MSCs are isolated by seeding onto plastic culture plates in specific culture conditions that can generate mesodermal, ectodermal, or endodermal lineages. MSCs are being studied for use in cancer immunotherapy as well as immunomodulating therapies for degenerative or autoimmune diseases. Currently there is considerable interest in using MSCs as either treatment for or prevention of graft-vs-host disease after allogeneic HCT (reviewed in Zhao et al. 2019).

6.2.7 Human-Induced Pluripotent Stem Cells (iPSCs)

Human iPSCs are not natural human cells but are mentioned here as these have been used to engineer BioDrugs. Human iPSCs are created by reprogramming a differentiated cell, such as a fibroblast, by insertion of genetic instructions (reviewed in Hockemeyer and Jaenisch 2016). This results in a personalized pluripotent cell that can then undergo differentiation by manipulating culture conditions to regenerate mature tissues, such as cardiac or neurologic tissues.

6.2.8 Target Tissues

Normal body tissues may be the target of genetic engineering in order to correct a genetic mutation within that specific cell. Examples include pulmonary epithelial cells in patients with cystic fibrosis, or retinal cells in patients with biallelic *RPE65* mutation-associated retinal dystrophy. Alternatively, an organ may play the role of host to new genetic machinery that produces a protein which functions elsewhere. The liver is a common target of in vivo gene therapy, because many viral vectors and nonviral particles that transport genetic material are hepatotropic. For example, the liver has been the target organ for expression of factor VIII in patients with hemophilia A (Pasi et al. 2020).

Abnormal tissues, such as solid tumors, are another type of target for gene or cell therapies. Tumors present challenges to effective drug delivery due to the heterogenous nature of the tumor and stromal cells. The tumor "ecosystem" results from interaction between tumor clones, stromal cells such as endothelial cells and fibroblasts, and host immune cells such as TAMs (Petty and Yang 2017). This symbiotic environment promotes tumorigenesis and creates an immunosuppressive tumor microenvironment (TME). Tumor heterogeneity poses a challenge to identify uniformly expressed tumor-specific antigens. Mechanisms to evade anti-tumor immune responses also vary within and between tumor types, resulting in a tumor-specific microenvironment that may be unique to the host (Hinshaw and Shevde 2019; Wu and Dai 2017).

6.3 BioDrug ToolKit: Genetic Material and Gene-Editing Machinery

The second important group of tools employed in the creation of a BioDrug are the genetic materials and machinery used for giving target cells new instructions or for correction of dysfunctional genes. The choice of genetic material depends upon whether gene replacement or gene editing is desired, whether long-term gene expression is desired, and the nature of the target tissue. Genetic information may be delivered to a cell as either mRNA or cDNA. cDNA must be transcribed into mRNA and therefore must enter the cell nucleus which contains the transcriptional machinery. Once in the nucleus, the genetic material of cDNA may become integrated into the host cell genome or can remain episomal, depending upon the approach used to deliver the cDNA into the cells. Integration of cDNA into the genome usually occurs randomly, although some vectors preferentially deliver the genetic material into specific genomic locations. The advantage of integrated cDNA is that the new genetic material will be replicated and carried into daughter cells during mitosis. Nonintegrated cDNA will be lost over time as its host cell undergoes mitosis. Accordingly, most cellular targets for nonintegrated cDNA are long-lived postmitotic cells in organs with low cell turnover, such as the liver, heart, or nervous system.

Protein expression from mRNA sequences requires just the intracellular translational machinery which can be found in the cytoplasm. However, protein expression is transient, persisting intracellularly for less than a month as mRNA will be degraded by intracellular RNase. Several techniques may increase the stability and durability of intracellular mRNA, for example, optimizing the non-translated genetic material at either end of the mRNA, such as 3′ untranslated regions (UTR) or the 5′ cap analogs (Orlandini von Niessen et al. 2019; Stepinski et al. 2001). The severe acute respiratory syndrome coronavirus 2 (SARS-CoV2) vaccine is an outstanding example of successful mRNA therapy that easily adapts to new viral mutations due to the relative ease of reprogramming the mRNA cassettes.

Transcription from either integrated or nonintegrated transgenes cannot occur without additional regulatory elements. Viral vectors used for episomal gene transfer may contain DNA replication and activation motifs sufficient to express the inserted mammalian genetic material (Van Craenenbroeck et al. 2000). Most vectors used in gene therapy con-

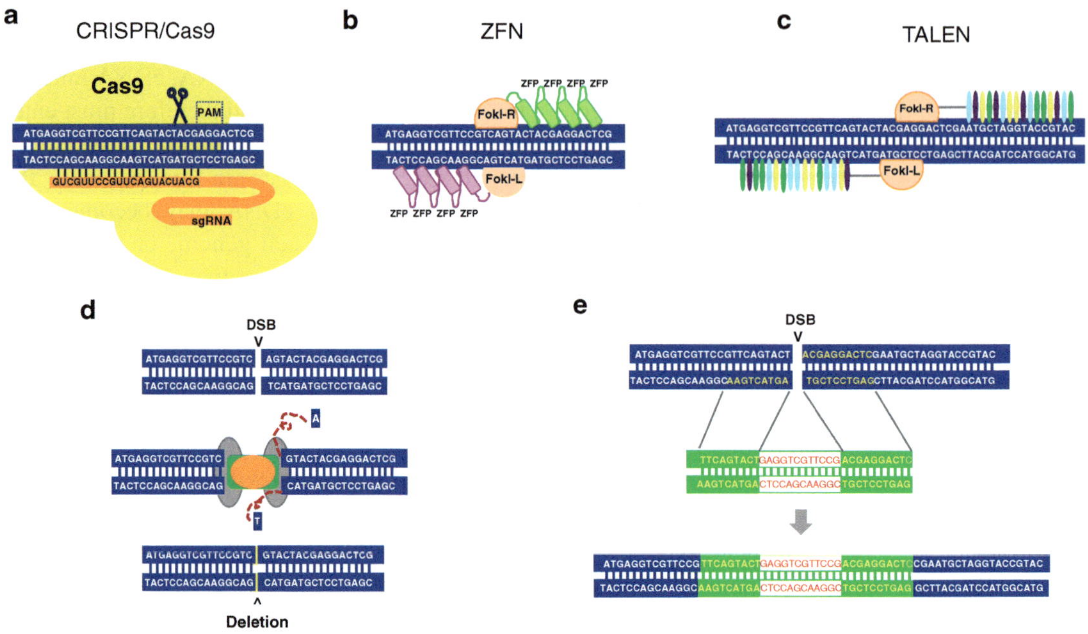

Fig. 6.3 Systems for gene editing in use most commonly include the clustered regularly interspaced short palindromic repeats (CRISPR)/CRISPR-associated (Cas) protein 9 or CRISPR/Cas9 system (panel **a**); zinc-finger nucleases (panel **b**); and transcription activator-like effector nucleases or TALENs (panel **c**). Each of these editing systems results in a double-strand DNA break. The broken strands are reunited by one of two natural repair pathways. The most common repair mechanism is nonhomologous end joining, in which the broken ends are directly ligated (panel **d**). Mistakes in the end ligation, such as a loss of a nucleotide, result in a deletion that can knock out the gene. Homology-directed repair (panel **e**) requires the presence of a homologous piece of DNA for religation. Insertion of new genetic sequence is accomplished by providing a length of DNA that has the new sequence, flanked by sections that are homologous the regions on either side of the double-strand break

tain an expression cassette, which consists of a promoter and a polyadenylation signal in addition to the therapeutic gene. DNA transcription is activated by a promoter within the cassette. The level of DNA transcription depends on promoter strength and tissue-specific activity. Elongation factor 1 alpha or cytomegalovirus (CMV) promoters are constitutively expressed and transactivate high levels of transgene expression (Kim et al. 2002; Teschendorf et al. 2002). In some situations, tissue-specific gene expression is desired, which requires knowledge of the natural promoter region and its location relative to the gene (Saukkonen and Hemminki 2004; Zheng and Baum 2008; Boulaire et al. 2009).

When gene editing is the desired objective, the BioDrug may be used to remove or inactivate a gene involved in the pathogenesis of a disease or to "fix" a gene by replacing a mutation with the correct genetic sequence. In either case, gene-editing "machinery" is delivered to the nucleus along with instructions for targeting the correct gene. The machinery includes a cutting device that causes a double-strand break followed by DNA repair by the endogenous repair mechanisms. The commonly used gene-editing machinery is described below (Fig. 6.3).

The clustered regularly interspaced short palindromic repeats (CRISPR)/CRISPR-associated (Cas) protein 9 system was first recognized as a bacterial defense against virus and phage infection (reviewed in Zhang et al. 2014). The CRISPR part of the system acts as a template to produce a sequence of RNA that is complementary to parts of the viral DNA. The Cas9 part of the system is an enzyme that cuts DNA producing double-strand breaks. Together the CRISPR RNA (crRNA) and a transactivating crRNA (tracrRNA) bind to Cas9 and guide it to sections of the DNA that contain a short protospacer adjacent motif (PAM). Once the PAM sequence is recognized, the CAS:RNA complex unwinds the DNA from the first 10–12 nucleotides after the PAM sequence. If that section of DNA is complementary to the crRNA sequence, the Cas9 produces a double-strand break (Jinek et al. 2012; Gasiunas et al. 2012).

The CRISPR/Cas9 system subsequently has been modified such that it can now be used to specifically target and cut precise areas in the human genome (reviewed in Thurtle-Schmidt and Lo 2018). The original bacterial crRNA and tracrRNA have been fused to create a single-guide RNA (Jinek et al. 2012; Gasiunas et al. 2012). Since PAM sequences occur approximately every 8 base pairs, CRISPR/Cas9 can interrogate the entire genome for a genetic sequence of interest. To target a specific gene, the crRNA is engineered to an RNA sequence of about 20 nucleotides complementary to the target gene. This engineered complex is termed the CRISPR/Cas9 site-specific endonuclease or sgRNA:Cas9. Once the sgRNA:Cas9 complex has bound at the target gene sequence, the Cas9 cuts both DNA strands. From that point, the native DNA machinery will repair the break by nonhomologous end joining. Since there are no overlapping homologous ends to form a template for repair, nonhomologous end joining frequently results in addition or subtraction of base pairs that effectively causes a disruption of the native gene. More sophisticated gene editing can be performed when two guide RNAs are used to target sites on either side of the mutation, resulting in loss of a segment of dsDNA. Nonhomologous repair can be used to replace the lost segment with an "inert" segment of dsDNA that essentially rejoins the cut ends. Alternatively, homology-directed repair can be used to substitute a section of dsDNA that contains the corrected genetic sequence, thus repairing the gene mutation and resulting in a functional gene.

Several challenges must be addressed for efficient and safe CRISPR/Cas9 gene editing. The design of the sgRNA must allow for the relatively short complementary RNA sequence to identify the correct part of the target gene for editing and at the same time avoid any chance of cutting at similar genetic sequences in nontarget genes (off-target cutting). Correction of genetic mutations remains more difficult than simply introducing a double-strand break that results in a deletion or mutation, because nonhomologous end joining is far more common than homology-directed repair (Maruyama et al. 2015). Optimization of Cas9 activity also must be achieved, for example, by using a Cas9 protein that recognizes a unique PAM sequence or other means to increase its enzymatic activity (Jinek et al. 2012).

Several other systems exist as alternative platforms for engineering customized DNA-binding nucleases. Meganucleases are homing endonucleases (enzymes that cut DNA) that recognize up to 40 base pairs of DNA sequence as binding sites for cleavage. In order to customize the meganuclease for gene editing, the DNA-binding sites of naturally occurring meganucleases are reengineered to target the desired DNA sequence (Ashworth et al. 2010). Meganucleases can be put together using selected protein units that have been created for this purpose (Smith et al. 2006; Arnould et al. 2006). Meganucleases potentially have less risk for off-target cleavage due to their very high specificity; however, other methods for creating double-strand DNA breaks are more easily customized.

Zinc-finger nucleases (ZFNs) are an engineered hybrid system that combines the DNA-cutting activity of the restriction endonuclease Fok1 with the DNA-binding specificity of zinc-finger proteins. A zinc-finger protein is a compact unit of approximately 30 amino acids arranged with as a double β-sheet linked to an α-helix that binds to DNA via surface amino acid side chains (Pavletich and Pabo 1991). An individual zinc finger will make contact with three to four base pairs in the major groove of DNA. Several zinc-finger proteins can be linked together in tandem to form domains that can bind to longer DNA sequences providing more specificity (Pabo et al. 2001). By combining zinc-finger proteins with unique DNA-binding specificity, ZFNs can be engineered to recognize specific genomic sequences for gene editing (reviewed in Gersbach et al. 2014). The second component of ZFNs, the restriction endonuclease Fok1, must be dimerized in order to cut DNA. To accomplish this, two ZFNs are delivered, each of which recognizes a sequence on opposite DNA strands that is 5–7 bp from the target cutting. This allows the Fok1 endonucleases to align, forming a dimer that allows cleavage of each strand resulting in a double-strand DNA break. ZFN-mediated double-strand breaks allow for homology-directed repair as well as nonhomologous end joining.

Transcription activator-like effector nucleases (TALENs) work in a similar manner by combining the endonuclease activity of the Fok1 restriction enzyme with a DNA-binding TALE proteins (Li et al. 2011a). TALE proteins have 33–35 amino acids that bind a single base pair in the major groove and wrap around the DNA in a superhelical structure. DNA-binding specificity can be engineered by assembling TALE repeats in a modular fashion to target almost any DNA sequence (Christian et al. 2010; Morbitzer et al. 2010). The TALE bonding domain is fused to the Fok1 endonuclease, which functions when dimerized in the same manner as in ZFNs. The two TALENs recognize sequences on opposite DNA strands 12–20 base pairs from the target cleavage site, inducing double-strand breaks for nonhomologous end joining or homology-directed repair (Li et al. 2011b). Advantages of TALEN-mediated gene editing include its limitless targeting capability and straightforward engineering; the disadvantage is the large size of TALE arrays which pose a significant barrier to using some in vivo delivery systems.

6.4 BioDrug ToolKit: Delivery Systems

The third important group of tools for creating a BioDrug are delivery systems to ensure the genetic materials or editing machinery are transferred into the target cells. Delivery systems fall into two broad categories: viral-based and nonviral-based delivery systems. Selection of a delivery system is dictated by the nature of the target tissue and whether the gene is to be transferred ex vivo or in vivo. The cellular targets for ex vivo gene transfer include HSC, T cells, and other hematopoietic cells that can be removed and kept healthy in culture before reintroduction into the body. In this case the delivery system should allow for transgene stability in dividing cells. Selection of a delivery system for in vivo gene therapy depends primarily on its cell tropism. This section describes the characteristics of the various delivery systems that can be used for building a BioDrug.

6.4.1 Viral-Based Delivery Systems

Viral vectors are used to infect target cells and then deliver genetic material into the nucleus or cytoplasm. Viral vectors used clinically are based on naturally occurring viruses known to infect human cells but rendered replication incompetent by removal of most of the native viral genes. Selection of a specific viral vector depends upon the target cell and whether the transferred genetic material is intended to be integrated into the genome. Integration of genetic material is important when the genetic information must not be lost during mitosis, such as when the target cells are HSC, other progenitor cells, or cells that expand in vivo such as T cells.

Factors that affect transgene expression within the target cell include the specific transgene being delivered and the *cis*-elements incorporated within the vector, such as the type of promoters and regulatory motifs and the orientation of the transgene within the vector. These elements influence the degree to which transgene expression may be repressed by the target cell silencing machinery or eliminated by host immune responses.

The optimal vector for gene therapy will result in stable and high-level transgene expression, high transfection efficiency, high carrying capacity of genetic material, no insertional mutagenesis, no host immune response, and no ability to transform and incite secondary malignancy. As yet, no viral delivery system has met all criteria, and each has specific advantages as well as carries specific risks for gene delivery into human cells. The most commonly employed viral vectors are described below.

Retroviral (RV) vectors are RNA viruses which require reverse transcription to generate cDNA for integration into the host genome (reviewed in Biasco et al. 2017). Although RV vectors are derived from wild-type retroviruses, substantial portions of the original viral genomes have been deleted or altered to render them acceptable for use in human gene therapy. RV vectors retain the genetic elements that encode for the reverse transcription machinery as well as the viral proteins required for integration into the host cell genome. These characteristics allow RV vectors to transfect dividing and sometimes non-dividing cells, resulting in stable long-term expression of the integrated transgene. RV-based gene transduction is primarily used in ex vivo gene delivery, such as gene transfer into HSC or lymphocytes.

Production of retroviral vectors occurs by transfecting a packaging cell line with the various components of the retrovirus required for host cell infection, delivered in separate cassettes that mitigate the possibility of generating replication-competent virus (reviewed in Cockrell and Kafri 2007). These components include (1) the envelope cassette that contains the viral genes required to form the envelope and which dictates the cell tropism and vector entry via endocytosis; (2) the packaging cassette that contains constitutive promoters that drive expression of packaging elements; (3) the vector cassette that contains the viral elements required for reverse transcription; and (4) the transgene expression cassette that includes the transgene sequence and promoter elements. Together these cassettes within the packaging cell line result in production of viral particles that contain the transgene. The viral particles can be harvested from the supernatant of the producer cells and purified. Target cells are then incubated with the virus at an optimal ratio of virus particles to cell, termed multiplicity of infection (MOI). The viral particle enters the cell through direct membrane fusion or attachment via a surface receptor. Once in the cell, the viral particle is uncoated to release the reverse transcription complex (RTC) which is transported to the chromosomal DNA where integration occurs (reviewed in Milone and O'Doherty 2018). The viral RNA is converted within the RTC into proviral DNA. The RV viral proteins deliver the proviral DNA into the nucleus where the RV integrase enzyme catalyzes the integration of the transgene DNA into the host genome. Each class of retrovirus has preferential DNA sequences for insertion. Following integration, the transgene is expressed by the host cellular transcription machinery.

The goal for most gene therapy using RV vectors is a single transduction event in the target cell genome that does not interfere with normal gene function and that results in stable high-level transgene expression. Producing a high-potency RV vector must take into consideration the incorporation of the specific envelope protein elements that dictate the appropriate RV pseudotype and the constitutive and tissue-specific promoters that dictate transgene expression. Additional considerations include the potential for transgene silencing by the host cell, which depends upon the *cis*-elements within the vector and the specific transgene being delivered (reviewed in Ellis 2005). Potential risks of all RV vectors include insertional mutagenesis, generation of replication-competent vectors, and germ-line transmission of vector sequences.

The first successful RV-based gene transduction was developed using the gamma retrovirus (γRV) murine leukemia virus (MLV). γRV vectors have a large capacity for transgenes, however, are restricted by the requirement for target cell mitosis for uptake. Thus, clinical use of γRV-based gene transfer has been limited to target cells that undergo cell division. A second limitation of γRV vectors is that genome integration is nonrandom with a preference for integration into actively transcribed loci near the initiation of transcription (Biasco et al. 2012, 2017). In clinical trials using γRV-based gene delivery, nonrandom integration has led to insertional mutagenesis resulting in leukemia (Hacein-Bey-Abina et al. 2008).

Lentiviral (LV) vectors have emerged as a potentially safer and more broadly applicable approach to delivering transgenes (reviewed in Cockrell and Kafri 2007; Kafri 2004; Escors and Breckpot 2010). LV vectors were initially derived from the human immunodeficiency virus-1 and are capable of infecting both dividing and nondividing cells (Lewis et al. 1992; Yamashita and Emerman 2006). Safety of LV vectors is enhanced by deletion of specific viral sequences that result in self-inactivating (SIN) vectors (Miyoshi et al. 1998; Zufferey et al. 1998). LV vectors have demonstrated high efficiency of infection and long-term stable expression in many tissues (Naldini et al. 1996; Kafri et al. 1997). Compared to γRV vectors, LV vectors appear to have a more favorable integration profile with less risk for insertional mutagenesis. Furthermore, LV vectors are less immunogenetic, which may decrease the risk for host cell silencing.

Foamy virus (FV) vectors have broad tropism and can carry large transgene cassettes (Trobridge 2009). The virus itself is not pathogenic in humans. FV vectors require cell division for efficient transduction and integration into the host genome. However, FV vectors can infect a quiescent cell and form a stable transduction intermediate that can then integrate into the host genome once the cell undergoes mitosis. Safety of FV vectors has been enhanced by deletion of sequences involved in viral replication. FV vectors have been used in both ex vivo and in vivo gene delivery (Liu et al. 2008; Simantirakis et al. 2020).

Other viral vector delivery systems have been developed that more effectively allow transgene delivery to nondividing cells and avoid the risks of insertional mutagenesis. These viral vectors may be used to deliver transgenes in vivo, without the requirement for ex vivo incubation with the target cell which offers an advantage over RV-based vectors.

Adenoviral vectors used for gene therapy can transfer large amounts of genetic material into both dividing and nondividing cells (Quantin et al. 1992; Athanasopoulos et al. 2017). Adenoviral vectors are nonintegrating dsDNA virus vectors capable of carrying payloads exceeding 30 kb (Youil et al. 2003). High transfection efficiency is achievable with adenoviral vectors, although transgene expression typically is transient. Because transgene expression may be lost when target cells undergo mitosis, the most appropriate target cells are stable nondividing cells such as hepatic or muscle cells. Since there is no need for target cells to undergo mitosis, adenoviral vectors can be administered directly in vivo by intravenous or other routes. Much of the native adenovirus genome has been deleted to render adenovirus vector replication incompetent; however, adenoviral vectors remain highly immunogenic since most humans have been exposed to wild-type adenoviruses (Nwanegbo et al. 2004). The immunogenicity of adenoviral vectors can result in target tissue inflammation and inhibition of transgene expression (Raper et al. 2003). Several engineering strategies have been developed to reduce immunogenicity such as the inclusion of adenoviral E3 genes that downregulate host cell MHC expression (Youil et al. 2003).

Adeno-associated virus (AAV) is a small non-enveloped virus that cannot self-replicate unless aided by an adenovirus (Lukashev and Zamyatnin 2016). AAV-based vectors do not integrate into the target cell genome, even though integration into a specific location on chromosome 19 has been observed for a very small proportion of wild-type AAV. Most AAV vectors are hepatotropic; moreover, depending on the serotype of the wild-type AAV, other tissue types can be targeted (Athanasopoulos et al. 2017; Balakrishnan and Jayandharan 2014). One constraint to AAV-based gene delivery is the limit to transgene capacity of approximately 4.5 kb. To overcome this capacity limitation, the genetic material may be divided into expression cassettes with complementary sequences that can anneal to form full-length dsDNA in the nuclei (Pasi et al. 2020). Compared to adenovirus, there is a lower likelihood for eliciting an immune response, as the proportion of humans previously exposed to AAV ranges from 10 to 50%, depending upon the serotype of AAV and the prevalence of AAV in the population (Louis Jeune et al. 2013).

Other viruses have been studied for gene delivery as episomal virus-derived vectors (reviewed in Van Craenenbroeck et al. 2000). These include vectors derived from BK virus, SV40 virus, bovine papilloma virus, and

EBV. Episomal vectors contain a viral origin of DNA replication and activation motifs, which allow replication of the inserted genetic material without the need for integration into cellular DNA. Persistence of episomal vectors in multiple copies in the nucleus allows for high transgene expression; however, long-term stability of transgene expression has not been established.

6.4.2 Nonviral Delivery Systems

Effective delivery of transgenes may also be accomplished through physical- or chemical-based systems. These systems tend to be less immunogenic than viral-based systems and have no limits to the transgene size. However, nonviral delivery systems are relatively inefficient compared to viral vectors.

6.4.2.1 Chemical Methods of Delivery

Nucleic acids are negatively charged, which allows genetic material to be packaged in cationic lipids or polymers forming a nanoparticle (Zhang et al. 2004). Nucleic acids within the complex are protected from degradation. Nanoparticle complexes are taken up by cells through endocytosis; subsequently the genetic material is released from the endosomes and translocated to the nucleus (Khalil et al. 2006). Nanoparticles are engineered to target specific cellular receptors by incorporating ligands in the lipid or polymer layer (Chiu et al. 2004; Hood et al. 2002). Advantages of chemical delivery systems include low risks for toxicity, immunogenicity, and insertional mutagenesis. The main disadvantage is the low efficiency of gene transduction.

Cationic liposomes form nanoparticles with DNA and can be used for ex vivo and in vivo gene delivery. The efficiency of delivery depends on the size, structure, charge ratio between transgenic DNA and cationic liposome, the cellular target, and whether a "helper lipid" is added (Birchall et al. 1999). Cationic liposome nanoparticles have been studied for delivery of the CRTR gene in patients with cystic fibrosis and shown to be well tolerated (Caplen et al. 1995; Alton et al. 1999). Cationic polymer nanoparticles also can be used for both in vitro and in vivo gene delivery. Particle engineering is critical to optimize gene delivery efficiency as well as toxicity (Tang and Szoka 1997; Tang et al. 2010).

6.4.2.2 Physical Methods of Delivery

There are a number of physical methods to deliver genetic material into target tissues; however, in most cases transduction efficiency is much lower than viral- or chemical-based delivery systems. It is possible for naked DNA to be transferred into cells via direct injection into cells or tissue (Herweijer and Wolff 2003). Electroporation is a procedure in which cells are placed in solution that contains the transgene and are subjected briefly to an electrical current. This allows the transgene to penetrate both cell and nuclear membranes (Heller et al. 2011). Magnetic fields also have been employed in combination with viral vectors to increase gene delivery to cells for which the virus has low tropism (Scherer et al. 2002). Other methods to penetrate the cell membrane include ultrasonic waves and mechanical forces, such as bombarding the tissue with DNA-coated metallic particles shot from a gene gun (Mahvi et al. 1997).

6.5 Building a BioDrug

Now that we understand the tools required for building a BioDrug, we can start putting them together. The following sections will focus on building BioDrugs for pediatric hematology/oncology patients.

6.5.1 Building Gene Therapies: Putting Together Genetic Material, Gene-Editing Machinery, Delivery Systems, and Target Cells

Gene therapy broadly covers a number of genetic engineering approaches aimed toward ameliorating human disease (Fig. 6.4). A gene therapy medicinal product contains a recombinant nucleic acid, the product of which is intended to regulate, repair, replace, delete, or augment an existing

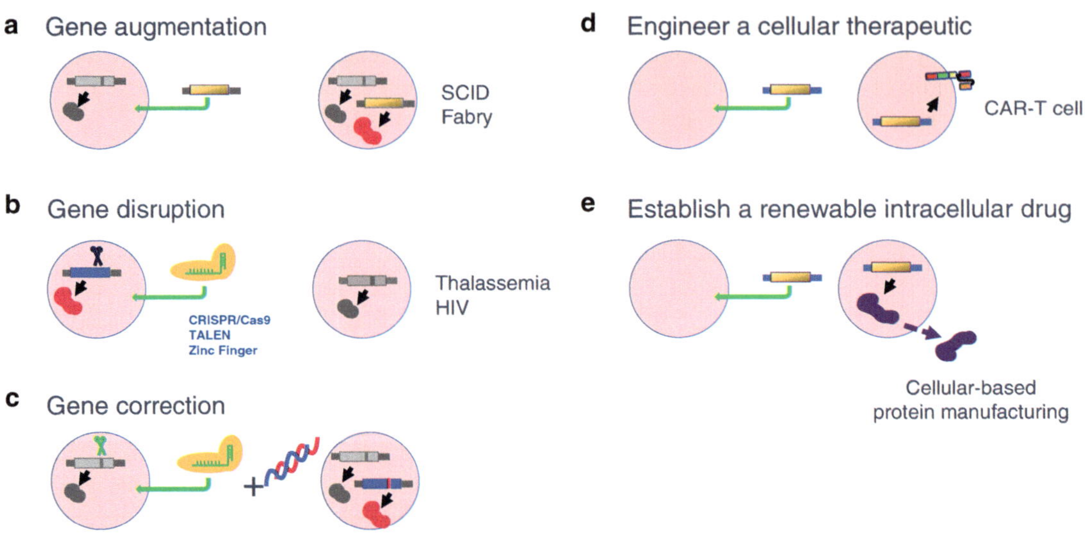

Fig. 6.4 Various genetic engineering strategies can be used to produce a BioDrug. In panels **a–c**, diseases are corrected using genetic engineering strategies that alter a protein product involved in the disease. In panel **a**, a new gene (yellow bar) that produces a normal protein (red globule) is transferred into the cell to replace a mutated gene (gray bar) and its abnormal protein product (gray globule). Examples of potentially treatable diseases using gene augmentation include inherited immunodeficiency disorders, which might be corrected using ex vivo transduction of hematopoietic stem cells (HSCs), or metabolic disorders, in which infusion of the gene therapy product for in vivo transduction might be effective. In panel **b**, a normal protein that may contribute to the disease is rendered dysfunctional using gene-editing machinery to delete part of its gene (gray bar). Examples of potential uses include disrupting the co-receptor required for HIV1 entry into CD4+ cells or disrupting the regulatory genes that silence HbF transcription in beta-thalassemia. In panel **c**, gene deletion is followed by homology-directed repair to replace the incorrect gene sequence (in gray) with the correct gene sequence (in red) to produce a normal protein. Sickle cell disease is an example of a disorder that might be amenable to this gene correction strategy. Genetic engineering strategies can also be used to turn cells into BioDrug products. In panel **d**, a T cell is transduced with a transgene construct that generates a chimeric antigen receptor (CAR). The CAR T cell is then used as a BioDrug to attack and destroy cancer cells. In panel **e**, a transgene construct that encodes a therapeutic protein, such as a cytokine, is introduced into a cell. The cell becomes an in vivo "manufacturing site" for the cytokine

human gene or genes. Gene therapies have been developed to correct inherited genetic defects, to interfere with acquired genetic mutations as might occur in a malignancy, or to artificially increase the amount of a gene product produced within a cell, such as a cytokine or functional protein, for therapeutic purposes.

The BioDrug ToolKit can be used to correct inherited genetic defects by delivering new genetic information into cells (gene augmentation) or by disabling genes that contribute to disease. The basic steps in building a gene therapy using the toolkit include:

1. Selection of the appropriate strategy for correcting the genetic disease, which can be gene replacement, gene editing, or a combination approach.
2. Engineering the transgene cassettes that includes the gene and regulatory elements or engineering the components of the gene-editing machinery.
3. Determination of the target cell, which dictates whether the gene transduction will be performed in vivo or ex vivo.
4. Selection of the optimal delivery system capable of carrying the genetic information to the targeted cell.

Building a gene therapy for correction of an inherited disorder begins with understanding the underlying pathophysiology of the genetic mutation. The design of the system must be based on knowledge of how the genetic mutation affects the resulting protein product as well as the factors important for the function of the protein. The following considerations will determine the type of genetic manipulation (e.g., gene replacement and/or gene editing), the type of vector, and the target tissue required for successful gene therapies.

How many mutations are involved in the disease? A disorder caused by a single nucleotide substitution, such as sickle cell anemia, might be treated by a gene-editing approach since the same gene-editing machinery could be used for every patient. However, for a disorder such as Wiskott-Aldrich syndrome in which there are over 100 known mutations, gene editing would be prohibitive, and a gene replacement strategy would be substantially more practical.

What is the consequence of the mutation? Premature termination codons or other nonsense mutations may abrogate production of the protein altogether, in which case a simple replacement therapy that provides genetic instructions for the normal protein may suffice. However, in many situations the mutation results in an aberrant protein that directly causes the disorder, such as in transthyretin amyloidosis, or that might interfere with the function of a normal protein. For example, the presence of β^S chains in red cells might lead to sickling even if a transgene were generating normalized β-chains, depending on the intracellular concentrations of each protein product (Mansilla-Soto et al. 2011). For these situations, the engineering approach might also include knocking out the function of the pathogenic gene.

What is the required level of gene expression for correction of symptoms? For any given disorder, there will be a level of protein expression that is required for amelioration of symptoms. Furthermore, there may be requirements for a given amount of protein expressed within a cell or for the overall number of cells that express any amount of protein. Lessons learned from treating nonmalignant diseases with allogeneic HCT illustrate disease-specific differences in requirements for the level of intracellular protein expression or for the proportion of cells with normal protein expression. For example, improvement in sickle cell vaso-occlusive symptoms and normalization of hemoglobin are feasible without achieving full donor chimerism and can also be achieved by transplantation of cells from a donor with sickle cell trait, i.e., donor cells with half normal levels of HbA per cell, provided full chimerism is achieved (Abraham et al. 2017; Eapen et al. 2019). In contrast, allogeneic HCT for correction of mucopolysaccharidosis type I must result in a normal level of α-l-iduronidase for disease response, which cannot be achieved with cells from a carrier donor because the intracellular protein expression is low, nor can normal donor cells produce sufficient enzyme levels if full donor chimerism is not attained (Peters et al. 1998).

Optimization of protein expression requires selection of the appropriate regulatory elements to include in the transgene cassette. The number of copies of the gene established within the cell also affects protein expression. The vector copy number (VCN) is a measurement of the average number of transgenes integrated into the genome. Too few integrated copies will result in low expression, whereas too many may increase the risk for insertional mutagenesis. Sensitive polymerase chain reaction (PCR) techniques are used to quantify VCN in preclinical studies as well clinically as a correlation with disease response (Lin et al. 2016; Thompson et al. 2018). Assessment of VCN in a clinical setting after gene therapy requires easily accessible tissue; thus, practically speaking it has been limited to monitoring results of gene-modified hematopoietic or lymphoid cells.

What is the requirement for tissue specificity of gene expression? The cell that expresses the transgene may not matter for normal function of some proteins. For example, hepatocytes or myocytes may express transgenes that encode for proteins normally made by other organs and which function systemically. The liver is the most easily targeted organ for in vivo delivery because hepatocytes take up nanoparticles through endocytosis and many of the viral vectors are hepatotropic. The size of the gene and regulatory elements in the transgene construct will dictate the options for in vivo delivery to hepatocytes, as transfer of large amounts of genetic material may not be feasible with rAAV vectors.

There are circumstances in which tissue-specific expression might be desired, such as expression of beta globin in erythrocytes; therefore, building a tissue-specific gene therapy will involve additional considerations. Design of the transgene cassette must include the appropriate regulatory elements, such as tissue-specific promoters. A delivery system can be selected to further optimize tissue targeting, based on tropism of viral vectors or the capability of transducing dividing or quiescent cells.

6.5.2 Building Gene Therapies: Progress and Challenges

Many of the early challenges to developing gene therapies have been overcome by progress made in improvement of gene delivery systems and gene-editing technologies, resulting in a plethora of clinical trials in patients with genetic disorders. While few gene therapy products have been approved to date, it is expected that many more will be approved within the next decade. This section summarizes the progress to date in gene therapy technologies that have led to gene therapies for pediatric patients with inherited hematologic or immunologic disorders.

Until recently, the mainstay for treatment of life-threatening inherited hematologic disorders has been allogeneic HCT, which can be viewed as a very crude form of gene therapy. In its simplest sense, replacement of the entire hematologic and immunologic system is done in order to correct a single mutation that may affect function of only one cell compartment. While often effective at correcting symptoms caused by the genetic defect, the immunologically mediated graft-versus-host and host-versus-graft reactions, and consequent risk for graft-versus-host disease or graft rejection, form major barriers to successful allogeneic HCT. Ex vivo gene therapy permits a more focused correction of the specific mutation within the affected autologous cells of an individual (Fig. 6.5).

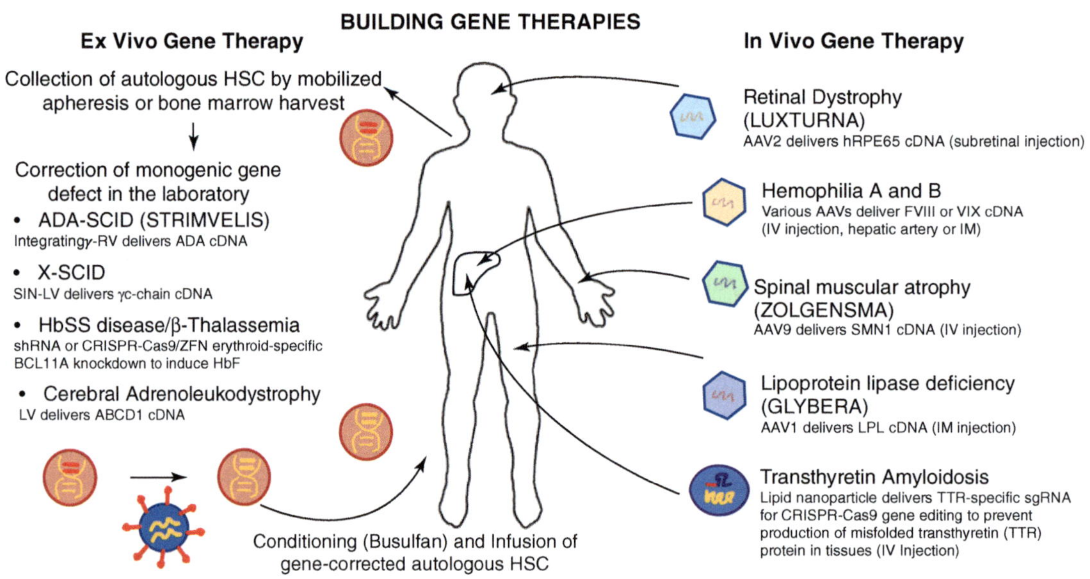

Fig. 6.5 Gene therapies can be distinguished based on "ex vivo" and "in vivo" approaches. "Ex vivo" gene therapy is utilized to correct monogenic gene defects in hematopoietic stem cells (HSCs). The patient's autologous HSCs are collected by apheresis following mobilization with G-CSF or Plerixafor (the latter being used in HbSS) or by bone marrow harvest. Cells are then placed in culture and gene-modified using the various approaches from the BioDrug ToolKit. After HSCs have been successfully corrected, the patient undergoes conditioning (typically busulfan-based), and gene-corrected autologous HSCs are reinfused intravenously with the goal of engraftment by the gene-corrected HSCs. In contrast, gene correction occurs in the patient's body rather than the laboratory when "in vivo" gene therapy approaches are utilized. Using elements of the BioDrug ToolKit such as adeno-associated virus and nanoparticles, cDNA or gene-editing tools are delivered via intravenous, intramuscular, or direct injection into the target organ

Introduction of a normal transgene into autologous HSC is especially relevant when a large number of possible mutations have been identified each of which can result in a nonfunctional gene product, such as occurs in many inherited immunodeficiency disorders (Bradford et al. 2017; Imai et al. 2003). Strimvelis is the first gene therapy product approved by the FDA for ex vivo gene augmentation of an inherited disorder, specifically to supersede mutations in the adenosine deaminase (ADA) gene that result in severe combined immunodeficiency (SCID) (https://www.ema.europa.eu/en/documents/product-information/strimvelis-epar-product-information_en.pdf). Components from the BioDrug ToolKit used to build Strimvelis include HSC as the target cells, adenosine deaminase cDNA as the genetic material, and a gamma retrovirus as the delivery system. Drug approval was based on safety and efficacy data from three trials with a combined total of 18 children. At 1 and 3 years following the procedure, genetically modified cells comprised a median of ~30% of CD19+ cells and ~70% of CD3+ cells, and by 8 years close to 100% of each subset were genetically modified. The 3-year overall survival was 100% and the rate of severe infection was reduced by 50% from baseline. There was a significant improvement in both the median number of T cells and the percent of dAXP in red blood cells. Adverse events related to Strimvelis included autoimmune reactions that were observed in 1–10% of patients, including autoimmune-mediated anemia, thrombocytopenia, thyroiditis, hepatitis, Guillain-Barré syndrome, and antineutrophil cytoplasmic antibodies. As would be expected, the most commonly observed adverse events in the clinical trials, such as anemia, neutropenia, and elevation of hepatic enzymes, were considered to be related to busulfan given to the children as conditioning before Strimvelis infusion.

Table 6.1 lists the ex vivo gene replacement trials currently in progress in patients with life-threatening hematologic or immunodeficiency disorders. A number of challenges remain for successful development of each of these BioDrugs, posed by complexities of disease indication as well as the limitations of current technologies available from the ToolKit. In addition to the issues that must be considered in designing a gene replacement therapy, such as strategies to avoid gene silencing or off-target cell expression, there remains an incomplete understanding of the variables involved in the cell engineering procedure that correlate with therapeutic efficacy, such as the optimal number of transduced HSC or the optimal VCN in the target cells. Furthermore, clinical toxicities have been observed in recipients of ex vivo genetically manipulated HSC, which may have relevance to BioDrug design.

The most serious toxicity observed to date has been the development of leukemia as a consequence of insertional mutagenesis. Initial trials that explored ex vivo gene replacement for X-SCID used a design strategy similar to

Table 6.1 Gene replacement and gene-editing trials for correction of inherited hematologic or immunodeficiency disorders (listed as open or recruiting on ClinicalTrials.gov as of April 2021)

Disorder	Trial
ADA-SCID	NCT03645460 NCT03765632
Artemis-SCID	NCT03538899
Beta-thalassemia	NCT03276455
Chronic granulomatous disease	NCT03645486
Fanconi anemia	NCT04248439 NCT03351868 NCT04069533
Hemophilia A	NCT04418414 NCT03818763 NCT03217032
Hemophilia B	NCT03961243
Infantile osteopetrosis	NCT04525352
Leukocyte adhesion deficiency	NCT03825783 NCT03812263
RAG1-SCID	NCT04797260
Sickle cell disease	NCT03964792 NCT04293185 NCT04443907 NCT04819841
X-linked SCID	NCT03311503 NCT01512888 NCT03601286 NCT04286815 NCT01306019 NCT03217617

ADA adenosine deaminase, *RAG* recombinant activating gene, *SCID* severe combined immunodeficiency

Strimvelis. Retroviral vectors based on the MLV were used to insert a copy of the common gamma chain (γ_c) cDNA into autologous CD34+ cells; expression of the γ_c cDNA was under control of the MLV promoter and enhancer within the retroviral long terminal repeat (LTR). The transduced CD34+ cells were reinfused into the patients without myeloablative conditioning. Of the 20 patients reported, reconstitution of normal T cell numbers and function were observed in 19, and normal B cell function was achieved in 8 (NCT01410019 and NCT01175239) (Hacein-Bey-Abina et al. 2010, 2014; Gaspar et al. 2004, 2011). However, five of the patients developed an acute T cell leukemia caused by insertion of the transgene near the LMO2 proto-oncogene. Oncogene activation was attributed to the activity of the strong T cell-tropic enhancer within the U3 region of the viral LTR. A similar experience occurred in patients with Wiskott-Aldrich syndrome after infusion of ex vivo transduced HSC using a γRV vector (Braun et al. 2014). Sustained engraftment and partial or full amelioration of immunodeficiency and thrombocytopenia were achieved in nine of ten patients; however, seven patients developed acute leukemia involving myeloid or T lymphocyte lineages.

To address this problem, LV vectors have supplanted γRV vectors as the preferred vector delivery system for ex vivo transduction of HSC. LV vectors have been further engineered to reduce the likelihood for replication-competent RV, termed self-inactivating (SIN), by removing viral transcriptional elements and including an enhancer-blocking element (Zhou et al. 2010; Morris et al. 2017). In 2019 the EMA approved betibeglogene autotemcel (Zynteglo) for treatment of non-β0/β0 beta-thalassemia (https://www.ema.europa.eu/en/documents/product-information/zynteglo-epar-product-information_en.pdf). Components from the BioDrug ToolKit used to build Zynteglo include mobilized HSC as the target cells and a LV vector delivery system (Thompson et al. 2018). The genetic material included an extended β-globin gene with regulatory segments of the locus control region. Drug approval was based on safety and efficacy data from 4 trials with a combined total of 32 adolescents and adults. Transfusion independence was demonstrated for 78–90% of patients at 24 months following infusion, and transfusion independence was maintained for at least 1 year following. Similar to the Strimvelis experience, the most commonly observed adverse events were related to the busulfan conditioning.

Transduction of autologous HSC using LV vectors also has shown early promise for delivering cDNA to replace the mutated *ABCD1* gene in patients with adrenal leukodystrophy and for delivering microRNA-adapted short hairpin RNA to interfere with expression of the HBB^s gene in patients with sickle cell disease (Eichler et al. 2017; Esrick et al. 2021). The clinical trials listed in Table 6.1 also employ LV vectors as the delivery system.

The degree of risk for development of leukemia after LV-mediated transduction of HSC remains unknown. In the Lentiglobin trial for sickle cell disease, in which a LV vector is used to transduce HSC with an anti-sickling β-globin, one patient has developed myelodysplastic syndrome approximately 3 years after gene therapy (Hsieh et al. 2020). Extensive analysis of the marrow found no clonal dominance of the insertion site in gene-modified cells, and there was no enrichment of the VCN in the MDS blasts compared to peripheral blood cells. In this case, leukemogenesis was considered to be caused by busulfan conditioning effects. However, long-term monitoring for insertional mutagenesis in all recipients of LV-transduced HSC will be essential, and the FDA has provided guidance for long-term follow-up of patients enrolled in trials of ex vivo transduced cell products (https://www.fda.gov/media/113768/download). In addition to insertional mutagenesis, gene therapy products based on retroviral vectors, including LV vectors, have the potential to transmit replication-competent retrovirus (RCR). While technologies for creating optimal vector designs and vector producing cells have markedly reduced the chance for transmission of RCR, the FDA has provided guidelines for RCR testing of both the product and the recipient of the gene-modified cells (https://www.fda.gov/media/113790/download).

Selection of the optimal target cell for ex vivo gene transduction also may pose a challenge. The initial trials of gene therapy for SCID used T lymphocytes as the target cell; however, long-term persistence of the gene-modified T cells was not achieved (Bordignon et al. 1995). The optimal target cell for ex vivo gene modification, whether for correction of disorders of hematopoiesis or immunodeficiency, is the HSC, which can provide a continual renewable source of lymphoid or myeloid lineage precursors. Because acquisition of high numbers of HSC may be critical to ensure a sufficient number of genetically modified cells for reinfusion, most studies utilize PBSC mobilized with G-CSF with or without plerixafor. However, G-CSF has been associated with severe adverse events in patients with sickle cell disease, and for these and other patient populations, alternative mobilization regimens such as plerixafor alone are being explored (Adler et al. 2001; Grigg 2001; Lagresle-Peyrou et al. 2018). It also may not be feasible to collect PBSC in very young infants due to the lack of vascular access for apheresis. Novel strategies to increase the total number of or to enrich the population of pluripotent HSC from harvested BM are being investigated (Radtke et al. 2020; Adair et al. 2018; Frangoul et al. 2007).

The early clinical trials of Strimvelis also showed that, despite optimal engineering and selection of appropriate vectors, engraftment of gene-modified HSC was impeded by competition from endogenous cells (Bordignon et al. 1995; Muul et al. 2003). Subsequent gene therapy trials included strategies to reduce in vivo completion by addition of conditioning with busulfan (BU) to create space for engraftment (Aiuti et al. 2002, 2009). Currently most trials include either sub-myeloablative or myeloablative Bu-based conditioning. Selection of dose intensity depends on the level of engraftment required for correction of the disease and comfort with the higher risk for toxicity associated with more intense conditioning. While myeloablative BU conditioning has been used for decades in conditioning for allogeneic HCT, it carries the risks of prolonged pancytopenia and liver toxicity. Sub-myeloablative BU dosing once daily for 1–2 days is preferable in most conditions (Mamcarz et al. 2019; Bradford et al. 2020). An additional concern associated with myelotoxic regimens is the potential for genotoxic effects on the host hematopoietic cells, which has been suggested by the development of myelodysplastic syndrome without evidence for insertional mutagenesis in recipients of LV-transduced HSC given BU conditioning (Hsieh et al. 2020). Improved conditioning regimens, such as antibodies that target CD34 or c-kit, are being explored as a method to decrease competition for marrow space while avoiding systemic toxicities and the risk for genotoxicity (Chandrasekaran et al. 2014; Srikanthan et al. 2020).

Gene-editing technologies, such as the CRISPR/Cas9 system, have the potential to overcome some of the limitations of gene replacement therapy. The ability to edit a mutation within the genome allows for the native transcriptional regulatory elements to control gene transcription, thus circumventing the need to engineer a transgene cassette with additional promoter elements. Gene-editing technology also can be used to knock out mutated genes that could interfere with gene replacement strategies or to knock out regulatory elements to reduce or enhance endogenous gene expression. For example, one strategy to improve hematopoiesis in patients with beta-thalassemia has been to "reawaken" fetal hemoglobin production by disrupting the regulatory genes that silence HbF transcription (Bauer et al. 2012). Some inherited disorders, such as transthyretin amyloidosis, are caused by gain-of-function mutations, in which case gene disruption has the potential to directly treat the disorder by knocking out production of the dysfunctional protein (Sekijima 2015; Gillmore et al. 2021). Currently there are multiple trials investigating gene-editing technology for correction of hematologic and immunodeficiency disorders (reviewed in Daniel-Moreno et al. 2019). Components from the BioDrug ToolKit used to build these products include HSC as the target cells, a selection of gene-editing machinery of which the CRISPR/Cas9 system is emerging as the most adaptable, and a selection of delivery systems that have included viral and nonviral methodologies. Given the rapid advances in gene-editing technologies, it is expected that approval of a gene-edited HSC BioDrug will occur in the near future.

Ex vivo gene modification of HSC is not suitable for treatment of genetic disorders that affect other tissue compartments, such as the nervous or musculoskeletal systems. For these disorders, delivery of the transgene must be targeted to the appropriate tissue via an in vivo delivery system (Fig. 6.5). Currently there are no approved in vivo gene therapy products for treatment of hematologic or immunodeficiency diseases; however, several have been approved for treatment of other inherited disorders. The first product for treatment of an inherited disorder was Glybera (alipogene tiparvovec) was approved by the EMA in 2012. Components from the BioDrug ToolKit used to build Glybera include human lipoprotein lipase (LPL) cDNA as the genetic material and the AAV1 viral vector as the delivery system, which has tropism for skeletal muscle and neurologic tissue (Scott 2015; Naso et al. 2017). Clinical trials demonstrated significant reductions in plasma triglyceride levels after a onetime series of intramuscular injections in patients with lipoprotein lipase deficiency, a rare autosomal recessive disorder which can cause severe pancreatitis. Luxturna (voretigene neparvovec-rzyl) was the first in vivo gene therapy approved in the USA for treatment of an inherited disorder, specifically to treat children and adults with an inherited retinal dystrophy resulting in vision loss. Components from the BioDrug ToolKit used to build Luxturna include *hRPE65* cDNA driven by a CMV enhancer and chicken beta actin (CβA) promoter as the genetic material and the AAV2 viral vector as the delivery system, which has broad tropism including retinal cells (Naso et al. 2017). In clinical trials, patients with biallelic *RPE65* mutation-associated retinal dystrophy who received subretinal injections of Luxturna showed a statistically significant clinical improvement compared to control patients over a period of 1–5 years, and adverse reactions were limited to ocular events (described in the FDA Summary Basis for Regulatory Action https://www.fda.gov/media/110141/download). The second US approval for in vivo gene therapy was for Zolgensma (onasemnogene abeparvovec-xioi), indicated for treatment of pediatric patients with spinal muscular atrophy caused by biallelic mutations in the *SMN1* gene, encoding for the SMN protein which is critical to the function and survival of motor neurons. Components from the BioDrug ToolKit used to build Zolgensma include *SMN1* cDNA under control of a CMV enhancer and CβA hybrid promoter as the genetic material and the AAV9 viral vector as the delivery system, which has broad tropism including for neurons (Foust et al. 2009). In clinical trials, a statistically significant improvement in survival and motor milestone achievement was observed for infants with SMA1 given a single intravenous infusion compared to natural history controls (described in the FDA Summary Basis for Regulatory Action https://www.fda.gov/media/127961/download) (Mendell et al. 2017; Al-Zaidy and Mendell 2019). In contrast to the experience with locally administered AAV-based gene therapy in the Glybera (i.e., intramuscular) and Luxturna (i.e., intraocular) trials, serious adverse reactions were observed, including severe liver toxicity in 6.8% of patients.

The studies supporting approval of these drugs provide several lessons for development of in vivo gene therapy for treatment of hematologic disorders. The target cells for each product were post-mitotic, thus allowing for sustained gene expression without genomic integration of the transgene. Selection of the delivery system was based on tropism of the AAV vector to achieve sufficient levels of gene product within the target tissue. Clinical studies of AAV-based gene replacement for hemophilia A and B have been underway over the last decade and show promising results (reviewed in Perrin et al. 2019). In these trials, the components from the BioDrug ToolKit include factor VIII or factor IX cDNA as the genetic material, AAV vectors as the delivery system, and the liver as the target organ for a systemically administered product (Pasi et al. 2020). Barriers to broader application of these therapies mainly are related to the immunogenicity of AAV vectors, which trigger both cytotoxic T lymphocyte (CTL) and humoral immune responses (reviewed in Mingozzi and High 2013). The presence of neutralizing antibodies (NAb) to the AAV capsid, even at low titers, can impede transduction of target tissues (Manno et al. 2006). The prevalence of NAb to AAV depends on the serotype and likely increases with age (Louis Jeune et al. 2013; Fu et al. 2017). Most clinical trials of AAV-based gene therapy require assessment of pre-existing NAb prior to enrollment of patients and take one of two general approaches in the management of NAb-positive patients. Exclusion of NAb-positive patients may improve interpretation of the dose-response data in early phase trials, as done in recent trials in patients with hemophilia B (Ertl and High 2017; Miesbach et al. 2018; Nathwani et al. 2011, 2014). However, depending on the serotype, this approach may exclude up to 50% of patients and seriously affect enrollment of the trial, particularly if focused on a rare disease. Several studies enrolled patients with detectable NAb, for example, the ZOLGENSMA clinical trials allowed anti-AAV9 titers ≤1:150 (Mendell et al. 2017; Al-Zaidy and Mendell 2019). Current trials that allow NAb-positive patients include a course of prophylactic immune suppression to block CTL responses, an approach taken in the clinical trials of Luxturna (Mingozzi and High 2013; Mingozzi et al. 2007; Jiang et al. 2006).

In NAb-negative patients, development of NAb also has been observed to occur weeks to months after receipt of AAV-based gene therapy, particularly when systemically administered. Therefore, AAV-based gene therapy protocols incorporate post-infusion monitoring for NAb and institution of immune suppression when detected (Nathwani et al. 2014). This phenomenon of post-infusion development of AAV-specific NAb also has implications for the design of early phase dose-escalation trials. Because any exposure to an AAV vector can elicit NAb, and because presence of NAb will exclude the patient from receiving AAV-based gene therapy in the future, it is important that the study minimize the number of patients exposed to a subtherapeutic dose (measured in vector genomes (vg) per kilogram recipient weight). For this reason, regulatory agencies have allowed dose escalation after demonstration of safety in a single patient, as reported in the initial hemophilia A trial (Rangarajan et al. 2017).

For systemic delivery of AAV-based gene therapy, the liver has become an ideal target tissue because it is a biosynthetic organ for which many AAV vectors have tropism and in which stable long-term transgene expression can be achieved (Mak et al. 2017). However, liver inflammation has emerged as a potential toxicity thought to be a consequence of the immune response to AAV (Miesbach et al. 2018; Nathwani et al. 2014). Clinical trials in patients with hemophilia observed elevations in liver transaminase levels that generally occurred between 6 and 16 weeks after infusion of AAV vectors. Current clinical trials require close monitoring of liver transaminase levels and prompt institution of a course of prednisolone given once levels exceed 1.5 times the upper limit of normal. Several recent trials have also incorporated a course of prophylactic corticosteroids during the first month or so after infusion, which could reduce the burden of monitoring transaminase levels.

Viral vector-based gene therapy products also raise the concern for vector shedding and the risk of transmission to untreated individuals. Vector viral shedding was observed in studies of AAV-based gene therapy for hemophilia B, with vector detected in nasal secretions, saliva, feces, urine, and semen for up to 48 weeks after systemic administration (Miesbach et al. 2018). The FDA has produced guidance for incorporating studies of vector shedding in clinical trials (https://www.fda.gov/regulatory-information/search-fda-guidance-documents/design-and-analysis-shedding-studies-virus-or-bacteria-based-gene-therapy-and-oncolytic-products).

The development of nanoparticles as delivery systems may help overcome the challenges of viral shedding and immune-mediated interference with transduction and transgene expression. Currently there are no approved nanoparticle-based gene therapies, but several clinical trials have commenced for study of local or systemic nanoparticle-based delivery of cDNA or mRNA in patients with solid tumors. Nanoparticles have been studied for delivery of the CFTR gene to the nasal epithelium in patients with cystic fibrosis

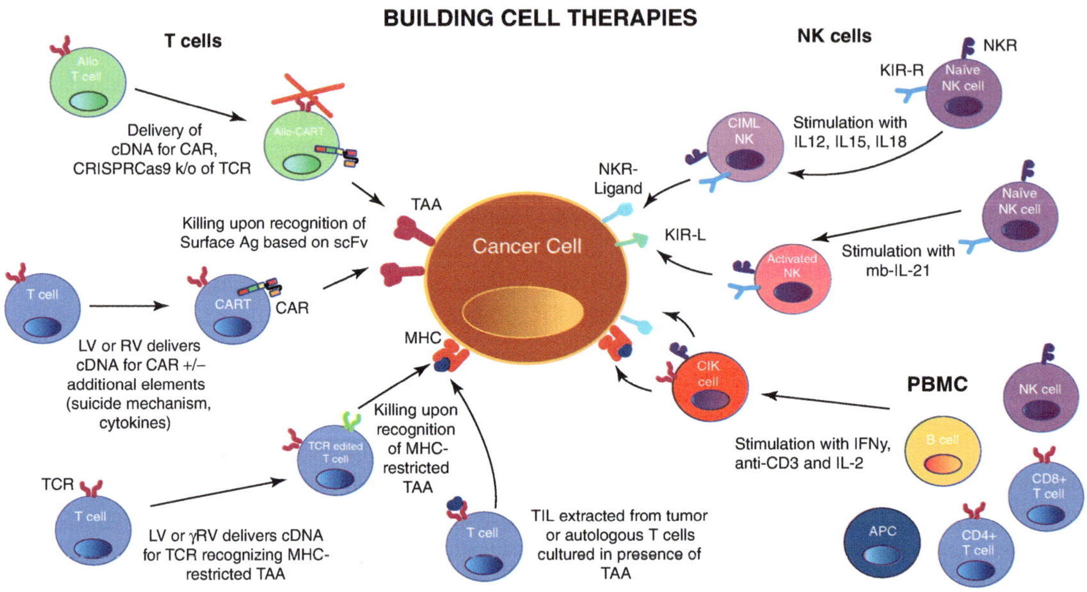

Fig. 6.6 The BioDrug ToolKit is also used to develop novel cellular immunotherapies to treat cancer. These strategies include non-engineered cells or gene-modified immune cells. Non-engineered approaches include extraction and ex vivo expansion of tumor-infiltrating lymphocytes (TILs) or peripheral blood T cells cultured in the presence of tumor-associated antigen (TAA), and ex vivo expansion and stimulation of NK cells with various approaches (IL-12, IL-15, IL-18 to generate cytokine-induced memory-like NK cells) or stimulation with membrane-bound IL-21, to generate NK cells with enhanced anti-tumor cytotoxicity. The stimulation of peripheral blood mononuclear cells with IFN-y, anti-CD3, and IL-2 generates cytokine-induced killer (CIK) cells equipped with TCR and NK-cell receptor recognition to eliminate cancer cells. Conversely, immune cells may be genetically modified in the laboratory, utilizing viral vectors from the BioDrug ToolKit to generate T cells expressing a chimeric antigen receptor (CAR). The CAR-binding domain (typically derived from a single-chain fragment variable region of an antibody) recognizes the cognate surface antigen in an MHC-independent fashion and can kill cancer cells in highly efficient fashion. While currently approved CART cell therapies are individualized to collect and gene-modify autologous T cells, CART cells derived from allogeneic donors for an off-the-shelf approach are increasingly explored in clinical trials. To prevent GVHD, the endogenous allogeneic T cell receptor has to be knocked out in this approach and is generally combined with additional strategies to minimize rejection of allogeneic T cells by the patient's immune system via MHC recognition on the allogeneic T cells. For recognition of intracellular tumor-associated proteins, introduction of a foreign high-affinity TCR recognizing an HLA-restricted peptide can be utilized

and have been studied for delivery of mRNA in preclinical models of inherited hematologic disorders for delivery of mRNA (Caplen et al. 1995; Russick et al. 2020).

6.5.3 Building Cell Therapies: Using the BioDrug ToolKit for Treatment of Malignancy

The BioDrug ToolKit provides a variety of cells that have been given for therapeutic purposes and additional tools that can be used to create highly engineered cells for treatment of advanced malignancies. This section provides examples of how the BioDrug ToolKit has been used to generate cell-based products for clinical trials in patients with malignancies (Fig. 6.6).

Non-engineered cells have been used as a "living drug product" for decades in treatment of hematologic malignancies, the classic example being transplantation of allogeneic HSC. Adoptive cell therapies (ACT) are good examples of more recent non-engineered BioDrugs that utilize the innate capabilities of T cells to provide the therapeutic effect. The goal of ACT is to exploit the capacity of endogenous T cells to generate an ongoing immune response to a tumor-associated antigen (TAA). TAA targeted by ACT can be neoantigens that arise from somatic mutations in cancer cells or may be normal tissue antigens that are overexpressed by malignant cells. Identification of targetable TAAs poses an enormous challenge that has been a significant barrier to the development of ACT.

The earliest studies of ACT avoided the problem of TAA identification by collecting and expanding lymphocytes found within the parenchyma of solid tumors, known as tumor-infiltrating lymphocytes (TILs) (Topalian et al. 1988). The presence of lymphocytes within tumor tissue has been shown to be a favorable prognostic biomarker for many tumors, and suggests the presence of an endogenous population of lymphocytes that recognize TAAs (Zhang et al. 2003; Djenidi et al. 2015). To generate the TIL product, small tumor sections are placed in culture medium with IL-2. The proliferating lymphocyte populations are harvested and placed in a second culture for rapid expansion in the presence of feeder cells, anti-CD3 antibody and IL-2 (Klapper et al. 2009; Dudley et al. 2003). The resulting product contains up to 1×10^{11} lymphocytes that have the potential to recognize a variety of TAAs. TIL therapy has been explored as an ACT for several tumor types (Dafni et al. 2019; Rohaan et al. 2018; Andersen et al. 2016). Infusion of TILs typically follows a lymphodepleting regimen, based on the hypothesis that reduction of the endogenous lymphocyte compartment decreases competition for homeostatic cytokines that support T cell function, such as IL-7 and IL-15. Post-infusion support with IL-2 also has shown to improve response in studies of melanoma-specific TIL therapy (Dafni et al. 2019). The FDA recently granted breakthrough status of a TIL product for advanced cervical cancer (https://ccr.cancer.gov/news/article/fda-grants-breakthrough-therapy-designation-of-new-til-therapy-for-advanced-cervical-cancer).

T cells also can be expanded ex vivo to generate cytotoxic T lymphocyte (CTL) lines to leverage the adaptive immune response to a specific antigen, such as viral protein or a TAA. The general steps in the production of an antigen-specific CTL product start with the establishment of a population of antigen-presenting cells derived from the patient, such as monocytes, dendritic cells, or an EBV-transformed B lymphocyte. Next the antigen-presenting cells are given the requisite antigen(s) for presentation, either by pulsing the cells with the peptide(s) or transfecting the cells with a vector that encodes the peptide sequence (Sili et al. 2012; Patel et al. 2018). Once the antigen-presenting stimulator cells have been established, peripheral blood mononuclear cells (PBMC) obtained from the patient are placed into the culture. T cells within the PBMC that recognize antigen become activated and expand in numbers. These T cells are collected and further expanded in culture to produce lines of CTLs that can be used for immunotherapy (Riddell and Greenberg 1990). Ex vivo expanded CTL lines have been studied for treatment of viral infections in immunocompromised patients and for malignancies, such as melanoma, for which TAAs have been defined (Sili et al. 2012; Hont et al. 2019; Weber et al. 2013). One advantage to this form of ACT is that T cell lines with a broader array of TCRs can be generated, which may increase the likelihood of antigen recognition. However, to date a limited number of TAA peptides have been identified. Furthermore, tumor cells may downregulate MHC, thus circumventing TCR recognition.

In contrast to T cell therapies, cells that comprise the innate immune system do not require antigen recognition in the context of MHC for activity. The potent anti-tumor activity of NK cells has prompted much interest in developing NK cell therapies for treatment of malignancy. One approach has been to exploit the "missing ligand" concept, which allows activation of NK cells when their inhibitory KIR fails to engage the cognate MHC class I inhibitory ligand. Much of this work has been done in the setting of HLA-haploidentical HCT, first brought to attention by Ruggeri and colleagues who reported a significantly lower risk for relapse among recipients who lacked the inhibitory HLA molecule for the donor NK cells (Ruggeri et al. 2002). Donor NK alloreactivity also has been utilized in HLA-matched HCT by selection of donors that have more favorable activating KIR phenotypes (Cooley et al. 2018; Hsu et al. 2006). Subsequently, alloreactive HLA-haploidentical

NK cells have been studied outside the setting of HCT for treatment of advanced myeloid malignancies (Kottaridis et al. 2015; Miller et al. 2005; Lee et al. 2016b; Curti et al. 2016). These studies obtained allogeneic NK cells from adult donors; however, allogeneic NK cell products have also been generated from umbilical cord blood (UBC) or established NK cell lines resulting in readily available "off-the-shelf" products (Spanholtz et al. 2011; Arai et al. 2008). Efforts also have been focused on enhancing NK cell activation, either by placing cells in culture with IL-12, IL-15, and IL-18, termed cytokine-induced memory-like (CIML) NK cells, or by in vivo activation of infused NK cells by administration of IL-2, IL-15, or membrane-bound IL-21 (Lee et al. 2016b; Uppendahl et al. 2019; Berrien-Elliott et al. 2015; Phillips et al. 1987; Romee et al. 2016). Tumor antigen-directed NK cells also have been engineered using genetic modification to generated chimeric antigen receptors, as described in the sections below (Liu et al. 2020).

Cells that have characteristics of both NK and T cells, including expression of both CD3 and CD56, capable of both MHC-restricted and non-restricted cytotoxicity, termed cytokine-induced killer (CIK) cells can be generated by incubating peripheral blood mononuclear cells with interferon gamma (IFNγ), IL-1, IL-2, and anti-CD3 (Lu and Negrin 1994; Pievani et al. 2011). The safety of CIK therapy has been shown in pilot studies, and efficacy is being assessed in patients with advanced malignancies (Rettinger et al. 2016; Introna et al. 2007; Schmeel et al. 2015).

6.5.4 Engineered Cell Therapy: Putting Together Cells, Genetic Material, Gene-Editing Machinery, and Delivery Systems to Target Malignant Cells

Cellular engineering strategies have evolved to overcome the biologic limits of the innate and adaptive immune systems by insertion of genetic instructions that direct the cells toward specific antigens and augment cellular immune responses. These technologies all rely on pre-identification of the tumor-associated antigen (TAA) for targeting tumor cells. This section describes the various approaches to genetic engineering of adaptive or innate immune responses to tumor antigens and the contributions of the various tools available from the BioDrug ToolKit.

The basic steps in building a tumor-directed BioDrug using the ToolKit include (1) selection of the appropriate TAA for targeting; (2) engineering the transgene cassettes to provide tumor-targeting genes and regulatory elements; (3) selection of the optimal delivery system capable of carrying the genetic information to the targeted cell; and (4) selection of the appropriate cell type as the best weapon to eradicate the tumor. To date, T cells have been the preferred cell for use in engineering a tumor-specific immune response. As described above, the endogenous adaptive immune response occurs when the TCR recognizes antigen in the context of MHC, which in concert with a co-stimulatory signal results in T cell activation. However, tumors that express self-antigens, even if overexpressed, are unlikely to be recognized by endogenous T cells, since these will have been deleted during thymic selection. Endogenous T cells may also fail to recognize tumor antigens due to inadequate presentation of TAA, downregulation of MHC, or lack of co-stimulatory signals within the tumor milieu. These limitations to endogenous TCR recognition of TAA have hampered the success of TIL and CTL therapies and led to the development of chimeric antigen receptor (CAR) T cells.

Building CAR T cells requires all the tool components in the BioDrug ToolKit, including cell culture systems, complex genetic material, and viral delivery systems. The genetic material is designed to express a long protein that links together a TAA-recognition domain expressed on the cell surface with intracellular signaling domains (Fig. 6.7). The TAA-recognition domain is most commonly a single-chain variable fragment (scFv) derived from a monoclonal antibody, linked to a "hinge" or transmembrane region that connects the surface antibody receptor to the intracellular signaling domains. The intracellular

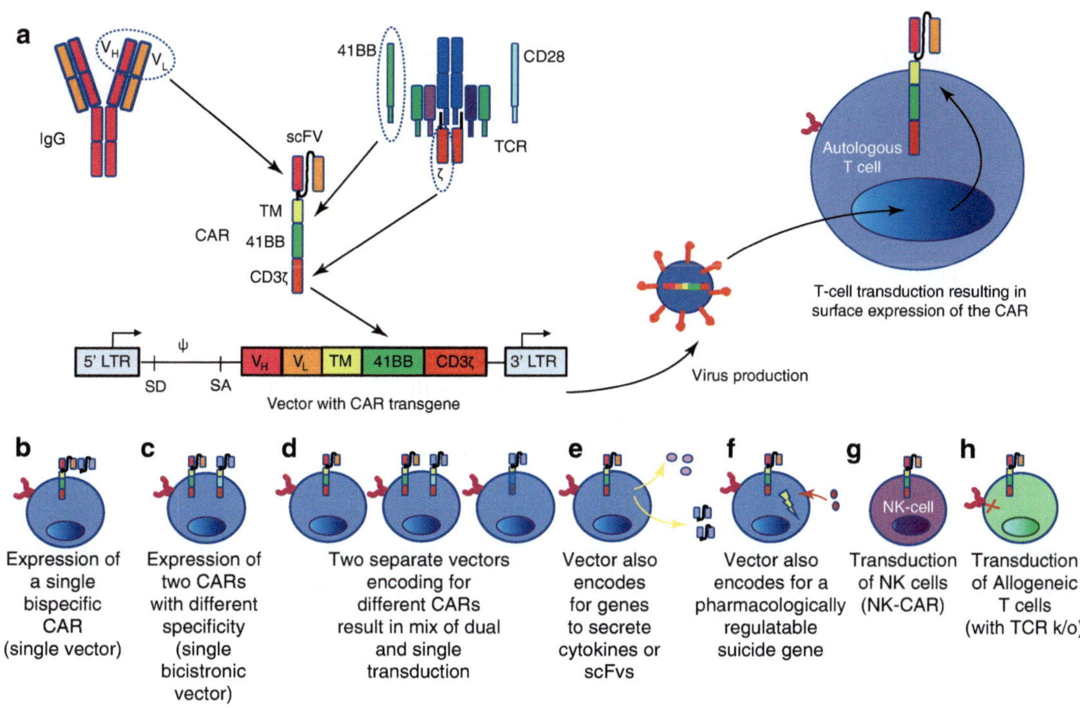

Fig. 6.7 (**a**) A typical CAR T cell configuration consists of a single-chain fragment variable region (scFV) derived from the variable chains of an IgG antibody as the antigen-recognition domain, a hinge/transmembrane (TM) region, a co-stimulatory moiety such as 41BB or CD28 and the CD3ζ chain derived from the T cell receptor (TCR). The CAR gene is cloned into a lentiviral or γ-retroviral vector. After production of replication-incompetent lentivirus or γ-retrovirus, these integrating viruses are used to transduce autologous T cells, leading to CAR expression on the cell surface. Several iterations of the classic CART approach are currently being explored. (**b**) To address antigen-escape mechanisms, CARs with dual antigen specificity have been developed. This may be achieved by inclusion of two separate scFVs in the transgene, resulting in a bi-specific CAR with a common signaling domain that is delivered by a single vector. (**c**) Alternatively, a single vector may encode for two separate CARs, each with their own signaling domain contained in the same transgene separated by a ribosomal skipping sequence such as T2A and delivered by a single bicistronic vector. (**d**) Dual specificity may also be achieved by utilizing two different vectors, each encoding for a different CAR to transduce T cells. This may result in a mixed T cell pool of cells expressing either one or both CARs. (**e**) In an effort to enhance CART efficacy, so-called "armored" CARs have been developed in which the transgene may include genes for cytokines or scFVs that can be secreted by the T cell. (**f**) In an effort to enhance the safety profile of CART cells, the transgene may include a suicide gene that can be activated by administering a drug to the patient. (**g**) CARs can also be introduced into autologous or allogeneic NK cells, which generally do not mediate graft-versus-host disease. (**h**) Approaches to develop universal off-the-shelf CAR T cells are underway, in which allogeneic T cells are transduced to express the CAR. However, this must be combined with a gene-editing approach to knock out the TCR to prevent GVHD. Additionally, it is frequently combined with strategies to minimize rejection of allogeneic CAR T cells based on HLA mismatch

signaling domains consist of the CD3ζ protein from the native TCR linked to one of the "second signal" proteins, either CD28 or 4-1BB. This entire construct artificially replicates the three important steps in the generation of an adaptive immune response. In step one the antibody domain engages the tumor antigen and replaces the need for TCR recognition of the antigen-MHC complex. Engagement of the antibody with antigen automatically stimulates both CD3ζ signaling and the second co-stimulatory signal, replacing both of these steps to initiate T cell activation. The engineered transgene construct may also include other linked domains for proteins that activate or modify cell migration, antigen recognition, or immune responses. In addition to the multiple transgenes, the CAR construct must include promoter regions that can drive expression of long RNA encoding multiple gene products (Rad et al. 2020). The choice of promoters currently is limited to more well-characterized promoters such as EF-1 and CMV, and depends on the level of desired CAR transgene expression. To generate the target cells, PBMC are collected by apheresis for initiation of T cell cultures. PBMC can be placed directly into T cell culture systems as described above, or T cell subsets can be selected from apheresis product prior to manufacturing (Shah et al. 2020; Turtle et al. 2016). Once the target T cells have been obtained and the CAR construct has been built, retroviral or lentiviral vectors are used for delivery of the genetic material for integration into the genome. The CAR T cells are expanded in culture and then cryopreserved for future administration. Several excellent reviews discuss the development of CAR T cell technology, including the stepwise incorporation of co-stimulatory domains (termed second-generation CARs) that have improved CAR T activation and efficacy (June et al. 2018; Boyiadzis et al. 2018).

To date, four CAR T cell products manufactured from autologous PDMC have gained FDA approval for treatment of hematologic malignancies (Table 6.2). In order to commercialize products originally conceived in academic laboratories, biotech companies were required to demonstrate that the manufacturing process and controls were capable of yielding a product with consistent quality and that chain of identity and chain of custody could be maintained throughout the manufacturing process. Kymriah (tisagenlecleucel) and Yescarta (axicabtagene ciloleucel) were the first CAR T cell products to be approved, and while both are directed at the CD19 antigen, they differ in the genetic material incorporated in the CAR construct and the vector delivery systems. Kymriah is generated from autologous T cells using a LV vector to deliver the CAR construct which contains the 4-1BB co-stimulatory domain, whereas the Yescarta CAR construct contains the CD28 co-stimulatory domain and is delivered by a RV vector. The latest CD19-directed CAR T cell product to be approved, Breyanzi (lisocabtagene maraleucel), also contains the 4-1BB co-stimulatory domain in its CAR construct but differs in its end composition which includes a fixed ratio of CD4+/CD8+ cells. Abecma (idecabtagene vicleucel) is the first CAR T cell approved for treatment of multiple myeloma. The CAR construct includes a B cell maturation antigen (BCMA) recognition single-chain variable fragment domain and the 4-BB and CD3ζ intracellular signaling domains, transduced into autologous T cells by a LV vector.

Approval of each of these products was based on results of multicenter, open-label, single-arm trials, and with respect to the CD19-directed CAR T cell products, there have not as yet been head-to-head comparisons (Grupp et al. 2013; Maude et al. 2014; Cappell et al. 2020; Locke et al. 2017, 2019; Wang et al. 2020; Neelapu et al. 2017; Schuster et al. 2019). However, these trials exhibited similar findings with lessons learned to

Table 6.2 Approved chimeric antigen receptor T cell products (of April 2021)

Cell therapy product	Indication	Target antigen	ORR CR
Abecma (idecabtagene vicleucel)	Multiple myeloma	BCMA	72% 28%
Breyanzi (lisocabtagene maraleucel)	Relapsed or refractory large B cell lymphoma	CD19	73% 54%
Kymriah (tisagenlecleucel)	Refractory B cell precursor acute lymphoblastic leukemia Relapsed or refractory large B cell lymphoma	CD19	50% 32%
Yescarta (axicabtagene ciloleucel)	Relapsed or refractory large B cell lymphoma	CD19	72% 51%

BCMA B cell maturation antigen, *CD* cluster of differentiation, *CR* complete remission, *ORR* overall response guide future trials. First, the median time from leukapheresis to final manufactured product was approximately 2–4 weeks, during which time the patient may need to receive bridging chemotherapy to maintain control of the malignancy. Second, both efficacy and toxicity correlated with the degree of in vivo expansion of the CAR T cells. Expansion typically peaked between 7 and 14 days after infusion, and the area under the curve within the first month was significantly higher in responding compared to non-responding patients. However, responding patients also had higher levels of cytokines, such as IL-6, associated with toxicity. Third, delivery of a lymphodepleting regimen before infusion of the CAR T cell product facilitated CAR T expansion, presumably by reducing competition and immunogenicity from endogenous T cells (Hirayama et al. 2019).

The speed at which the CD19-directed CAR T cells have been shown to be effective illustrates the promise of this therapy when a tumor expresses an antigen on its surface that can be directly recognized by the CAR T cell receptor, and when elimination of cells that express the surface antigen does not result in serious off-tumor effects. CD19 expression is limited to malignant and nonmalignant B cells; thus, CD19-directed CAR T cell therapy typically causes profound B cell aplasia. The on-target off-tumor consequence of hypogammaglobulinemia is treatable by administration of gamma globulin. Development of CAR T cells for other tumor types is made more challenging by the fact that tumor antigens may be internally expressed, therefore only "visible" to a T cell when processed peptides are expressed in the context of MHC.

For this reason, investigators are exploring alternatives to CAR T cells that exploit the entire TCR complex for TAA recognition in the context of self-MHC (Fig. 6.6). Compared to CARs, TCRs can target virtually every tumor protein, independent of their cellular localization, and are reactive at lower antigen densities than CARs (Harris et al. 2018). This process starts by identification of the T cells that recognize the desired peptide in the context of MHC, which in and of itself is a challenge, since MHC genes are highly polymorphic. Most studies use peptides restricted to HLA-A*02, because it is the most common HLA allele, present in up to 50% of the population depending on the ethnic background. Several systems can be used to isolate T cells with the desired TCRs, such as affinity-enhanced phage display (Varela-Rohena et al. 2008). Once identified, the TCRα and TCRβ chains can be cloned and inserted into viral vectors for delivery into T cells. The engineering can become more sophisticated by using CRISPR/Cas9 or other gene-editing tools to knock out the native TCRα and TCRβ chains so as not to interfere with the transgenic TCRαβ complex. The engineered T cells can be expanded in culture similar to the process for CAR T cells. Theoretically, by infusing T cells with an intact, albeit engineered, TCR complex, intracellular signaling occurs through the six TCR subunits in contrast to the single CD3ζ signal from CAR T cells, which exploits the full potential of TCR-driven T cell activation, effector function, and regulation. A hybrid system has also been developed that combines the MHC-unrestricted antigen recognition properties of CAR T cells with the native TCR signaling. T cells are transduced with a construct containing an antigen recognition domain, such as an scFv, which is connected to a transmembrane spacer domain and then to the CD3ε chain. These hybrid constructs overcome the limitation of HLA-A*02 restriction, however, may be limited by the need for surface expression of the antigen.

6.5.4.1 Toxicities of Engineered T cell Therapy

Clinical trials have brought to attention unique toxicities related to the biologic activity of engineered T cells (Neelapu et al. 2018). It is not yet known whether the toxicities observed in trials of CD19- and BCMA-directed T cells will be observed with T cells directed toward other TAA, or with TCR-engineered T cell therapies, since these toxicities may be driven by the antigen in addition to the biology of T cell activation. Specific to the individual TAA will be the potential for on-target off-tumor effects, such as the B cell aplasia observed with CD19-directed therapy. To the extent that TAA expression is unique to the tumor cells, off-tumor effects will be minimized.

Toxicities that result from T cell activation and proliferation become a potential concern for any engineered T cell. In the studies that supported approval of CAR T cell products, a dose-toxicity relationship was observed, such that a greater proportion of patients and a higher grade of toxicity was observed in patients given higher CAR T cell doses. The most important toxicities reported in these patients include cytokine release syndrome (CRS), immune effector cell-associated neurotoxicity (ICANS), macrophage activation syndrome (MAS), and prolonged cytopenias (Neelapu et al. 2018). CRS represents the double-edged sword of T cell therapies, because it is associated with T cell activity and is observed to some extent in most patients who have tumor response. Onset of the symptoms correlates with in vivo expansion and proliferation of activated T cells and usually occurs within a week after infusion of the T cell product. The hallmark of CRS is fever (>38.0 °C) which occurs in all patients. CRS can progress to a state of vasodilation and capillary leak, resulting in hypotension, and respiratory distress (Acharya et al. 2019). A standardized grading system is used to aid in diagnosis and management of patients (Lee et al. 2019). The symptoms are caused by release of inflammatory cytokines from activated T cells, including interleukin (IL)-6, IL-2, IL-10, IL-15, and IL-18 (Hay et al. 2017). Markers of inflammation are often elevated, including ferritin, C-reactive protein, lactic acid dehydrogenase, interferon gamma (IFNγ), and soluble IL-2 receptor. Management of CRS involves supportive care and judicious medical intervention guided by staging criteria and accepted algorithms (Lee et al. 2014, 2019). The primary treatment is tocilizumab, an IL-6 receptor antagonist that is approved by the FDA for treating CRS (Le et al. 2018; Gardner et al. 2019). Dexamethasone can be added for patients who do not respond to tocilizumab or other anti-IL-6 agents. MAS is another potentially life-threatening complication of CAR T cell therapy, observed in 1–5% of CAR T cell recipients, and may be difficult to differentiate from CRS, as a markedly elevated serum ferritin is associated in both disorders. Treatment of MAS typically includes etoposide; however, its role in treatment of CAR T cell recipients has not been established (reviewed in Sandler et al. 2020).

ICANS has been defined as a disorder characterized by a pathologic process involving the central nervous system following any immunotherapy that results in the activation or engagement of endogenous or infused T cells and/or other immune effector cells (Lee et al. 2019; Sheth and Gauthier 2021). ICANS was observed initially in trials of CD19 CAR T cells and later in the BCMA CAR T cell trials (Raje et al. 2019). ICANS is characterized by speech difficulties, tremor, dysgraphia, cognitive difficulties, and/or altered level of consciousness (reviewed in Rice et al. 2019). Symptoms typically occur within the first week after infusion of CAR T cells and range from mild to severe. Similar to CRS, a standardized grading system has been developed to aid in diagnosis and management of ICANS (Lee et al. 2019). While it is likely that inflammatory cytokines play an important role in the development of ICANs, it appears treatment aimed toward inhibiting IL-6 may not be sufficient for control, some evidence even suggests that tocilizumab paradoxically contributes to worsening ICANS; therefore, treatment relies upon supportive care, control of seizures, and corticosteroids (Rice et al. 2019; Gust et al. 2020).

Building a less toxic cell T cell therapy must take into consideration that almost all patients with tumor response also develop some degree of CRS; thus, strategies must not interfere with TAA recognition and T cell activation. Engineering strategies include cloning in suicide genes such as inducible caspase 9, which was shown capable of "turning off" alloimmune T cell activation in recipients of HLA-haploidentical HCT (Di Stasi et al. 2011), or genes that express cell surface molecules that can be targeted with monoclonal antibodies (Fig. 6.7). Others have proposed developing a "universal CAR" that recognizes one moiety on a bi-specific engager, which recruits the CAR T cell to the tumor via its TAA engager (Yu et al. 2019). Alternatively, nonintegrating vectors such as AAV might be used to deliver constructs that would be expressed for a limited timeframe (Rotolo et al. 2018).

6.5.4.2 Building a More Effective T cell BioDrug: Remaining Challenges

The recent approval of several CAR T cell BioDrugs and the proliferation of clinical trials for engineered immunotherapeutic cell products speak to the progress and promise of tumor-directed cell therapies. The studies that have supported development of the currently approved CAR T cell products unequivocally demonstrated the power of T cells not only for killing malignant cells but for maintaining tumor surveillance and preventing relapse. Currently approved T cell products achieve disease response in 50–75% of patients and complete remission in 28–54%. However, the success in targeting B cell malignancies has not yet translated to solid tumors. Building a T cell BioDrug for treatment of a solid tumor begins with identifying the barriers to success, and the design of the system must be based on knowledge of the interactions between T cells and the TME. The difficulties must be overcome along with potential approaches to build improved cellular therapy for solid tumors. Some of the obstacles to current cellular therapies and strategies for building improved tumor-targeting BioDrugs are outlined below and shown in Figs. 6.6 and 6.7.

How can we improve tumor cell targeting? In contrast to CD19 and BCMA, many tumor antigens are also expressed by a variety of normal cells, resulting in the potential for significant off-tumor toxicity, and expression is heterogenous within the tumor, resulting in inadequate recognition of tumor cells. Furthermore, overexpressed TAA may be intracellular antigens not normally found on the cell surface, such as NY-ESO-1 or WT1. As described above, engineered TCR approaches were developed to recognize TAA presented in the context of HLA. However, much of the improvement in solid tumor antigen recognition will come through complex genetic engineering to enable T cells to recognize patterns of gene or protein expression that differentiate malignant cells from normal cells (Springuel et al. 2019). Examples of proposed strategies include multi-specific CAR constructs that recognize different TAA, with a specific recognition pattern required to initiate T cell activation or that recognize TAA in the context of other signals expressed by tumor cells, such as stress-induced ligands in the TME.

How can we prevent antigen negative escape? Approximately 60% of patients with relapsed disease after treatment with CD19-directed CAR T cells had a recurrence with a CD19-negative malignancy. Antigen-negative relapse results from the pressure that CAR Ts place on leukemic cells that leads to natural selection of alternatively spliced variants of the CD19 molecule (Sotillo et al. 2015). Strategies proposed to reduce the risk for antigen-negative relapse include administration of CAR T cells with different specificity (CAR pools), for example, coadministration of CD19- and CD20-directed CAR T products, based on the idea that there is a lower probability of losing two different antigen targets (reviewed in Ruella et al. 2016). Others have proposed developing multi-antigen specific CAR constructs allowing each T cell to recognize multiple TAAs. An alternative approach is based on the success of bi-specific T cell engagers (BiTEs), wherein the CAR construct has a universal recognition site activated by antibodies or other molecules bound to the tumor surface. Various antibodies can be delivered independently, each capable of activating the universal CAR T cells (Ayyappan and Maddocks 2019; Darowski et al. 2019).

How can we build a stronger BioDrug? T cell exhaustion caused by continual antigen stimulation results in impaired in vivo proliferation and lack of persistence, both correlated with lower anti-tumor efficacy. One strategy to strengthen the overall BioDrug product is to consider the optimal cell to engineer. For example, investigators have proposed to start with T cells that are less prone to exhaustion by upfront selection of less differentiated naïve or central memory phenotypes and/or to modify culture conditions that support T cell persistence (Gattinoni et al. 2011; Ghassemi et al. 2018; Ceppi and Gardner 2019).

Alternatively, collection of T cells from healthy donors not previously exposed to cancer therapy might improve T cell fitness. Gene-editing machinery, such as CRISPR/Cas9, has been used to remove the endogenous TCR and/or HLA molecules that could lead to alloimmune responses. Alternatives to T cells, such as NK cells or MΦs, also are being explored as optimal cells for overcoming the immunosuppressive TME (Fig. 6.6). In addition to novel cell selection, genetic engineering may contribute to strengthening cellular products. One example is the advance made by the addition of co-stimulatory genes to the first-generation CAR constructs, now termed "second-generation" CAR T cells, which led to improved T cell activation and proliferation products. Genetic engineering strategies proposed to improve T cell persistence include the addition of genes for cytokines that support T cell proliferation, such as IL-2, or precisely target the insertion of the transgene next to endogenous T cell regulatory elements using gene-editing machinery by using gene editing such as CRISPR/Cas9 (Perales et al. 2018).

How can we overcome the immunosuppressive TME? The main obstacle to successful TIL therapy has been the immunosuppressive nature of the TME, which presumably will pose a challenge to even the most potent T cell products. The TME combines the interactions of stromal cells, secretory factors, tumor vasculature, and immune regulatory cells such as Tregs, myeloid-derived suppressor cells, and TAMs within a hostile hypoxic and nutritionally depleted environment, each part of which can form a barrier to T cell function (reviewed in Ye et al. 2018). Lessons from the development of immuno-oncology drugs, such as the checkpoint inhibitors that have radically changed the treatment of solid tumors, will need to be incorporated into cellular therapy strategies to ensure a potent anti-tumor response. The simplest approaches have proposed to administer checkpoint inhibitors, IL-12, or other immuno-oncology drugs alongside cell therapy products; however, these strategies may increase the risks for added systemic toxicities from the additional agents. More complex strategies seek to incorporate these genes within the transgene constructs, resulting T cells capable of locally secreting pro-inflammatory cytokines within the TME (Springuel et al. 2019).

6.6 Summary

The future holds bright promise for new curative therapies for life-threatening malignancies and inherited blood disorders in children based on BioDrug technology. Building better BioDrugs in the future will incorporate many of the strategies outlined in this chapter, and the components in the Toolkit will be utilized. Undoubtedly the ToolKit will expand to include technologies and components not yet imagined for BioDrug development. The resources provided here are meant to provide pediatric hematologist/oncologists with the knowledge to understand current and future developments so that they can better inform their patients and guide them through clinical trials and complex therapies aimed toward permanently correcting genetic disorders and eradicating childhood malignancies.

References

Abraham A, Hsieh M, Eapen M, Fitzhugh C, Carreras J, Keesler D et al (2017) Relationship between mixed donor-recipient chimerism and disease recurrence after hematopoietic cell transplantation for sickle cell disease. Biol Blood Marrow Transplant 23(12):2178–2183

Acharya UH, Dhawale T, Yun S, Jacobson CA, Chavez JC, Ramos JD et al (2019) Management of cytokine release syndrome and neurotoxicity in chimeric antigen receptor (CAR) T cell therapy. Expert Rev Hematol 12(3):195–205

Adair JE, Chandrasekaran D, Sghia-Hughes G, Haworth KG, Woolfrey AE, Burroughs LM et al (2018) Novel lineage depletion preserves autologous blood stem cells for gene therapy of Fanconi anemia complementation group A. Haematologica 103(11):1806–1814

Adler BK, Salzman DE, Carabasi MH, Vaughan WP, Reddy VV, Prchal JT (2001) Fatal sickle cell crisis after granulocyte colony-stimulating factor administration. Blood 97(10):3313–3314

Aiuti A, Slavin S, Aker M, Ficara F, Deola S, Mortellaro A et al (2002) Correction of ADA-SCID by stem cell gene therapy combined with nonmyeloablative conditioning. Science 296(5577):2410–2413

Aiuti A, Cattaneo F, Galimberti S, Benninghoff U, Cassani B, Callegaro L et al (2009) Gene therapy for immunodeficiency due to adenosine deaminase deficiency. N Engl J Med 360(5):447–458

Alcover A, Alarcón B, Di Bartolo V (2018) Cell biology of T cell receptor expression and regulation. Annu Rev Immunol 36:103–125

Alton EW, Stern M, Farley R, Jaffe A, Chadwick SL, Phillips J et al (1999) Cationic lipid-mediated CFTR gene transfer to the lungs and nose of patients with cystic fibrosis: a double-blind placebo-controlled trial. Lancet 353(9157):947–954

Al-Zaidy SA, Mendell JR (2019) From clinical trials to clinical practice: practical considerations for gene replacement therapy in SMA type 1. Pediatr Neurol 100:3–11

Andersen R, Donia M, Ellebaek E, Borch TH, Kongsted P, Iversen TZ et al (2016) Long-lasting complete responses in patients with metastatic melanoma after adoptive cell therapy with tumor-infiltrating lymphocytes and an attenuated IL2 regimen. Clin Cancer Res 22(15):3734–3745

Arai S, Meagher R, Swearingen M, Myint H, Rich E, Martinson J et al (2008) Infusion of the allogeneic cell line NK-92 in patients with advanced renal cell cancer or melanoma: a phase I trial. Cytotherapy 10(6):625–632

Arnould S, Chames P, Perez C, Lacroix E, Duclert A, Epinat JC et al (2006) Engineering of large numbers of highly specific homing endonucleases that induce recombination on novel DNA targets. J Mol Biol 355(3):443–458

Ashworth J, Taylor GK, Havranek JJ, Quadri SA, Stoddard BL, Baker D (2010) Computational reprogramming of homing endonuclease specificity at multiple adjacent base pairs. Nucleic Acids Res 38(16):5601–5608

Athanasopoulos T, Munye MM, Yáñez-Muñoz RJ (2017) Nonintegrating gene therapy vectors. Hematol Oncol Clin North Am 31(5):753–770

Ayyappan S, Maddocks K (2019) Novel and emerging therapies for B cell lymphoma. J Hematol Oncol 12(1):82

Azuma M (2019) Co-signal molecules in T-cell activation: historical overview and perspective. Adv Exp Med Biol 1189:3–23

Balakrishnan B, Jayandharan GR (2014) Basic biology of adeno-associated virus (AAV) vectors used in gene therapy. Curr Gene Ther 14(2):86–100

Bauer DE, Kamran SC, Orkin SH (2012) Reawakening fetal hemoglobin: prospects for new therapies for the β-globin disorders. Blood 120(15):2945–2953

Berrien-Elliott MM, Wagner JA, Fehniger TA (2015) Human cytokine-induced memory-like natural killer cells. J Innate Immun 7(6):563–571

Biasco L, Baricordi C, Aiuti A (2012) Retroviral integrations in gene therapy trials. Mol Ther 20(4):709–716

Biasco L, Rothe M, Schott JW, Schambach A (2017) Integrating vectors for gene therapy and clonal tracking of engineered hematopoiesis. Hematol Oncol Clin North Am 31(5):737–752

Birchall JC, Kellaway IW, Mills SN (1999) Physico-chemical characterisation and transfection efficiency of lipid-based gene delivery complexes. Int J Pharm 183(2):195–207

Bordignon C, Notarangelo LD, Nobili N, Ferrari G, Casorati G, Panina P et al (1995) Gene therapy in peripheral blood lymphocytes and bone marrow for ADA-immunodeficient patients. Science 270(5235):470–475

Boulaire J, Balani P, Wang S (2009) Transcriptional targeting to brain cells: engineering cell type-specific promoter containing cassettes for enhanced transgene expression. Adv Drug Deliv Rev 61(7–8):589–602

Boyiadzis MM, Dhodapkar MV, Brentjens RJ, Kochenderfer JN, Neelapu SS, Maus MV et al (2018) Chimeric antigen receptor (CAR) T therapies for the treatment of hematologic malignancies: clinical perspective and significance. J Immunother Cancer 6(1):137

Bradford KL, Moretti FA, Carbonaro-Sarracino DA, Gaspar HB, Kohn DB (2017) Adenosine deaminase (ADA)-deficient severe combined immune deficiency (SCID): molecular pathogenesis and clinical manifestations. J Clin Immunol 37(7):626–637

Bradford KL, Liu S, Krajinovic M, Ansari M, Garabedian E, Tse J et al (2020) Busulfan pharmacokinetics in adenosine deaminase-deficient severe combined immunodeficiency gene therapy. Biol Blood Marrow Transplant 26(10):1819–1827

Brandes M, Willimann K, Moser B (2005) Professional antigen-presentation function by human gammadelta T Cells. Science 309(5732):264–268

Braun CJ, Boztug K, Paruzynski A, Witzel M, Schwarzer A, Rothe M et al (2014) Gene therapy for Wiskott-Aldrich syndrome—long-term efficacy and genotoxicity. Sci Transl Med 6(227):227ra33

Bryceson YT, March ME, Ljunggren HG, Long EO (2006) Activation, coactivation, and costimulation of resting human natural killer cells. Immunol Rev 214:73–91

Caligiuri MA (2008) Human natural killer cells. Blood 112(3):461–469

Campbell KS, Hasegawa J (2013) Natural killer cell biology: an update and future directions. J Allergy Clin Immunol 132(3):536–544

Caplen NJ, Alton EW, Middleton PG, Dorin JR, Stevenson BJ, Gao X et al (1995) Liposome-mediated CFTR gene transfer to the nasal epithelium of patients with cystic fibrosis. Nat Med 1(1):39–46

Cappell KM, Sherry RM, Yang JC, Goff SL, Vanasse DA, McIntyre L et al (2020) Long-term follow-up of anti-CD19 chimeric antigen receptor T-cell therapy. J Clin Oncol 38(32):3805–3815

Ceppi F, Gardner RA (2019) Chimeric antigen receptor T cells for B-cell acute lymphoblastic leukemia. Cancer J 25(3):191–198

Chandrasekaran D, Nakamoto B, Watts KL, Kiem HP, Papayannopoulou T (2014) Modeling promising nonmyeloablative conditioning regimens in nonhuman primates. Hum Gene Ther 25(12):1013–1022

Chiu SJ, Ueno NT, Lee RJ (2004) Tumor-targeted gene delivery via anti-HER2 antibody (trastuzumab, Herceptin) conjugated polyethylenimine. J Control Release 97(2):357–369
Christian M, Cermak T, Doyle EL, Schmidt C, Zhang F, Hummel A et al (2010) Targeting DNA double-strand breaks with TAL effector nucleases. Genetics 186(2):757–761
Cockrell AS, Kafri T (2007) Gene delivery by lentivirus vectors. Mol Biotechnol 36(3):184–204
Collin M, Bigley V (2018) Human dendritic cell subsets: an update. Immunology 154(1):3–20
Cooley S, Parham P, Miller JS (2018) Strategies to activate NK cells to prevent relapse and induce remission following hematopoietic stem cell transplantation. Blood 131(10):1053–1062
Curti A, Ruggeri L, Parisi S, Bontadini A, Dan E, Motta MR et al (2016) Larger size of donor alloreactive NK cell repertoire correlates with better response to NK cell immunotherapy in elderly acute myeloid leukemia patients. Clin Cancer Res 22(8):1914–1921
Dafni U, Michielin O, Lluesma SM, Tsourti Z, Polydoropoulou V, Karlis D et al (2019) Efficacy of adoptive therapy with tumor-infiltrating lymphocytes and recombinant interleukin-2 in advanced cutaneous melanoma: a systematic review and meta-analysis. Ann Oncol 30(12):1902–1913
Daniel-Moreno A, Lamsfus-Calle A, Raju J, Antony JS, Handgretinger R, Mezger M (2019) CRISPR/Cas9-modified hematopoietic stem cells-present and future perspectives for stem cell transplantation. Bone Marrow Transplant 54(12):1940–1950
Darowski D, Kobold S, Jost C, Klein C (2019) Combining the best of two worlds: highly flexible chimeric antigen receptor adaptor molecules (CAR-adaptors) for the recruitment of chimeric antigen receptor T cells. MAbs 11(4):621–631
Davis MM, Bjorkman PJ (1988) T-cell antigen receptor genes and T-cell recognition. Nature 334(6181):395–402
De Rosa SC, Herzenberg LA, Herzenberg LA, Roederer M (2001) 11-color, 13-parameter flow cytometry: identification of human naive T cells by phenotype, function, and T-cell receptor diversity. Nat Med 7(2):245–248
Di Stasi A, Tey SK, Dotti G, Fujita Y, Kennedy-Nasser A, Martinez C et al (2011) Inducible apoptosis as a safety switch for adoptive cell therapy. N Engl J Med 365(18):1673–1683
Djenidi F, Adam J, Goubar A, Durgeau A, Meurice G, de Montpréville V et al (2015) CD8+CD103+ tumor-infiltrating lymphocytes are tumor-specific tissue-resident memory T cells and a prognostic factor for survival in lung cancer patients. J Immunol 194(7):3475–3486
Dudley ME, Wunderlich JR, Shelton TE, Even J, Rosenberg SA (2003) Generation of tumor-infiltrating lymphocyte cultures for use in adoptive transfer therapy for melanoma patients. J Immunother 26(4):332–342
Eapen M, Brazauskas R, Walters MC, Bernaudin F, Bo-Subait K, Fitzhugh CD et al (2019) Effect of donor type and conditioning regimen intensity on allogeneic transplantation outcomes in patients with sickle cell disease: a retrospective multicentre, cohort study. Lancet Haematol 6(11):e585–e596
Eichler F, Duncan C, Musolino PL, Orchard PJ, De Oliveira S, Thrasher AJ et al (2017) Hematopoietic stem-cell gene therapy for cerebral adrenoleukodystrophy. N Engl J Med 377(17):1630–1638
Ellis J (2005) Silencing and variegation of gammaretrovirus and lentivirus vectors. Hum Gene Ther 16(11):1241–1246
Ertl HCJ, High KA (2017) Impact of AAV capsid-specific T-cell responses on design and outcome of clinical gene transfer trials with recombinant adeno-associated viral vectors: an evolving controversy. Hum Gene Ther 28(4):328–337
Escors D, Breckpot K (2010) Lentiviral vectors in gene therapy: their current status and future potential. Arch Immunol Ther Exp (Warsz) 58(2): 107–119
Esrick EB, Lehmann LE, Biffi A, Achebe M, Brendel C, Ciuculescu MF et al (2021) Post-transcriptional genetic silencing of BCL11A to treat sickle cell disease. N Engl J Med 384(3):205–215
Foust KD, Nurre E, Montgomery CL, Hernandez A, Chan CM, Kaspar BK (2009) Intravascular AAV9 preferentially targets neonatal neurons and adult astrocytes. Nat Biotechnol 27(1):59–65
Frangoul H, Nemecek ER, Billheimer D, Pulsipher MA, Khan S, Woolfrey A et al (2007) A prospective study of G-CSF primed bone marrow as a stem-cell source for allogeneic bone marrow transplantation in children: a Pediatric Blood and Marrow Transplant Consortium (PBMTC) study. Blood 110(13):4584–4587
Fu H, Meadows AS, Pineda RJ, Kunkler KL, Truxal KV, McBride KL et al (2017) Differential prevalence of antibodies against adeno-associated virus in healthy children and patients with mucopolysaccharidosis III: perspective for AAV-mediated gene therapy. Hum Gene Ther Clin Dev 28(4):187–196
Gardner RA, Ceppi F, Rivers J, Annesley C, Summers C, Taraseviciute A et al (2019) Preemptive mitigation of CD19 CAR T-cell cytokine release syndrome without attenuation of antileukemic efficacy. Blood 134(24):2149–2158
Gasiunas G, Barrangou R, Horvath P, Siksnys V (2012) Cas9-crRNA ribonucleoprotein complex mediates specific DNA cleavage for adaptive immunity in bacteria. Proc Natl Acad Sci U S A 109(39):E2579–E2586
Gaspar HB, Parsley KL, Howe S, King D, Gilmour KC, Sinclair J et al (2004) Gene therapy of X-linked severe combined immunodeficiency by use of a pseudotyped gammaretroviral vector. Lancet 364(9452):2181–2187
Gaspar HB, Cooray S, Gilmour KC, Parsley KL, Adams S, Howe SJ et al (2011) Long-term persistence of a polyclonal T cell repertoire after gene therapy for

X-linked severe combined immunodeficiency. Sci Transl Med 3(97):97ra79
Gattinoni L, Lugli E, Ji Y, Pos Z, Paulos CM, Quigley MF et al (2011) A human memory T cell subset with stem cell-like properties. Nat Med 17(10):1290–1297
Gersbach CA, Gaj T, Barbas CF 3rd. (2014) Synthetic zinc finger proteins: the advent of targeted gene regulation and genome modification technologies. Acc Chem Res 47(8):2309–2318
Gertner-Dardenne J, Castellano R, Mamessier E, Garbit S, Kochbati E, Etienne A et al (2012) Human Vγ9Vδ2 T cells specifically recognize and kill acute myeloid leukemic blasts. J Immunol 188(9):4701–4708
Ghassemi S, Nunez-Cruz S, O'Connor RS, Fraietta JA, Patel PR, Scholler J et al (2018) Reducing ex vivo culture improves the antileukemic activity of chimeric antigen receptor (CAR) T cells. Cancer Immunol Res 6(9):1100–1109
Gillmore JD, Gane E, Taubel J, Kao J, Fontana M, Maitland ML et al (2021) CRISPR-Cas9 in vivo gene editing for transthyretin amyloidosis. N Engl J Med 385(6):493–502
Giralt S, Costa L, Schriber J, Dipersio J, Maziarz R, McCarty J et al (2014) Optimizing autologous stem cell mobilization strategies to improve patient outcomes: consensus guidelines and recommendations. Biol Blood Marrow Transplant 20(3):295–308
Grigg AP (2001) Granulocyte colony-stimulating factor-induced sickle cell crisis and multiorgan dysfunction in a patient with compound heterozygous sickle cell/beta+ thalassemia. Blood 97(12):3998–3999
Groh V, Rhinehart R, Secrist H, Bauer S, Grabstein KH, Spies T (1999) Broad tumor-associated expression and recognition by tumor-derived gamma delta T cells of MICA and MICB. Proc Natl Acad Sci U S A 96(12):6879–6884
Grupp SA, Kalos M, Barrett D, Aplenc R, Porter DL, Rheingold SR et al (2013) Chimeric antigen receptor-modified T cells for acute lymphoid leukemia. N Engl J Med 368(16):1509–1518
Gust J, Ponce R, Liles WC, Garden GA, Turtle CJ (2020) Cytokines in CAR T cell-associated neurotoxicity. Front Immunol 11:577027
Hacein-Bey-Abina S, Garrigue A, Wang GP, Soulier J, Lim A, Morillon E et al (2008) Insertional oncogenesis in 4 patients after retrovirus-mediated gene therapy of SCID-X1. J Clin Invest 118(9):3132–3142
Hacein-Bey-Abina S, Hauer J, Lim A, Picard C, Wang GP, Berry CC et al (2010) Efficacy of gene therapy for X-linked severe combined immunodeficiency. N Engl J Med 363(4):355–364
Hacein-Bey-Abina S, Pai SY, Gaspar HB, Armant M, Berry CC, Blanche S et al (2014) A modified γ-retrovirus vector for X-linked severe combined immunodeficiency. N Engl J Med 371(15):1407–1417
Harris DT, Hager MV, Smith SN, Cai Q, Stone JD, Kruger P et al (2018) Comparison of T cell activities mediated by human TCRs and CARs that use the same recognition domains. J Immunol 200(3):1088–1100
Hay KA, Hanafi LA, Li D, Gust J, Liles WC, Wurfel MM et al (2017) Kinetics and biomarkers of severe cytokine release syndrome after CD19 chimeric antigen receptor-modified T-cell therapy. Blood 130(21):2295–2306
Heller R, Shirley S, Guo S, Donate A, Heller L (2011) Electroporation based gene therapy—from the bench to the bedside. Annu Int Conf IEEE Eng Med Biol Soc 2011:736–738
Herweijer H, Wolff JA (2003) Progress and prospects: naked DNA gene transfer and therapy. Gene Ther 10(6):453–458
Hinshaw DC, Shevde LA (2019) The tumor microenvironment innately modulates cancer progression. Cancer Res 79(18):4557–4566
Hirayama AV, Gauthier J, Hay KA, Voutsinas JM, Wu Q, Gooley T et al (2019) The response to lymphodepletion impacts PFS in patients with aggressive non-Hodgkin lymphoma treated with CD19 CAR T cells. Blood 133(17):1876–1887
Hockemeyer D, Jaenisch R (2016) Induced pluripotent stem cells meet genome editing. Cell Stem Cell 18(5):573–586
Hont AB, Cruz CR, Ulrey R, O'Brien B, Stanojevic M, Datar A et al (2019) Immunotherapy of relapsed and refractory solid tumors with ex vivo expanded multi-tumor associated antigen specific cytotoxic T lymphocytes: a phase I study. J Clin Oncol 37(26):2349–2359
Hood JD, Bednarski M, Frausto R, Guccione S, Reisfeld RA, Xiang R et al (2002) Tumor regression by targeted gene delivery to the neovasculature. Science 296(5577):2404–2407
Hornberger K, Yu G, McKenna D, Hubel A (2019) Cryopreservation of hematopoietic stem cells: emerging assays, cryoprotectant agents, and technology to improve outcomes. Transfus Med Hemother 46(3):188–196
Hsieh MM, Bonner M, Pierciey FJ, Uchida N, Rottman J, Demopoulos L et al (2020) Myelodysplastic syndrome unrelated to lentiviral vector in a patient treated with gene therapy for sickle cell disease. Blood Adv 4(9):2058–2063
Hsu KC, Gooley T, Malkki M, Pinto-Agnello C, Dupont B, Bignon JD et al (2006) KIR ligands and prediction of relapse after unrelated donor hematopoietic cell transplantation for hematologic malignancy. Biol Blood Marrow Transplant 12(8):828–836
Imai K, Nonoyama S, Ochs HD (2003) WASP (Wiskott-Aldrich syndrome protein) gene mutations and phenotype. Curr Opin Allergy Clin Immunol 3(6):427–436
Introna M, Borleri G, Conti E, Franceschetti M, Barbui AM, Broady R et al (2007) Repeated infusions of donor-derived cytokine-induced killer cells in patients relapsing after allogeneic stem cell transplantation: a phase I study. Haematologica 92(7):952–959
Italiani P, Boraschi D (2014) From monocytes to M1/M2 macrophages: phenotypical vs. functional differentiation. Front Immunol 5:514

Jiang H, Couto LB, Patarroyo-White S, Liu T, Nagy D, Vargas JA et al (2006) Effects of transient immunosuppression on adenoassociated, virus-mediated, liver-directed gene transfer in rhesus macaques and implications for human gene therapy. Blood 108(10):3321–3328

Jinek M, Chylinski K, Fonfara I, Hauer M, Doudna JA, Charpentier E (2012) A programmable dual-RNA-guided DNA endonuclease in adaptive bacterial immunity. Science 337(6096):816–821

June CH, O'Connor RS, Kawalekar OU, Ghassemi S, Milone MC (2018) CAR T cell immunotherapy for human cancer. Science 359(6382):1361–1365

Kafri T (2004) Gene delivery by lentivirus vectors an overview. Methods Mol Biol 246:367–390

Kafri T, Blömer U, Peterson DA, Gage FH, Verma IM (1997) Sustained expression of genes delivered directly into liver and muscle by lentiviral vectors. Nat Genet 17(3):314–317

Khalil IA, Kogure K, Akita H, Harashima H (2006) Uptake pathways and subsequent intracellular trafficking in nonviral gene delivery. Pharmacol Rev 58(1):32–45

Kim SY, Lee JH, Shin HS, Kang HJ, Kim YS (2002) The human elongation factor 1 alpha (EF-1 alpha) first intron highly enhances expression of foreign genes from the murine cytomegalovirus promoter. J Biotechnol 93(2):183–187

Klapper JA, Thomasian AA, Smith DM, Gorgas GC, Wunderlich JR, Smith FO et al (2009) Single-pass, closed-system rapid expansion of lymphocyte cultures for adoptive cell therapy. J Immunol Methods 345(1–2):90–99

Klichinsky M, Ruella M, Shestova O, Lu XM, Best A, Zeeman M et al (2020) Human chimeric antigen receptor macrophages for cancer immunotherapy. Nat Biotechnol 38(8):947–953

Kottaridis PD, North J, Tsirogianni M, Marden C, Samuel ER, Jide-Banwo S et al (2015) Two-stage priming of allogeneic natural killer cells for the treatment of patients with acute myeloid leukemia: a phase I trial. PLoS One 10(6):e0123416

La Gruta NL, Gras S, Daley SR, Thomas PG, Rossjohn J (2018) Understanding the drivers of MHC restriction of T cell receptors. Nat Rev Immunol 18(7):467–478

Lagresle-Peyrou C, Lefrère F, Magrin E, Ribeil JA, Romano O, Weber L et al (2018) Plerixafor enables safe, rapid, efficient mobilization of hematopoietic stem cells in sickle cell disease patients after exchange transfusion. Haematologica 103(5):778–786

Lazarus HM, Kan F, Tarima S, Champlin RE, Confer DL, Frey N et al (2009) Rapid transport and infusion of hematopoietic cells is associated with improved outcome after myeloablative therapy and unrelated donor transplant. Biol Blood Marrow Transplant 15(5):589–596

Le RQ, Li L, Yuan W, Shord SS, Nie L, Habtemariam BA et al (2018) FDA approval summary: tocilizumab for treatment of chimeric antigen receptor T cell-induced severe or life-threatening cytokine release syndrome. Oncologist 23(8):943–947

Lee DW, Gardner R, Porter DL, Louis CU, Ahmed N, Jensen M et al (2014) Current concepts in the diagnosis and management of cytokine release syndrome. Blood 124(2):188–195

Lee S, Kivimäe S, Dolor A, Szoka FC (2016a) Macrophage-based cell therapies: the long and winding road. J Control Release 240:527–540

Lee DA, Denman CJ, Rondon G, Woodworth G, Chen J, Fisher T et al (2016b) Haploidentical natural killer cells infused before allogeneic stem cell transplantation for myeloid malignancies: a phase I trial. Biol Blood Marrow Transplant 22(7):1290–1298

Lee DW, Santomasso BD, Locke FL, Ghobadi A, Turtle CJ, Brudno JN et al (2019) ASTCT consensus grading for cytokine release syndrome and neurologic toxicity associated with immune effector cells. Biol Blood Marrow Transplant 25(4):625–638

Lewis P, Hensel M, Emerman M (1992) Human immunodeficiency virus infection of cells arrested in the cell cycle. EMBO J 11(8):3053–3058

Li T, Huang S, Jiang WZ, Wright D, Spalding MH, Weeks DP et al (2011a) TAL nucleases (TALNs): hybrid proteins composed of TAL effectors and FokI DNA-cleavage domain. Nucleic Acids Res 39(1):359–372

Li T, Huang S, Zhao X, Wright DA, Carpenter S, Spalding MH et al (2011b) Modularly assembled designer TAL effector nucleases for targeted gene knockout and gene replacement in eukaryotes. Nucleic Acids Res 39(14):6315–6325

Lin HT, Okumura T, Yatsuda Y, Ito S, Nakauchi H, Otsu M (2016) Application of droplet digital PCR for estimating vector copy number states in stem cell gene therapy. Hum Gene Ther Methods 27(5):197–208

Liu K, Nussenzweig MC (2010) Origin and development of dendritic cells. Immunol Rev 234(1):45–54

Liu W, Liu Z, Liu L, Xiao Z, Cao X, Cao Z et al (2008) A novel human foamy virus mediated gene transfer of GAD67 reduces neuropathic pain following spinal cord injury. Neurosci Lett 432(1):13–18

Liu E, Marin D, Banerjee P, Macapinlac HA, Thompson P, Basar R et al (2020) Use of CAR-transduced natural killer cells in CD19-positive lymphoid tumors. N Engl J Med 382(6):545–553

Locke FL, Neelapu SS, Bartlett NL, Siddiqi T, Chavez JC, Hosing CM et al (2017) Phase 1 results of ZUMA-1: a multicenter study of KTE-C19 anti-CD19 CAR T cell therapy in refractory aggressive lymphoma. Mol Ther 25(1):285–295

Locke FL, Ghobadi A, Jacobson CA, Miklos DB, Lekakis LJ, Oluwole OO et al (2019) Long-term safety and activity of axicabtagene ciloleucel in refractory large B-cell lymphoma (ZUMA-1): a single-arm, multicentre, phase 1-2 trial. Lancet Oncol 20(1):31–42

Louis Jeune V, Joergensen JA, Hajjar RJ, Weber T (2013) Pre-existing anti-adeno-associated virus antibodies as a challenge in AAV gene therapy. Hum Gene Ther Methods 24(2):59–67

Lu PH, Negrin RS (1994) A novel population of expanded human CD3+CD56+ cells derived from T cells with potent in vivo antitumor activity in mice with severe combined immunodeficiency. J Immunol 153(4):1687–1696

Lukashev AN, Zamyatnin AA Jr (2016) Viral vectors for gene therapy: current state and clinical perspectives. Biochemistry (Mosc) 81(7):700–708

Mahvi DM, Sheehy MJ, Yang NS (1997) DNA cancer vaccines: a gene gun approach. Immunol Cell Biol 75(5):456–460

Mak KY, Rajapaksha IG, Angus PW, Herath CB (2017) The adeno-associated virus—a safe and promising vehicle for liverspecific gene therapy of inherited and non-inherited disorders. Curr Gene Ther 17(1):4–16

Mamcarz E, Zhou S, Lockey T, Abdelsamed H, Cross SJ, Kang G et al (2019) Lentiviral gene therapy combined with low-dose busulfan in infants with SCID-X1. N Engl J Med 380(16):1525–1534

Manno CS, Pierce GF, Arruda VR, Glader B, Ragni M, Rasko JJ et al (2006) Successful transduction of liver in hemophilia by AAV-Factor IX and limitations imposed by the host immune response. Nat Med 12(3):342–347

Mansilla-Soto J, Rivière I, Sadelain M (2011) Genetic strategies for the treatment of sickle cell anaemia. Br J Haematol 154(6):715–727

Maruyama T, Dougan SK, Truttmann MC, Bilate AM, Ingram JR, Ploegh HL (2015) Increasing the efficiency of precise genome editing with CRISPR-Cas9 by inhibition of nonhomologous end joining. Nat Biotechnol 33(5):538–542

Maude SL, Frey N, Shaw PA, Aplenc R, Barrett DM, Bunin NJ et al (2014) Chimeric antigen receptor T cells for sustained remissions in leukemia. N Engl J Med 371(16):1507–1517

Mendell JR, Al-Zaidy S, Shell R, Arnold WD, Rodino-Klapac LR, Prior TW et al (2017) Single-dose gene-replacement therapy for spinal muscular atrophy. N Engl J Med 377(18):1713–1722

Miesbach W, Meijer K, Coppens M, Kampmann P, Klamroth R, Schutgens R et al (2018) Gene therapy with adeno-associated virus vector 5-human factor IX in adults with hemophilia B. Blood 131(9):1022–1031

Miller JS, Soignier Y, Panoskaltsis-Mortari A, McNearney SA, Yun GH, Fautsch SK et al (2005) Successful adoptive transfer and in vivo expansion of human haploidentical NK cells in patients with cancer. Blood 105(8):3051–3057

Mills CD, Kincaid K, Alt JM, Heilman MJ, Hill AM (2000) M-1/M-2 macrophages and the Th1/Th2 paradigm. J Immunol 164(12):6166–6173

Milone MC, O'Doherty U (2018) Clinical use of lentiviral vectors. Leukemia 32(7):1529–1541

Mingozzi F, High KA (2013) Immune responses to AAV vectors: overcoming barriers to successful gene therapy. Blood 122(1):23–36

Mingozzi F, Hasbrouck NC, Basner-Tschakarjan E, Edmonson SA, Hui DJ, Sabatino DE et al (2007) Modulation of tolerance to the transgene product in a nonhuman primate model of AAV-mediated gene transfer to liver. Blood 110(7):2334–2341

Miyoshi H, Blömer U, Takahashi M, Gage FH, Verma IM (1998) Development of a self-inactivating lentivirus vector. J Virol 72(10):8150–8157

Morbitzer R, Römer P, Boch J, Lahaye T (2010) Regulation of selected genome loci using de novo-engineered transcription activator-like effector (TALE)-type transcription factors. Proc Natl Acad Sci U S A 107(50):21617–21622

Morris EC, Fox T, Chakraverty R, Tendeiro R, Snell K, Rivat C et al (2017) Gene therapy for Wiskott-Aldrich syndrome in a severely affected adult. Blood 130(11):1327–1335

Muul LM, Tuschong LM, Soenen SL, Jagadeesh GJ, Ramsey WJ, Long Z et al (2003) Persistence and expression of the adenosine deaminase gene for 12 years and immune reaction to gene transfer components: long-term results of the first clinical gene therapy trial. Blood 101(7):2563–2569

Naldini L, Blömer U, Gage FH, Trono D, Verma IM (1996) Efficient transfer, integration, and sustained long-term expression of the transgene in adult rat brains injected with a lentiviral vector. Proc Natl Acad Sci U S A 93(21):11382–11388

Naso MF, Tomkowicz B, Perry WL 3rd, Strohl WR (2017) Adeno-associated virus (AAV) as a vector for gene therapy. BioDrugs 31(4):317–334

Nathwani AC, Tuddenham EG, Rangarajan S, Rosales C, McIntosh J, Linch DC et al (2011) Adenovirus-associated virus vector-mediated gene transfer in hemophilia B. N Engl J Med 365(25):2357–2365

Nathwani AC, Reiss UM, Tuddenham EG, Rosales C, Chowdary P, McIntosh J et al (2014) Long-term safety and efficacy of factor IX gene therapy in hemophilia B. N Engl J Med 371(21):1994–2004

Neelapu SS, Locke FL, Bartlett NL, Lekakis LJ, Miklos DB, Jacobson CA et al (2017) Axicabtagene ciloleucel CAR T-cell therapy in refractory large B-cell lymphoma. N Engl J Med 377(26):2531–2544

Neelapu SS, Tummala S, Kebriaei P, Wierda W, Gutierrez C, Locke FL et al (2018) Chimeric antigen receptor T-cell therapy—assessment and management of toxicities. Nat Rev Clin Oncol 15(1):47–62

Nwanegbo E, Vardas E, Gao W, Whittle H, Sun H, Rowe D et al (2004) Prevalence of neutralizing antibodies to adenoviral serotypes 5 and 35 in the adult populations of The Gambia, South Africa, and the United States. Clin Diagn Lab Immunol 11(2):351–357

Orlandini von Niessen AG, Poleganov MA, Rechner C, Plaschke A, Kranz LM, Fesser S et al (2019) Improving mRNA-based therapeutic gene delivery by expression-augmenting 3′ UTRs identified by cellular library screening. Mol Ther 27(4):824–836

Owen DL, Sjaastad LE, Farrar MA (2019) Regulatory T cell development in the thymus. J Immunol 203(8):2031–2041

Pabo CO, Peisach E, Grant RA (2001) Design and selection of novel Cys2His2 zinc finger proteins. Annu Rev Biochem 70:313–340

Pasi KJ, Rangarajan S, Mitchell N, Lester W, Symington E, Madan B et al (2020) Multiyear follow-up of

AAV5-hFVIII-SQ gene therapy for hemophilia A. N Engl J Med 382(1):29–40
Patel S, Chorvinsky E, Albihani S, Cruz CR, Jones RB, Shpall EJ et al (2018) HIV-specific T cells generated from naive T cells suppress HIV in vitro and recognize wide epitope breadths. Mol Ther 26(6):1435–1446
Paul S, Singh AK, Shilpi LG (2014) Phenotypic and functional plasticity of gamma-delta (γδ) T cells in inflammation and tolerance. Int Rev Immunol 33(6):537–558
Pavletich NP, Pabo CO (1991) Zinc finger-DNA recognition: crystal structure of a Zif268-DNA complex at 2.1 A. Science 252(5007):809–817
Perales MA, Kebriaei P, Kean LS, Sadelain M (2018) Building a safer and faster CAR: seatbelts, airbags, and CRISPR. Biol Blood Marrow Transplant 24(1):27–31
Perrin GQ, Herzog RW, Markusic DM (2019) Update on clinical gene therapy for hemophilia. Blood 133(5):407–414
Peters C, Shapiro EG, Anderson J, Henslee-Downey PJ, Klemperer MR, Cowan MJ et al (1998) Hurler syndrome: II. Outcome of HLA-genotypically identical sibling and HLA-haploidentical related donor bone marrow transplantation in fifty-four children. The Storage Disease Collaborative Study Group. Blood 91(7):2601–2608
Petty AJ, Yang Y (2017) Tumor-associated macrophages: implications in cancer immunotherapy. Immunotherapy 9(3):289–302
Phillips JH, Gemlo BT, Myers WW, Rayner AA, Lanier LL (1987) In vivo and in vitro activation of natural killer cells in advanced cancer patients undergoing combined recombinant interleukin-2 and LAK cell therapy. J Clin Oncol 5(12):1933–1941
Pievani A, Borleri G, Pende D, Moretta L, Rambaldi A, Golay J et al (2011) Dual-functional capability of CD3+CD56+ CIK cells, a T-cell subset that acquires NK function and retains TCR-mediated specific cytotoxicity. Blood 118(12):3301–3310
Quantin B, Perricaudet LD, Tajbakhsh S, Mandel JL (1992) Adenovirus as an expression vector in muscle cells in vivo. Proc Natl Acad Sci U S A 89(7):2581–2584
Rad SMA, Poudel A, Tan GMY, McLellan AD (2020) Promoter choice: who should drive the CAR in T cells? PLoS One 15(7):e0232915
Radtke S, Pande D, Cui M, Perez AM, Chan YY, Enstrom M et al (2020) Purification of human CD34(+) CD90(+) HSCs reduces target cell population and improves lentiviral transduction for gene therapy. Mol Ther Methods Clin Dev 18:679–691
Raje N, Berdeja J, Lin Y, Siegel D, Jagannath S, Madduri D et al (2019) Anti-BCMA CAR T-cell therapy bb2121 in relapsed or refractory multiple myeloma. N Engl J Med 380(18):1726–1737
Rangarajan S, Walsh L, Lester W, Perry D, Madan B, Laffan M et al (2017) AAV5-factor VIII gene transfer in severe hemophilia A. N Engl J Med 377(26):2519–2530
Raper SE, Chirmule N, Lee FS, Wivel NA, Bagg A, Gao GP et al (2003) Fatal systemic inflammatory response syndrome in a ornithine transcarbamylase deficient patient following adenoviral gene transfer. Mol Genet Metab 80(1–2):148–158
Rettinger E, Huenecke S, Bonig H, Merker M, Jarisch A, Soerensen J et al (2016) Interleukin-15-activated cytokine-induced killer cells may sustain remission in leukemia patients after allogeneic stem cell transplantation: feasibility, safety and first insights on efficacy. Haematologica 101(4):e153–e156
Rice J, Nagle S, Randall J, Hinson HE (2019) Chimeric antigen receptor T cell-related neurotoxicity: mechanisms, clinical presentation, and approach to treatment. Curr Treat Options Neurol 21(8):40
Riddell SR, Greenberg PD (1990) The use of anti-CD3 and anti-CD28 monoclonal antibodies to clone and expand human antigen-specific T cells. J Immunol Methods 128(2):189–201
Rohaan MW, van den Berg JH, Kvistborg P, Haanen J (2018) Adoptive transfer of tumor-infiltrating lymphocytes in melanoma: a viable treatment option. J Immunother Cancer 6(1):102
Romee R, Rosario M, Berrien-Elliott MM, Wagner JA, Jewell BA, Schappe T et al (2016) Cytokine-induced memory-like natural killer cells exhibit enhanced responses against myeloid leukemia. Sci Transl Med 8(357):357ra123
Rotolo A, Karadimitris A, Ruella M (2018) Building upon the success of CART19: chimeric antigen receptor T cells for hematologic malignancies. Leuk Lymphoma 59(9):2040–2055
Ruella M, Barrett DM, Kenderian SS, Shestova O, Hofmann TJ, Perazzelli J et al (2016) Dual CD19 and CD123 targeting prevents antigen-loss relapses after CD19-directed immunotherapies. J Clin Invest 126(10):3814–3826
Ruggeri L, Capanni M, Urbani E, Perruccio K, Shlomchik WD, Tosti A et al (2002) Effectiveness of donor natural killer cell alloreactivity in mismatched hematopoietic transplants. Science 295(5562):2097–2100
Russick J, Delignat S, Milanov P, Christophe O, Boros G, Denis CV et al (2020) Correction of bleeding in experimental severe hemophilia A by systemic delivery of factor VIII-encoding mRNA. Haematologica 105(4):1129–1137
Sabado RL, Balan S, Bhardwaj N (2017) Dendritic cell-based immunotherapy. Cell Res 27(1):74–95
Sandler RD, Tattersall RS, Schoemans H, Greco R, Badoglio M, Labopin M et al (2020) Diagnosis and management of secondary HLH/MAS following HSCT and CAR-T cell therapy in adults; a review of the literature and a survey of practice within EBMT Centres on Behalf of the Autoimmune Diseases Working Party (ADWP) and Transplant Complications Working Party (TCWP). Front Immunol 11:524
Saukkonen K, Hemminki A (2004) Tissue-specific promoters for cancer gene therapy. Expert Opin Biol Ther 4(5):683–696
Scherer F, Anton M, Schillinger U, Henke J, Bergemann C, Krüger A et al (2002) Magnetofection: enhancing

and targeting gene delivery by magnetic force in vitro and in vivo. Gene Ther 9(2):102–109
Schmeel LC, Schmeel FC, Coch C, Schmidt-Wolf IG (2015) Cytokine-induced killer (CIK) cells in cancer immunotherapy: report of the international registry on CIK cells (IRCC). J Cancer Res Clin Oncol 141(5):839–849
Schuster SJ, Bishop MR, Tam CS, Waller EK, Borchmann P, McGuirk JP et al (2019) Tisagenlecleucel in adult relapsed or refractory diffuse large B-cell lymphoma. N Engl J Med 380(1):45–56
Scott LJ (2015) Alipogene tiparvovec: a review of its use in adults with familial lipoprotein lipase deficiency. Drugs 75(2):175–182
Sekijima Y (2015) Transthyretin (ATTR) amyloidosis: clinical spectrum, molecular pathogenesis and disease-modifying treatments. J Neurol Neurosurg Psychiatry 86(9):1036–1043
Shah NN, Highfill SL, Shalabi H, Yates B, Jin J, Wolters PL et al (2020) CD4/CD8 T-cell selection affects chimeric antigen receptor (CAR) T-cell potency and toxicity: updated results from a phase I anti-CD22 CAR T-cell trial. J Clin Oncol 38(17):1938–1950
Sharpe AH, Freeman GJ (2002) The B7-CD28 superfamily. Nat Rev Immunol 2(2):116–126
Sheth VS, Gauthier J (2021) Taming the beast: CRS and ICANS after CAR T-cell therapy for ALL. Bone Marrow Transplant 56(3):552–566
Sili U, Leen AM, Vera JF, Gee AP, Huls H, Heslop HE et al (2012) Production of good manufacturing practice-grade cytotoxic T lymphocytes specific for Epstein-Barr virus, cytomegalovirus and adenovirus to prevent or treat viral infections post-allogeneic hematopoietic stem cell transplant. Cytotherapy 14(1):7–11
Simantirakis E, Tsironis I, Vassilopoulos G (2020) FV vectors as alternative gene vehicles for gene transfer in HSCs. Viruses 12(3):332
Smith J, Grizot S, Arnould S, Duclert A, Epinat JC, Chames P et al (2006) A combinatorial approach to create artificial homing endonucleases cleaving chosen sequences. Nucleic Acids Res 34(22):e149
Smith-Garvin JE, Koretzky GA, Jordan MS (2009) T cell activation. Annu Rev Immunol 27:591–619
Smyth MJ, Cretney E, Takeda K, Wiltrout RH, Sedger LM, Kayagaki N et al (2001) Tumor necrosis factor-related apoptosis-inducing ligand (TRAIL) contributes to interferon gamma-dependent natural killer cell protection from tumor metastasis. J Exp Med 193(6):661–670
Sotillo E, Barrett DM, Black KL, Bagashev A, Oldridge D, Wu G et al (2015) Convergence of acquired mutations and alternative splicing of CD19 enables resistance to CART-19 immunotherapy. Cancer Discov 5(12):1282–1295
Spanholtz J, Preijers F, Tordoir M, Trilsbeek C, Paardekooper J, de Witte T et al (2011) Clinical-grade generation of active NK cells from cord blood hematopoietic progenitor cells for immunotherapy using a closed-system culture process. PLoS One 6(6):e20740
Springuel L, Lonez C, Alexandre B, Van Cutsem E, Machiels JH, Van Den Eynde M et al (2019) Chimeric antigen receptor-T cells for targeting solid tumors: current challenges and existing strategies. BioDrugs 33(5):515–537
Srikanthan MA, Humbert O, Haworth KG, Ironside C, Rajawat YS, Blazar BR et al (2020) Effective multi-lineage engraftment in a mouse model of Fanconi anemia using non-genotoxic antibody-based conditioning. Mol Ther Methods Clin Dev 17:455–464
Stepinski J, Waddell C, Stolarski R, Darzynkiewicz E, Rhoads RE (2001) Synthesis and properties of mRNAs containing the novel "anti-reverse" cap analogs 7-methyl(3′-O-methyl)GpppG and 7-methyl (3′-deoxy)GpppG. RNA 7(10):1486–1495
Sun JC, Beilke JN, Lanier LL (2009) Adaptive immune features of natural killer cells. Nature 457(7229):557–561
Tang MX, Szoka FC (1997) The influence of polymer structure on the interactions of cationic polymers with DNA and morphology of the resulting complexes. Gene Ther 4(8):823–832
Tang R, Palumbo RN, Nagarajan L, Krogstad E, Wang C (2010) Well-defined block copolymers for gene delivery to dendritic cells: probing the effect of polycation chain-length. J Control Release 142(2):229–237
Teschendorf C, Warrington KH Jr, Siemann DW, Muzyczka N (2002) Comparison of the EF-1 alpha and the CMV promoter for engineering stable tumor cell lines using recombinant adeno-associated virus. Anticancer Res 22(6a):3325–3330
Thompson AA, Walters MC, Kwiatkowski J, Rasko JEJ, Ribeil JA, Hongeng S et al (2018) Gene therapy in patients with transfusion-dependent β-thalassemia. N Engl J Med 378(16):1479–1493
Thurtle-Schmidt DM, Lo TW (2018) Molecular biology at the cutting edge: a review on CRISPR/CAS9 gene editing for undergraduates. Biochem Mol Biol Educ 46(2):195–205
Topalian SL, Solomon D, Avis FP, Chang AE, Freerksen DL, Linehan WM et al (1988) Immunotherapy of patients with advanced cancer using tumor-infiltrating lymphocytes and recombinant interleukin-2: a pilot study. J Clin Oncol 6(5):839–853
Trobridge GD (2009) Foamy virus vectors for gene transfer. Expert Opin Biol Ther 9(11):1427–1436
Turtle CJ, Hanafi LA, Berger C, Gooley TA, Cherian S, Hudecek M et al (2016) CD19 CAR-T cells of defined CD4+:CD8+ composition in adult B cell ALL patients. J Clin Invest 126(6):2123–2138
Ullah I, Subbarao RB, Rho GJ (2015) Human mesenchymal stem cells—current trends and future prospective. Biosci Rep 35(2):e00191
Uppendahl LD, Felices M, Bendzick L, Ryan C, Kodal B, Hinderlie P et al (2019) Cytokine-induced memory-like natural killer cells have enhanced function, proliferation, and in vivo expansion against ovarian cancer cells. Gynecol Oncol 153(1):149–157

Van Craenenbroeck K, Vanhoenacker P, Haegeman G (2000) Episomal vectors for gene expression in mammalian cells. Eur J Biochem 267(18): 5665–5678

Varela-Rohena A, Molloy PE, Dunn SM, Li Y, Suhoski MM, Carroll RG et al (2008) Control of HIV-1 immune escape by CD8 T cells expressing enhanced T-cell receptor. Nat Med 14(12):1390–1395

Wagner W, Wein F, Seckinger A, Frankhauser M, Wirkner U, Krause U et al (2005) Comparative characteristics of mesenchymal stem cells from human bone marrow, adipose tissue, and umbilical cord blood. Exp Hematol 33(11):1402–1416

Wang GG, Calvo KR, Pasillas MP, Sykes DB, Häcker H, Kamps MP (2006) Quantitative production of macrophages or neutrophils ex vivo using conditional Hoxb8. Nat Methods 3(4):287–293

Wang M, Munoz J, Goy A, Locke FL, Jacobson CA, Hill BT et al (2020) KTE-X19 CAR T-cell therapy in relapsed or refractory mantle-cell lymphoma. N Engl J Med 382(14):1331–1342

Weber G, Caruana I, Rouce RH, Barrett AJ, Gerdemann U, Leen AM et al (2013) Generation of tumor antigen-specific T cell lines from pediatric patients with acute lymphoblastic leukemia—implications for immunotherapy. Clin Cancer Res 19(18):5079–5091

Wu T, Dai Y (2017) Tumor microenvironment and therapeutic response. Cancer Lett 387:61–68

Yamashita M, Emerman M (2006) Retroviral infection of non-dividing cells: old and new perspectives. Virology 344(1):88–93

Ye B, Stary CM, Li X, Gao Q, Kang C, Xiong X (2018) Engineering chimeric antigen receptor-T cells for cancer treatment. Mol Cancer 17(1):32

Youil R, Toner TJ, Su Q, Casimiro D, Shiver JW, Chen L et al (2003) Comparative analysis of the effects of packaging signal, transgene orientation, promoters, polyadenylation signals, and E3 region on growth properties of first-generation adenoviruses. Hum Gene Ther 14(10):1017–1034

Yu S, Yi M, Qin S, Wu K (2019) Next generation chimeric antigen receptor T cells: safety strategies to overcome toxicity. Mol Cancer 18(1):125

Zhang L, Conejo-Garcia JR, Katsaros D, Gimotty PA, Massobrio M, Regnani G et al (2003) Intratumoral T cells, recurrence, and survival in epithelial ovarian cancer. N Engl J Med 348(3):203–213

Zhang S, Xu Y, Wang B, Qiao W, Liu D, Li Z (2004) Cationic compounds used in lipoplexes and polyplexes for gene delivery. J Control Release 100(2):165–180

Zhang F, Wen Y, Guo X (2014) CRISPR/Cas9 for genome editing: progress, implications and challenges. Hum Mol Genet 23(R1):R40–R46

Zhao L, Chen S, Yang P, Cao H, Li L (2019) The role of mesenchymal stem cells in hematopoietic stem cell transplantation: prevention and treatment of graft-versus-host disease. Stem Cell Res Ther 10(1):182

Zheng C, Baum BJ (2008) Evaluation of promoters for use in tissue-specific gene delivery. Methods Mol Biol 434:205–219

Zhou S, Mody D, DeRavin SS, Hauer J, Lu T, Ma Z et al (2010) A self-inactivating lentiviral vector for SCID-X1 gene therapy that does not activate LMO2 expression in human T cells. Blood 116(6):900–908

Zufferey R, Dull T, Mandel RJ, Bukovsky A, Quiroz D, Naldini L et al (1998) Self-inactivating lentivirus vector for safe and efficient in vivo gene delivery. J Virol 72(12):9873–9880

The Pharma/Biotech Model for Drug Development: Implications for Pediatric Cancer Therapeutics

7

Peter T. C. Ho

Contents

7.1 The Old: Large Pharma

7.1.1 Background and History

We are all familiar with big drug companies and what they do. The drug and biological products developed and marketed by biopharmaceutical companies have contributed to improved quality of life and longer life expectancy that in the United States has increased from an average of 47 years in 1850 to 79 years in 2020. During the COVID-19 pandemic of 2020 that continues into 2022, large, multinational pharmaceutical companies such as Pfizer, Johnson & Johnson, and AstraZeneca have leveraged their considerable scientific, manufacturing, and logistical might to develop vaccines quickly and efficiently for an anxiously awaiting global public. Most large pharma companies have a long history, but the biopharmaceutical industry as a whole along with the large and small players, e.g., biotechs, that comprise it live within a very fluid environment with a plethora of foreseeable and unpredicted challenges such that the business credo "change or die" is very apt.

Today's pharma industry is rooted in small European apothecaries from the 1800s that

P. T. C. Ho (✉)
Phase One Advisors LLC, Newton Centre, MA, USA
e-mail: peter@oncologytx.com

J. DiMartino et al. (eds.), *Pediatric Cancer Therapeutics Development*, Pediatric Oncology,
https://doi.org/10.1007/978-3-031-06357-2_7

evolved to produce large quantities of drugs such as morphine and quinine and in the dye and chemical companies that discovered medicinal uses for their products (Daemmrich and Bowden 2005). For example, Merck began as an apothecary shop in Darmstadt, Germany, in 1668 that transformed into a wholesale manufacturer of drugs by the 1840s. Similarly, Schering in Germany, Hoffmann-La Roche in Switzerland, and Burroughs Wellcome in England all derived from apothecaries and drug producers from that era. The ensuing decades saw the discovery of new drugs accelerate as companies forged research collaborations with academic laboratories while synthetic chemistry and pharmacology matured as scientific disciplines. Researchers applied the theory of structure-activity relationships to chemicals and began generating experimental data in animals and humans to systematically discover new drugs. Despite these advances, most medicines sold in the United States by 1930 were without a prescription with almost half compounded by local pharmacists rather than produced by a central manufacturer.

With World War II came the demand for mass production of a variety of drugs needed by soldiers, including penicillin and antimalarials. This served to stimulate the growth of US pharmaceutical companies. In the post-war era, pharma companies in the United States, Europe, and Japan grew rapidly in the areas of research and development (R&D) and global marketing. Over the next several decades, large pharmas invested their rising revenues to build expansive state-of-the-art research campuses to drive innovation using a host of new technologies such as spectroscopy, high-pressure liquid chromatography, genetic engineering for protein production, and combinatorial chemistry. The advent of high-throughput screening technologies combined with massive chemical libraries collected and curated over decades by large pharma chemists expedited the testing of millions of chemical compounds against multiple molecular targets. This served to further advance the tradition of empirical drug discovery that began in the 1800s. It was only when high-throughput X-ray crystallography, nuclear magnetic spectroscopy, and computational biology were married in the 1980s that molecular modeling became the workhorse for the rational design of small molecule drugs that exists today.

7.1.2 Profile of a Large Pharma: Merck & Co.

Every large pharma is unique, but there are common threads with respect to their mission, organizational structure, and tactical operations. For those unfamiliar with the characteristics of a large pharma, Merck & Company, more commonly known as Merck, is profiled below as an illustrative example.

Merck was founded in the United States in 1891 by George Merck who at age 23 established the company to distribute fine chemicals throughout the New York City region. It currently describes itself as "a global health care company that delivers innovative health solutions through its prescription medicines, vaccines, biologic therapies, and animal health products." In 2020, Merck had approximately 71,000 employees worldwide of whom 26,000 were in the United States (Merck 2019). Its corporate headquarters are in Kenilworth, NJ; however, its geographic reach extends throughout the world. Merck's main pharmaceutical R&D campuses are in Rahway, NJ; West Point and Upper Gwynedd, PA; South San Francisco, CA; Boston, MA; and London, UK. Its headquarters for manufacturing is in Whitehouse Station, NJ, but Merck maintains production facilities at numerous locations all over the world including the United States, Puerto Rico, Japan, Singapore, South Africa, and countries in Western Europe, Central and South America, and Asia.

Its pharmaceutical division encompasses pharmaceutical and vaccine products that are generally sold by prescription. Merck sells their pharmaceutical products primarily to drug wholesalers and retailers, physicians, hospitals, government agencies and managed healthcare providers such as health maintenance organizations, pharmacy benefit managers, and other institutions. Its Animal Health division discovers, develops, manufactures, and markets a wide range of veterinary pharmaceutical products, vaccines, and services for the prevention, treatment, and control of disease in all major livestock and companion animal species. These products are marketed to veterinarians, distributors, and animal producers.

As reported in its 2019 Annual Report, Merck's R&D groups employed approximately 15,600 people worldwide and spent $9.9 billion ($9.9B) in 2019. Merck's R&D programs are described as prioritizing drug candidates that represent breakthrough science for patients and payers. Its clinical pipeline includes candidate molecules for a variety of disease areas including cancer, cardiovascular diseases, diabetes, and other metabolic diseases, infectious diseases, neurosciences, pain, respiratory diseases, and vaccines. As of November 2020, Merck disclosed publicly that it had 31 programs in phase 2 development, 25 programs in phase 3, and 3 programs under regulatory review for approval. Of note, pharmas and biotechs typically define a program as a single drug candidate under clinical testing for a single disease indication. Thus, a company that is testing a single drug candidate for three different types of cancers would count that as three programs. Given the scientific and commercial success of Merck's Keytruda® (pembrolizumab), an immune checkpoint monoclonal antibody that binds to and acts through the PD-1 receptor on T lymphocytes, it is not surprising that the overwhelming majority of Merck's programs were for oncologic indications. As such, 23 of its 31 phase 2 programs, 22 of 25 phase 3, and 1 of 3 programs under regulatory review were directed at various cancers. However, of these 46 programs for oncology diseases, only one program was specifically directed at a childhood tumor indication. Koselugo® (selumetinib), an inhibitor of MEK1 and MEK2 kinases originally discovered by and developed in collaboration with AstraZeneca, was approved in 2020 by the US Food and Drug Administration (FDA) for pediatric neurofibromatosis and under review for the same indication in Europe. Like many large pharmas, Merck does not publicly disclose the number of programs in the discovery phase or phase 1 trials, but it would be reasonable to expect that programs in each of these categories would far exceed the total number of phase 2 programs.

Table 7.1 Merck's 2019 sales by top pharma products and sales of animal health products (Merck 2019)

Category	Product or subcategory	2019 Sales (in millions)
Total		$46,840
Pharmaceutical		$41,751
	Keytruda®	$11,084
	Januvia®/Janumet®	$5524
	Gardasil®/Gardasil 9®	$3737
	ProQuad/M-M-R II/ Varivax®	$2275
	Bridion®	$1131
	Isentress®/Isentress HD®	$975
	Pneumovax 23®	$926
	NuvaRing®	$879
	Zetia®/Vytorin®	$874
	Simponi®	$830
Animal health		$4393
	Livestock	$2784
	Companion animals	$1609
Other revenues		$696

All large pharmas tout their scientific prowess and commitment to patients, but as corporate entities, they are all ultimately judged on their financial performance and indeed define their own success based on their yearly top line and bottom line. In 2019, Merck generated sales of $46.8B which represented an 11% increase over that of 2018. Sales within the United States accounted for 43% ($20.3B) of this total, while the remaining 57% of sales came from outside the United States. At $11.1B Keytruda® accounted for nearly 24% of Merck's total sales (Table 7.1), and this represented a 55% increase over its sales in 2018. Januvia®/Janumet® (sitagliptin), a drug for type 2 diabetes, recorded $5.5B in sales, but this represented a 7% decline compared with that of 2018. Finally, vaccines led by Gardasil®, a vaccine against human papillomavirus ($3.7B in sales), accounted for a total of $6.8B or 14.5% of Merck's total sales.

Merck's major outlays in 2019 came from the costs of sales and general and administrative expenses which totaled $24.7B. As noted above Merck spent $9.9B in R&D that same year or

21% of their total sales. Across the industry, most large pharmas have R&D spends that equate to 15–22% of their annual sales. This range has been invariant over time, and it is extremely rare for a pharma to have R&D spending above 25% of annual sales. It is a common refrain from large pharma that high R&D costs are the primary reason for the high cost of drugs. However, as is seen for Merck, and every other major large pharma, R&D expenses typically account for only one-fifth of total sales revenues every year. Merck reported an income of $11.5B in 2019 for which it paid taxes of $1.7B for an effective corporate tax rate of 14.7%. For reference, a married couple in the United States filing jointly in 2019 would need to have an annual income of $113,466 to qualify for an effective federal tax rate as low as 14.7%. Any income above this amount for this couple would result in a higher effective tax rate than what Merck paid for earning nearly $47B. This seems rather inequitable for the average American taxpayer.

7.2 The New: Biotech

The 1980s and 1990s saw dramatic advances in molecular biology, genomics, and genetic engineering. These innovations sparked the advent of synthetic protein-based therapeutics, exemplified by insulin, interferons, interleukins, and hematopoietic growth factors, that ushered in the era of biotechnology to complement small molecule (chemical) drugs in the therapeutic armamentarium. Moreover, these "large molecule drugs" which were developed by small biotechs, such as Genentech and Amgen, served as a bellwether that large pharma's monopoly on the creation of medicines was over. Indeed, the early scientific and financial successes of California-based Genentech and Amgen paved the way for the eventual formation of thousands of biotech start-ups funded by venture capital (VC) hungry to replicate this success. The early history of these two shining stars is illustrative of the growth of the biotech sector as a whole.

In the early 1970s, Herbert Boyer at the University of California San Francisco successfully spliced genes in his laboratory using newly discovered restriction endonucleases. Confident that genetic recombination had significant commercial potential, Robert Swanson from the VC firm Kleiner Perkins convinced Boyer in 1976 to start a company that Boyer named Genentech, an amalgam of the words "genetic engineering technology." Boyer and Swanson each invested $500 to start Genentech. Within a year, they produced the human peptide, somatostatin. By 1978, Genentech successfully synthesized human insulin using the same laboratory techniques and entered into a critical R&D collaboration with Eli Lilly to develop human insulin as a replacement for porcine insulin which was extracted from pigs (Pisano 2006). This resulted in the FDA approval of Humulin®, the first genetically engineered therapeutic, in 1982. Over the next nearly 30 years, Genentech successfully developed and commercialized a host of protein therapeutics including human growth hormone (Protropin®), recombinant DNase (Pulmozyme®) for cystic fibrosis, anti-CD20 monoclonal antibody (Rituxan®) for lymphoma, anti-Her2 monoclonal antibody (Herceptin®) for breast cancer, anti-IgE monoclonal antibody (Xolair®) for asthma, and the anti-VEGF monoclonal antibody (Avastin®) for several cancers.

Genentech also broke ground by being the first biotech to transition into a public company. It raised $35 million ($35M), equivalent to $110M in 2020, in its initial public offering (IPO) in 1980 that was underwritten by the investment bank Hambrecht & Quist. Moreover, Genentech's stock price jumped from $35 to $88 in only its first hour of public trading. Genentech's subsequent track record of R&D, regulatory approvals, and commercial success along with its culture of scientific excellence made it an attractive target for pharmaceutical companies. Hoffmann-La Roche which had been collaborating with Genentech on several projects bought a controlling interest (56%) of Genentech for $2.1B in 1990. In 2009, Roche completed its acquisition, some would say "ingestion," of Genentech by buying its remaining outstanding shares for approximately $46.8B, a far cry from the initial $1000 start-up investment by Boyer and Swanson in 1976.

Amgen is another archetype of a successful biotech. It was founded a few years after Genentech in 1980 with several million dollars of VC funding and originally called Applied Molecular Genetics. Its name was shortened to Amgen in 1983 when it raised $40M (equivalent to $104M in 2020) in its IPO that year. In its early days, Amgen, like Genentech, focused on exploiting recombinant DNA technology which it applied to cloning the human erythropoietin gene. By doing so, they created their first drug Epogen® which was approved by FDA in 1989 to treat anemia associated with chronic renal failure. Amgen received its second FDA approval in 1991 for Neupogen® (filgrastim) to prevent chemotherapy-related infections.

By 2019 Amgen recorded sales of $23.4B with eight products generating the bulk of this revenue. Enbrel® (etanercept), an anti-TNF fusion protein approved to treat arthritis and other inflammatory diseases, was Amgen's biggest seller with sales of $5.2B or 30% of Amgen's annual revenue. Neulasta®, the successor to Neupogen®, was second in sales with $3.2B or 19% of total revenue. Unlike Genentech, Amgen today remains an independent corporate entity. Reflective of its financial success, $1000 invested in Amgen at the time of its IPO would have grown to be $780,692 as of April 2020 even without having reinvested dividends. This represents a consistent annual return on investment of nearly 20% over 37 years.

The founding and early success of Genentech and Amgen stimulated the creation of many other biotech start-ups. San Francisco, San Diego, and Boston served as their most common birthplaces as opposed to Philadelphia, New York, New Jersey, and the Midwest which served as the headquarters for most pharmas in the United States. The growth of biotech was made possible only through the financial investment from VC firms and investment banks which saw the opportunity for massive returns resulting from the successful development of promising new medicines. Although there were bumps in the road, e.g., the financial crisis of 2008, the marriage of VC with biotech entrepreneurs ultimately proved to be extremely financially rewarding to both and to biotech investors as a whole. From the beginning of 2009 to the end of 2020, the NASDAQ Biotechnology Index rose 6.67-fold which is nearly 60% higher than the benchmark S&P 500 Index which increased by 4.22-fold over the same period.

Fueled by investment banks that underwrote IPOs and public market investors who did not want to miss out, biotechs claiming to be the "next Genentech" positioned themselves to leverage science and their "secret sauce" to create the next big medicines. Those that eventually succeeded such as Biogen, Chiron, Genetics Institute, Genzyme, and Gilead experienced meteoric growth to become vertically integrated companies with sales and marketing capabilities just like Genentech. For some their scientific and financial success made them attractive takeover targets, e.g., Novartis's acquisition of Chiron, Sanofi's purchase of Genzyme, and Wyeth's acquisition of Genetics Institute. Others, like Biogen and Gilead, remain independent companies even today. But the high likelihood of failure inherent to drug discovery and development more commonly translates into the collapse of most biotech start-ups usually within their first few years.

However, it is precisely this high-risk, high-reward feature of biotech investment that makes it so attractive to VC firms like Kleiner Perkins, New Enterprise Associates, OrbiMed Advisors, Third Rock Ventures, and many others that excel at playing the investment game for the benefit of themselves and their investors. VC firms offset the high risk of failure for biotech start-ups with the expectation that the small fraction (10–15%) of companies that ultimately succeed will provide a 10–50-fold return on their initial investment. For example, to offset the cost of the many failures that it funds, a VC that invests $50M in a start-up biotech through several rounds of private financing before the biotech's IPO 3–5 years later will look to recoup $500M or more through the IPO and future growth in the company's market valuation when its stock becomes traded on the public markets.

The growth of the biopharmaceutical industry is fueled by interdependencies and interactions between large pharma, biotech, VC, investment bankers, and Wall Street analysts. There is no greater evidence of this than at the annual JP Morgan Healthcare Conference held every January in San Francisco. For those in the industry, this convocation's invitation-only participation makes a pilgrimage to "JPM," as it is commonly called, the essential place to go, be seen, and make business deals. Absence from JPM is viewed as a negative sign that you and your organization are irrelevant players in biopharma. JPM had humble beginnings when in the early 1980s Hambrecht & Quist along with a few other investment banks saw great profitability in raising capital for biotechnology. In 1983, to highlight new technologies, showcase companies, and stimulate further investment in biotechs such as Genentech, Hambrecht & Quist (later acquired by Chase Manhattan Bank, a predecessor of JP Morgan) held its first conference which lasted just half a day in San Francisco. JPM has since grown into a 20,000 attendee behemoth that spans nearly an entire week. The conference consumes virtually all hotels in downtown San Francisco and results in even substandard hotel room rates rising to over $1000 per night. Even companies that are not invited to present at JPM feel the need to be in town to have an endless series of 30-minute "speed-dating" meetings with a seemingly endless list of investors and analysts that stretch from early morning to late evening every day.

7.2.1 Biotech Financing: From Birth to Adulthood

From a financial perspective, a typical start-up biotech comes into being when a VC buys into its concept and leads a "consortium" of other VCs to assemble an initial investment of $20–$50M, termed a Series A financing. This allows the biotech to hire people, buy equipment, rent labs and/or offices, and begin R&D work. Over the next several years, this invested sum is spent by the biotech necessitating subsequent rounds (Series B, C, etc.) of private financing that not only involves the original consortium but also includes an expanded set of newer investors who see opportunity in the interim R&D progress demonstrated. Since transforming a scientific concept into an investigational therapeutic becomes more expensive with every progressive step, these subsequent financing rounds generally raise progressively larger sums of money such that the aggregate amount invested in the biotech can easily reach well over $200M.

At a certain point, if the biotech makes sufficient R&D progress and the external stock market conditions are favorable, the company can "go public," as Genentech did in 1980, in an IPO. The timing of an IPO varies according to the company. For biotechs developing therapeutics, an IPO is frequently timed to coincide with its lead molecule entering a first-in-human clinical trial or demonstrating a clear path to enter the clinic in the near future. Going public achieves several financial objectives for all parties involved. It allows the VCs to cash in on their investment(s) and make an "exit." Despite the public pronouncements from VC that their biotech investments are made to drive innovation for the greater healthcare good of society, the overriding objective of VC firms is to generate a large return on investment for their investors and themselves so they can repeat the cycle with the next set of start-ups. This has proven to be a very lucrative positive feedback loop for VC firms. A successful IPO also delivers large fees, ranging from $10–$20M per IPO, for investment banks, like JP Morgan and Cowen, who underwrite the public offering. Going public provides the biotech access to capital from the public markets which can provide much larger sums of invested capital to fund clinical trials that are much more expensive to conduct than laboratory-based research. Finally, for investors in the public markets that can include mutual funds and institutional and individual investors, an IPO opens up the opportunity to invest in the biotech.

However, transitioning from a private to a public company comes at a significant cost, both literally and metaphorically, to every biotech. The company now spends a smaller fraction of its precious funds on R&D as it must hire more finance and administrative staff to handle the legal and financial reporting obligations, e.g., Security and Exchange Commission requirements, that come with being traded on a stock exchange. Being public also imposes a veil of confidentiality over the company and its employees. Experimental data and results, especially those involving clinical trials, that previously were discussed freely among staff are now restricted to those on a need-to-know basis because it is considered "material information." If inadvertently leaked to public investors which can now include anyone outside the company, it could affect the stock price. Perhaps, the greatest cost for a biotech's going public is that it brings daily scrutiny from the external world over the goings-on within the company. Public perception can be immediately reflected in the rise and fall of the biotech's stock price. Experimental setbacks that were once simply accepted and dealt with as an R&D obstacle to be overcome now become potentially material information that must be reviewed by lawyers, described in a carefully massaged press release as part of a "communication plan," and discussed ad nauseam with nervous investors and financial analysts who demand to understand why the stock price is dropping and what the company will do about it… today.

As a result, a public biotech is forced to focus increasingly on short-term goals and milestones that are reported in its quarterly SEC filings and "earnings calls." The former is a regulatory requirement, but the latter is not. This results in perhaps one of the more inane oddities for biotechs post-IPO. Pharma companies, like Merck and GlaxoSmithKline (GSK), use quarterly earnings calls with investors and industry analysts to actually report on their top-line sales and earnings to guide future financial expectations. However, biotechs that may be years away from having their first product on the market have no profit or even earnings to report. Rather they only generate quarter after quarter of losses through their R&D expenditures. Nevertheless, it remains commonplace for biotechs to host these "quarterly earnings calls" that in the absence of any earnings to speak of usually devolve into shadow puppetry theater of analysts and investors asking about the company's R&D progress and the biotech's management dodging these questions that they cannot or will not answer.

One consequence of this focus on near-term milestones and financials is the prioritization of clinical trials over laboratory research when the two activities compete for a limited R&D budget. Biotechs generally are 100% focused on laboratory research in their early years while they aim to bring forth a molecule into clinical trials. The initiation of phase 1 studies and the transition of the biotech into a clinical-stage company are defining milestones that bring pride and joy to the biotech's employees and financial returns to its investors. However, this landmark event is frequently the beginning of the end for the laboratory research that carried the company to this same milestone.

The conduct of clinical trials is exceptionally expensive, and their costs increase every year. A single phase 1 trial in cancer typically costs $5–$15M, and a phase 2 trial can total up to $50M. These R&D expenditures easily overshadow, figuratively and fiscally, that of the laboratory research that will bring forth the next molecule from the preclinical pipeline. The biotech's investors and analysts tend to be singularly focused on the progress of the molecule(s) in clinical trials rather than on earlier discovery programs since the former will generate data necessary for an eventual FDA submission. Thus, the clinical programs of a biotech become the greatest near-term value drivers of its stock price. As such, it is common for biotechs to make resourcing and budgetary trade-offs by constricting laboratory research when their first molecule(s) enters clinical trials. In more extreme cases, a biotech may completely cease further discovery work on new or next-generation molecules in order to focus entirely on advancing their clinical portfolio. This is particularly unfortunate when the clinical-stage molecules have clear liabilities that could be solved with follow-on compounds that are a few years behind in the laboratory. This reduction or termination of discovery research means that the laboratory scientists whose hard work created the molecules behind the biotech's success in its early years are less valued or no longer needed.

Thus, the start-up biotech that began with the promise of a portfolio of molecules that leverage its technological "secret sauce" frequently transforms itself into a one or two molecule clinical development company that bets its future on one molecule achieving FDA approval and hitting the market. Sometimes, that bet pays off handsomely for the biotech and its investors. More often than not, a highly anticipated pivotal trial fails, and there are either no other molecules left in the cupboard or not enough money in the bank, or both, to rescue the biotech facing its first major clinical failure. As a result, the landscape is dotted with shuttered biotechs that faced withering punishment to their stock price from disappointed and skeptical investors.

Recognizing that the expense of clinical trials to bring a molecule to the market is substantial, the time required is long, and the probability of failure remains high, some biotechs are content to advance their portfolio to a certain point, usually in phase 2 or phase 3 clinical trials, at which time they become an attractive acquisition target for large pharma. Earlier selling of a biotech to a pharma will generate a lower return on investment to the biotech's investors compared with when a biotech attempts to go all the way to an FDA-approved New Drug Application (NDA) or Biologics License Application (BLA). However, the risk of seeing the biotech's market value fall to near zero after a late-stage clinical trial failure and walking away with no return on investment is eliminated. The acquiring pharma assumes the risk of future failure but gains ownership of the candidate drug, portfolio, or technology platform at a much lower cost than what it might otherwise have to pay if it waits for clarity from a positive pivotal trial result. A recent example of this is Gilead's $4.9B acquisition in 2020 of Forty Seven, Inc. for the latter's magrolimab, an anti-CD47 monoclonal antibody in clinical development for myelodysplastic syndrome (MDS), acute myeloid leukemia (AML), and diffuse large B-cell lymphoma. Gilead's purchase came after Forty Seven reported interim results from a phase 1B trial of magrolimab and azacitidine wherein overall response rates of 92% and 64% were observed in 24 patients with high-risk MDS and 22 patients with untreated AML, respectively (Sallman et al. 2019).

7.3 The Drive for Pharmaceutical Innovation

It is often cited by the pharmaceutical industry that the cost of discovering a new drug in the laboratory, taking it through clinical trials, and ultimately gaining FDA approval is exorbitant and can run up to several billion dollars. Part of this calculus is based on the high failure rates in both laboratory and clinical trial phases of a new drug's gestation resulting in no financial return for most programs within a company's R&D portfolio. Even for a molecule that survives the preclinical gauntlet to enter into a phase 1 trial, the remaining probability of success for FDA approval of a cancer drug is generally considered to be only 5–10%. Although all of these probability calculations are predicated on assumptions that may be reasonably questioned, drug discovery and clinical development are nevertheless expensive and high-risk propositions that are beyond the fiscal scope of an individual or most companies in other fields of business.

The drive for ever-increasing revenues in the setting of the high cost and low success rates of pharmaceutical R&D has resulted in three phenomena that are diametrically opposed to enhancing R&D investment of new therapeutics for pediatric cancers. First, to offset financial expense and risk, large pharmas and arguably many, if not most, biotechs have evolved to focus their attention on "blockbuster drugs" that are generally defined as those that generate annual sales revenues of $1B or more. This strategy drives pharmas to work on drugs for diseases of higher prevalence in the population and for which treatment is chronic or at least longer term. Childhood cancers are thankfully quite uncommon such that even the predominant pediatric solid tumors and leukemias have annual incidences in the United States of a few hundred to two thousand. Besides, treatment for these diseases ranges from several months to 2 years rather than a lifetime. Thus, childhood cancers do not and will never meet the blockbuster criteria that large pharma seeks. It should be emphasized that a commercial sales forecast is just as important for project progression as a scientific assessment when pharmas evaluate early-stage R&D projects and decide where to place their bets. One might argue that higher drug pricing may offset lower patient numbers to generate the desired financial return. Indeed, Cerezyme®, an enzyme replacement therapy for patients with Gaucher's disease, is frequently cited as an example whereby high pricing compensates for an extremely low disease incidence. However, it must be remembered that drugs like Cerezyme® are administered for the lifetime of a patient in contradistinction to that of the treatments given to children with cancer. Even so, one may reasonably question whether pricing that amounts to $200,000 or more per year represents a sustainable solution to rising societal healthcare costs in the United States and developed world, to say nothing of the developing world.

The second consequence of the drive for pharmas to lower R&D costs and risk is to merge with or acquire other pharmas. Since 1999, over 45 mergers or acquisitions (M&A) with a value of over $10B have been consummated by large pharma resulting in companies of ever-increasing size. Take GSK as an example. Like Merck, GSK had its origins as an apothecary shop in London in 1715. This pharmacy was eventually acquired by Glaxo Labs which was established in 1935 in England. Burroughs Wellcome was started in 1880 in London. Glaxo merged with Wellcome in 1995 to form GlaxoWellcome. Across the Atlantic, Smith, Kline & French (SKF) Company, itself a product of an acquisition, was formed in 1871 in Philadelphia. SKF merged with Beecham Group to form SmithKline Beecham in 1989. GlaxoWellcome merged with SmithKline Beecham in 2000 to form GSK, a global giant of over 100,000 employees. Likewise, the Pfizer of today was founded in New York in 1849 but over its life has acquired either directly or indirectly Wyeth, Ayerst, Warner-Lambert, Parke-Davis, Pharmacia, and Upjohn pharmaceutical companies.

The rationale for M&A in the pharmaceutical industry is the same as that for corporate mergers in other industries. The annual sales of the combined entity will be much greater than either of the pre-M&A companies. Indeed, the annual revenues in 2019 for the top ten pharmas ranged from $23B to $52B (Table 7.2). Conversely, the number of employees, whether they be in R&D, sales/marketing, or administrative functions, needed to sustain the combined organization is expected to be fewer than the sum total of both at least according to the bean counters and MBAs who drive these corporate shotgun marriages. These "efficiencies" or "synergies" touted when a pharma M&A occurs typically mean early retirements or layoffs for at least some of the employees when the dust settles from the corporate fusion.

The third reaction to the challenge of bringing innovative medicines to the market in light of large pharma's desire to control R&D costs is the increasingly frequent practice of in-licensing or acquiring molecules discovered in biotech companies. Frequently, large pharma focuses on buying molecules that have met criteria demonstrating clinical proof of concept (PoC) usually comprised of positive phase 2A clinical data. The rationale for this is that it is preferable from a financial and risk management perspective to buy someone else's "de-risked" molecule than to invest money and people resources in one's own laboratory discovery efforts with no guarantees that expected innovative molecules will emanate years in the future. Pharmas are quite willing to

Table 7.2 Largest pharmaceutical companies (by revenue as of December 2020) (Anderson 2020)

Rank	Company	Annual revenue (in billions)
1	Pfizer	$51.9
2	Roche	$50.0
3	Novartis	$47.5
4	Merck & Co.	$46.8
5	GlaxoSmithKline	$43.5
6	Johnson & Johnson	$42.1
7	AbbVie	$33.3
8	Sanofi	$27.8
9	Bristol Myers Squibb	$26.2
10	AstraZeneca	$23.6

pay even a premium price for these clinical-stage molecules because they have presumptively already met the considerable hurdles of laboratory and animal studies and that of initial clinical safety, pharmacokinetic, and early efficacy data from phase 1 trials that can cause termination of numerous other molecules along the way. In essence, pharmas are willing to pay more for these molecules because the risk of failure to this point has been borne by the biotech and the attrition of other unsuccessful molecules has already occurred.

Large pharmas' acquisitions of promising molecules from biotech through a variety of means have differing financial and corporate implications on biotech. The least intrusive is when a pharma in-licenses the molecule or, in other words, buys the molecule with all of its patent rights and assumes all further responsibilities to develop and market the molecule. This maneuver leaves the biotech independent and intact with the other molecules in its portfolio. The biotech generally receives (1) an upfront licensing fee upon transfer of rights to the pharma; (2) future milestone payments when the molecule reaches certain prespecified events, such as the start of a phase 3 trial or the filing of an NDA or BLA with the FDA; and (3) royalties as a percentage of future sales achieved by the pharma.

As an example of this theme, Novartis in early 2021 licensed BeiGene's tislelizumab, an anti-PD-1 monoclonal antibody approved in China in 2019, after the clinical failure of Novartis's own immune checkpoint inhibitor spartalizumab in a phase 3 trial in melanoma. Novartis obtained the commercial rights to tislelizumab in major markets outside China, including the United States, Europe, and Japan, in return for an upfront payment of $650M and up to $1.55B in future milestones to BeiGene. While the upfront licensing payment was sizable for most industries other than biopharma, it was relatively modest for an approved biological drug for cancer. Likely this resulted because the landscape of FDA-approved immunomodulatory agents was already dotted with established monoclonal antibodies such as ipilimumab (2011), nivolumab (2014), pembrolizumab (2014), atezolizumab (2016), avelumab (2017), durvalumab (2017), and cemiplimab (2018). Thus, the commercial potential of tislelizumab in Novartis's hands was limited.

A second mechanism is a collaboration in which the pharma and biotech agree to work together to develop the molecule through late-stage trials and registration. Upon regulatory approval, the sales and marketing of the new drug will be shared between the two partners. A common way to divide the future revenues is to split the geographic rights for sales and marketing. For example, the biotech retains commercial responsibilities and revenues in the United States while the global pharma gains that for Europe and the rest of the world. This type of business arrangement is preferred by biotechs that wish to transform themselves from a pure R&D organization to a vertically integrated mini-pharma with both R&D and sales and marketing capabilities. The advantage of this strategy, and one taken by Amgen and Genentech, is that the biotech maintains control over its future sales revenues which can be much larger than a percentage royalty of the pharma's sales in the first example. Another advantage to the biotech is that it retains its corporate independence while receiving an infusion of cash or resource investment and assistance from the pharma to complete late phase clinical trials that can be large, lengthy, and expensive.

A recent example of this type of R&D arrangement is AstraZeneca's 2020 collaboration with Accent Therapeutics on the latter's discovery-stage molecules targeting RNA-modifying proteins for the treatment of cancer. Under the terms of their agreement, Accent is responsible for R&D activities for a predetermined preclinical program through to the end of phase 1 clinical trials. AstraZeneca will then lead development and commercialization activities from phase 2 onward with Accent retaining an option to jointly develop and commercialize the molecule with AstraZeneca in the United States. AstraZeneca will also have the exclusive option to license worldwide rights to two additional programs that will be prosecuted by Accent through the preclinical stage. In return Accent received an upfront payment of $55M and can receive up to $1.1B in additional success-based payments across all three programs in the form of option fees and milestone payments, as well as royalties on future sales.

The final mechanism is acquisition or the outright purchase of the biotech by the pharma which by definition transfers the rights for the biotech's entire portfolio of molecules to the pharma. This swallowing whole of the biotech also results in the transfer of all the biotech's physical assets (labs, equipment, buildings), people, and remaining cash to the pharma. Although there are instances when the biotech's staff are retained by the pharma, more often than not many if not most of the biotech's employees move onto other companies, whether by their own choice or their new employer's. The driver for most biotech acquisitions is its assets (molecules and intellectual property) rather than its people. A relevant example to the contrary is Eli Lilly's $8.0B acquisition of Loxo Oncology in 2019 for the latter's Vitrakvi® (larotrectinib), a TRK inhibitor that had recently received FDA approval for adults and children with solid tumors having a neurotrophic receptor tyrosine kinase gene fusion, along with LOXO-292, a RET kinase inhibitor, and LOXO-305, a BTK inhibitor. In this case, many of Loxo's employees were retained at Lilly including Loxo's CEO, Josh Bilenker, who later assumed leadership of Lilly's oncology R&D franchise.

There are countless variations of pharma/biotech in-licenses, collaborations, and acquisitions that are beyond the scope of this high-level overview. The aforementioned examples are representative but not meant to be comprehensive for all of the different business arrangements that can be made when pharma and biotech work together to create and develop innovative new medicines.

An acquisition of a company or in-license of several investigational molecules from a biotech's portfolio may yield unexpected value from molecules that were not perceived originally as the value driver. In 2009, Bristol Myers Squibb (BMS) acquired Medarex for $2.1B. In its press release announcing the purchase, BMS touted that it was gaining full ownership and rights to ipilimumab, an anti-CTLA-4 monoclonal antibody in phase 3 trials at the time, rights to ten additional clinical-stage antibodies, and Medarex's fully human antibody technology platform. At the time, the most prized asset of this transaction was ipilimumab which became the first immune checkpoint inhibitor approved for cancer treatment. However, by 2019, Yervoy® (ipilimumab) generated sales of $1.5B for BMS, while Opdivo® (nivolumab), an anti-PD-1 monoclonal that turned out to be one of the hidden gems in the ten other Medarex antibodies that BMS acquired in 2009, generated sales of $8.1B. The Medarex acquisition proved to be highly valuable for BMS not only financially but by paving the way for its becoming a leading pharma in the area of immuno-oncology with nivolumab ultimately becoming the unanticipated jewel of this acquisition.

One consequence of pharma's strategy of sourcing candidate molecules from biotech is that the size and scope of large pharma R&D groups have been steadily reduced over the past two decades as large pharmas have increasingly turned to biotech to discover the molecules in their pipelines. The initial layoffs or "reductions in force" in R&D generally involved the biologists, chemists, and pharmacologists within large pharma laboratory discovery groups charged with identifying and characterizing molecules that would be brought to a first-in-human clinical trial. Then large pharma clinical pharmacology groups that conducted phase 1 studies in healthy volunteers were downsized or eliminated along with the hospital-based clinical pharmacology units that many pharmas owned and operated in the past. For example, GSK in 2002 had three clinical pharmacology units (Philadelphia, PA; Cambridge, UK; Sydney, Australia) that performed healthy volunteer phase 1 studies on the company's portfolio. By 2020, only the Addenbrooke's Hospital site in Cambridge remained operative as the others were closed or sold to contract research organizations (CROs). Finally, clinical scientists, in particular those responsible for the planning and conduct of early phase clinical trials in patients, were made redundant as pharmas increasingly relied on biotechs to generate early clinical trials data for them.

7.4 Current Trends in Pharmaceutical R&D

Although successful R&D has powered scientific innovation and financial success in the pharmaceutical industry for decades, there has been increasing concern about declining R&D productivity since the late 1990s. This is so despite consistent rising annual investment. For example, R&D spending by the pharmaceutical industry totaled $186B globally in 2019 compared with $136B in 2012 (Mikulic 2020). As evidenced above with Merck, it is common for a large pharma to spend several billion dollars each year on R&D. Moreover, R&D productivity as reflected by the simple (but simplistically flawed) ratio of total R&D annual expenses of a pharma divided by its number of new molecular entities (NMEs) approved has resulted in a steady increase of this already shockingly high benchmark. For example, in the 1990s this calculated metric was generally accepted as $1B per NME, but more recent analyses have determined this to be as much as $5B per NME for large pharmas (Harper 2013). Beyond expenditures, R&D productivity loss can also be reflected in employees and time. A typical large pharma company may employ tens of thousands of scientists and support staff at multiple research campuses around the world. The road to getting a new drug approved from the time of its first discovery in the lab is inordinately long, averaging 14 years (Paul et al. 2010) compared to product development cycles as short as a few months in other industries such as high tech and software.

Finally, "attrition" or the sequential reduction in the size of a pharma's R&D portfolio resulting from project failures due to insufficient efficacy, unacceptable toxicity, technical challenges of manufacture, or changes in the competitive landscape is an inescapable consequence of the high-risk nature of pharmaceutical R&D. In an analysis of 4451 drugs from 835 companies in clinical development from 2003 to 2011, the aggregate probability of successfully turning a phase 1 molecule into an approved drug is only 10.4% (Hay et al. 2014). All of these factors have contributed to the leadership and investors of large pharmas questioning the traditional model of pharmaceutical R&D in which a large pharma is staffed with a stable of the best scientists, performs cutting-edge R&D inside the company, generates its own intellectual property (IP), and successfully drives regulatory approval of innovative first-to-market or best-in-class medicines.

In response, large pharmas have faced the challenge of declining R&D productivity by reducing their internal R&D budgets and staffing while seeking creative methods of conducting R&D. These may be categorized into three primary strategies: "open innovation"; restructuring to create smaller entrepreneurial R&D units; and virtualization/outsourcing.

7.4.1 Open Innovation

Led by Chief Scientific Officer Paul Stoffels (Mullard 2013), Janssen, the pharmaceutical arm of Johnson & Johnson, has pushed the concept of "open innovation" since the mid-2000s with a variety of R&D initiatives designed to grow Janssen's commercial product lines (Wang 2009). Janssen studiously avoids the "not-invented-here" syndrome that resides in many pharma R&D organizations. Its historically poor productivity from its internal drug discovery apparatus (excepting for its Centocor unit) may be one reason for Janssen's embrace of open innovation. Over the past two decades, Janssen's oncology unit has been arguably more successful than its peers at in-licensing or partnering molecules discovered by much smaller biotechs. For example, its 2020 commercial product line for oncology includes treatments for myeloma (Darzalex® [daratumumab], Velcade® [bortezomib]), prostate cancer (Zytiga® [abiraterone], Erleada® [apalutamide]), lymphoma/leukemia (Imbruvica® [ibrutinib]), ovarian cancer (Doxil® [liposomal doxorubicin]), sarcoma (Yondelis® [trabectedin]), Castleman's disease (Sylvant® [siltuximab]), and bladder cancer (Balversa® [erdafitinib]). Of note, all of these except for Sylvant® and Balversa® are molecules discovered by biotech companies who partnered with or were bought outright by Janssen. Nevertheless, Janssen maintains large research campuses replete with scientists and labs in the United

States, the United Kingdom, Belgium, the Netherlands, France, Spain, and Switzerland.

Janssen has also aggressively advanced the concept of "innovation centers" as globally located life science hubs situated to capture externally derived ideas and technology that can eventually become Janssen products of the future (Robaczewska et al. 2019). Located in San Francisco, Boston, London, and Shanghai, these centers provide laboratory and office space to entrepreneurial scientists to nurture collaborations between them and co-located Janssen scientific and business staff who can follow their technology as it develops and be ready to execute licensing or partnership deals to advance these programs for the benefit of both parties.

7.4.2 Small Entrepreneurial Units

GlaxoSmithKline took the approach of restructuring its R&D organization into smaller units to emulate the entrepreneurial risk-taking, autonomy, and ownership spirit characteristic of smaller biotechs, but absent from large pharma. In 2001, then Chairman of R&D Tachi Yamada decentralized GSK's R&D organization to create six "Centres of Excellence for Drug Discovery" (CEDDs) (Huckman and Strick 2005). These CEDDs were charged with discovering new drug candidates within targeted therapeutic areas and taking their molecules through phase 2 "proof-of-concept" (PoC) clinical trials. CEDDs, comprised of medicinal chemists, biologists, pharmacologists, toxicologists, and physicians, could number no more than 350 to operate nimbly and autonomously from that of the rest of GSK R&D. Their limited size and multidisciplinary integration were designed to remove the bureaucratic layers and processes that frequently strangle scientific innovation in the traditional centralized "command and control" R&D units typical of large pharmas (Naik 2003).

Yamada's rationale was that the critical bottleneck to pharma R&D productivity was the scarcity of molecules that successfully demonstrate clinical PoC and advance to large phase 3 registrational trials. By freeing up the scientists and physicians who conduct discovery and early clinical development (phase 1 and phase 2A trials), GSK hoped to see a dramatic increase in molecules that advance to late development. In hindsight, the CEDD experiment was a mixed success. Led initially by Allen Oliff (Whalen 2006), GSK's Oncology CEDD in just 5 years generated several molecules that achieved PoC and were eventually approved by FDA and European regulators. These included the erbB2 kinase inhibitor Tykerb® (lapatinib), VEGF receptor kinase inhibitor Votrient® (pazopanib), thrombopoietin receptor agonist Promacta® (eltrombopag), B-Raf kinase inhibitor Tafinlar® (dabrafenib), MEK inhibitor Mekinist® (trametinib), and the prolyl hydroxylase inhibitor Duvroq® (daprodustat). Together these products account for nearly $4B in sales revenues in 2020 (Novartis 2020).

However, many of GSK's other CEDDs did not come close to achieving this same degree of success as judged by the number and quality of clinical PoCs. In hindsight, there were several reasons for the variable output between different CEDDs. For example, the psychiatry and cardiovascular CEDDs were working in areas where scientific advances at that time did not reliably translate into successful drug discovery programs—not just at GSK but throughout the industry. Another differentiating factor was the degree to which the heads of each CEDD manifest the triumvirate leadership requisites of scientific insight, experimental creativity, and out-of-the-box thinking that proved to be the critical determinants of success.

In a further effort to mimic start-up biotechs, GSK R&D under Patrick Vallance extended the "smaller-is-better" approach in 2008 and replaced the CEDDs with Discovery Performance Units (DPU) (Vallance 2010). These much smaller groups of only 50–60 scientists still covered the same disciplines—biology, chemistry, and clinical research—as the CEDDs but were even more narrowly focused. For example, instead of being responsible for an entire therapeutic area, e.g., oncology, a DPU worked solely in one area of disease biology, e.g., cancer epigenetics. In retrospect, this experiment was a dismal failure, and GSK's oncology R&D productivity declined dramatically over the next several years. The inherent advantages of vast scientific and technological resources that large pharmas can bring to bear on novel drug discovery were partitioned into too many small and ineffectual groups with each competing against the others for the same pot of resources rather than working collaboratively. Moreover, the breadth of a typical large pharma therapeutic area portfolio consisting of 10–20 programs running simultaneously allows for projects deserving to be abandoned to be terminated thus freeing people and budget to be redeployed onto other projects that are progressing more favorably. The DPUs were so small that they could run only a few projects at a time such that to give up on any single project could result in the dissolution of the DPU and unemployment for its members (Torsoli 2011). Lastly, the DPUs did not and could not incentivize GSK researchers with the same opportunity for substantial individual wealth creation through equity that scientists in real biotechs can experience through an IPO or bringing a drug to market. Thus, GSK R&D could not be transformed into a biotech simply by replicating the staffing and portfolio size of a start-up. The DPU experiment ended in 2017 when GSK disbanded the DPUs, significantly trimmed its R&D portfolio by 30 programs, and restructured itself back to a more typical R&D organization (Pagliarulo 2017).

7.4.3 Virtualization and Outsourcing

Another major evolution in how pharma and biotech conduct discovery and development to create innovative new medicines while reducing R&D expenditures is to outsource R&D activities that were previously performed within their own walls (Schuhmacher et al. 2016). This strategy results in lower fixed costs to the pharma or biotech in the form of fewer R&D employees, lower capital investment on R&D, and fewer, smaller, or even no research campuses. Pharmas began the trend of outsourcing their synthetic chemistry activities to specialty chemistry companies in the 1990s as a way to expand their capacity for discovery research without having to hire additional staff and open new laboratories. Synthetic chemistry was considered to be straightforward to do and required less scientific creativity than medicinal chemistry which remained a prized discipline within pharma and was retained as an in-house function. When that proved to be successful, pharmas began experimenting with outsourcing medicinal chemistry in the early 2000s mostly as a means of expanding their throughput but now with the added goal of reducing R&D costs. Whereas a team of 15–20 medicinal chemists might have worked on a single discovery program in the past, it was now run instead by 2 or 3 internal chemists directing a team of medicinal chemists at one or more chemistry CROs. It proved far more cost-effective to hire a contingent of medicinal chemists at a CRO, especially when that CRO was located in a lower-cost country such as China or India, to do what was previously conducted solely by a pharma's own chemists. This industry-wide practice led to a proliferation of CROs such as Charles River Laboratories, WuXi AppTec, Evotec, Covance, and countless others that can perform virtually any R&D activity needed by pharmas and biotechs. These R&D activities range from chemistry to biology to animal toxicology to biopharmaceutical processing to clinical trials support to biostatistics and data management to regulatory affairs. The list is endless.

The outsourcing of a myriad of pharma R&D functions continues to grow in large part because outsourcing expenditures do not entail long-term budgetary commitments and can be flexed from year to year unlike R&D spends for internal headcount and research campuses which are generally fixed over time. Pressured by its investors, large pharmas have been willing to reduce their R&D headcount and physical footprint to improve the bottom line while maintaining or even increasing total R&D spends through outsourcing. For example, in 2005 GSK's R&D organization consisted of 14,963 employees which represented 15% of its total global workforce (GlaxoSmithKline 2005). By 2017, GSK's R&D staffing was reduced to 11,576 or 11.6% of its total workforce (GlaxoSmithKline 2017). By contrast, GSK's R&D spending during this period was relatively stable at \$5.71B (£3.13B) in 2005 compared with \$5.77B (£4.47B) in 2017.

Eli Lilly took a very innovative and radical approach to outsourcing when it virtualized an entire segment of its development portfolio. In 2002, it created the Chorus unit, a small, operationally independent clinical development organization that was separate from the rest of its sizable R&D organization (Owens et al. 2015). Chorus focused strictly on advancing molecules from late preclinical stages (roughly 1 year from entry into phase 1 trials) through clinical proof of concept which was typically a phase 2A trial. Chorus's mission was to achieve proof of concept rapidly and at a low cost using a "quick-win, fail-fast" model. Successful projects from Chorus would then return to the larger Lilly clinical development organization to complete late-stage (phase 2B or 3) clinical trials. At its peak, Chorus was able to sustain a portfolio of 15–17 active projects with approximately 40 full-time staff members who were selected for being experienced drug developers. This small group utilized an extensive network of CROs and other external vendors to design and implement activities in biology, preclinical toxicology, manufacturing, and phase 1 and 2 clinical trials in a diverse range of therapeutic areas including neuroscience, endocrine, inflammatory, oncologic, and cardiovascular diseases. From 2002 through 2012, the Chorus group prosecuted 41 molecules ranging from small molecules, synthetic peptides, engineered proteins, and monoclonal antibodies that originated from Lilly's discovery research. Of 35 molecules that completed clinical development within Chorus, 8 (23%) reached a positive outcome consisting of 5 that demonstrated a positive proof of mechanism and 3 that provided evidence of PoC. Although not an apples-to-apples comparison, the progression of a molecule to a phase 2A decision point by the Chorus approach was estimated on average to be faster and cheaper (28 months, $6.3M/molecule) than a more traditional large pharma approach to arrive at phase 2B decision (48 months, $42M/molecule).

In contrast to large pharma, biotechs, especially start-up or early-stage ones, do not have an option and must outsource its R&D liberally. Absent the armies of scientists and acres of laboratories that reside within large pharma, biotechs must conduct their laboratory and clinical research mostly, if not entirely, through CROs and their drug manufacturing through contract manufacturing organizations (CMOs). The voracious appetite from both large pharmas and biotechs for CROs and CMOs to conduct pharmaceutical R&D has resulted in their global revenues reaching $39B in 2018 with expected growth to $44B in 2021. This insatiable demand for their services is reflected by growth both in the number and organizational size of CROs and CMOs. In the areas of preclinical biology and medicinal chemistry, two of the leading CROs are Charles River Laboratories ($2.6B revenues in 2019, 17,000 employees) and WuXi AppTec ($1.8B revenues in 2019, 21,000 scientists). Catalent ($2.5B revenues in 2019, 15,000 employees) and Lonza ($6.6B revenues in 2019 15,000 employees) represent the largest CMOs in the areas of small molecules and biologicals, respectively.

Due to many clinical trials having substantial logistical complexity, worldwide reach, and requisite adherence to regulatory requirements, CROs that primarily support clinical development can be multinational enterprises with broad therapeutic area capabilities like Covance ($11.5B in 2019 revenues, >75,000 employees) or IQVIA ($11.1B in 2019 revenues, >67,000 employees). Frequently these large CROs are favored by large pharma that must conduct phase 3 clinical trials involving thousands of subjects across many continents. Biotechs, however, frequently prefer to work with mid-sized clinical CROs like Medpace ($861M in 2019 revenues, 2500 employees) or small regional companies like Quotient Sciences (2019: $138M in revenues, 850 employees) that focus on therapeutic areas such as oncology or specialty disciplines like clinical pharmacology and formulation development.

7.5 Implications for Pediatric Cancer Therapeutics

Given that large pharma and biotechs have R&D infrastructures that have a track record for scientific successes, especially in oncology, over several decades and have grown dramatically as an industry, it is reasonable to ask why the discovery and development of novel medicines to treat pediatric cancers have not paralleled that of adult malignancies. A retrospective review of FDA approvals over a prior 20-year period through 2002 revealed a striking paucity of New Drug Application submissions for pediatric cancer indications (Hirschfeld et al. 2003). In fact, of over 100 drugs approved by the FDA at that time for the treatment of cancer, only 15 had any pediatric use information in their labeling with the majority of these drugs having been approved in the 1950s and 1960s. Furthermore, from 1979 to 1997, there were only six NDA or BLA submissions to the FDA for pediatric oncology indications of which just three received regulatory approvals.

The number of new drugs and biologics approved for use in childhood cancers, usually in concert with an approval for an adult malignancy but occasionally without a parallel adult indication, has without question improved since 2005. For example, since 2015, dinutuximab beta was approved for high-risk neuroblastoma, blinatumomab and tisagenlecleucel were approved for both adult and pediatric B-cell precursor acute lymphoblastic leukemia (ALL), and larotrectinib was approved for any adult or pediatric solid tumor having an NTRK gene fusion. However, there remains a substantial disparity in R&D activities and regulatory submissions and approvals from the biopharmaceutical industry when it comes to pediatric vs. adult oncology. There are many systemic reasons for the relative inattention by industry to pediatric cancer therapeutics.

The first and foremost reason is the projected financial return on investment. Both VCs when making their decisions to invest in start-up and early-stage companies and large pharma when determining which programs within its R&D portfolios to continue funding closely evaluate and model the commercial potential for every investigational drug. At its simplest distillation, these decisions are driven by a few key variables. First is the epidemiology, in particular the incidence, of the disease in question since that provides the number of new patients with the disease who may be prescribed the drug. Second is how long a patient will take the drug since the revenue from a drug taken for a few days like an antibiotic is far less than one taken indefinitely for a chronic condition like rheumatoid arthritis. And third is the price that the payors will agree to pay for the new drug. New drug pricing frequently reduces down to "what the market will bear" based on the competitive landscape of other drugs used to treat the disease, the therapeutic advance offered by the new drug, and once again the number of patients involved. All of these factors are quantified and placed into financial models that generate a net present value calculation that represents the profitability of the R&D investment based on what needs to be spent to get the drug to market vs. the future projected revenues of the new drug.

The critical limitation for pediatric cancers is their far lower disease incidence compared to commonly occurring adult cancers. For example, the American Cancer Society estimates that the annual US incidence of osteosarcoma and pediatric AML is only 1000 and 750, respectively. Even pediatric ALL, the most common childhood cancer, has an annual US incidence of only 2400. Compared to lung cancer and breast cancer with their respective US incidences of >235,000 and >281,000, respectively, it becomes obvious why adult cancers have been and remain the focus of VCs and large pharma when it comes to R&D investment decisions. Recall that the high-risk, high-reward strategy of VCs demands a projected 10- to 50-fold return on investment. This further underscores that childhood cancers with relatively small numbers of patients are severely disadvantaged when it comes to VC funding to create a start-up biotech or for a large pharma to invest in a discovery program that is 10 years or more from arriving at the FDA as an NDA or BLA submission.

The competition for R&D investment dollars extends beyond the decision to initiate a pediatric program but persists through the program's life in R&D. For example, Epizyme was advancing tazemetostat, an EZH2 inhibitor, in clinical trials targeting both follicular lymphoma, a common adult cancer, and atypical teratoid rhabdoid tumor (ATRT), a rare pediatric brain tumor. The clinical program reached the point of needing R&D investment to develop an approvable liquid oral formulation since infants and toddlers are diagnosed with ATRT. Upon learning the cost of creating an oral suspension for tazemetostat, Epizyme's chief operating officer not only proposed stopping the formulation work but also all pediatric trials because the return on ATRT paled in comparison to follicular lymphoma, a more lucrative adult indication. When questioned about the ethics of potentially depriving children of a new drug for this rare cancer, he offered to "just give away" the adult-sized tablets after the drug would be approved for lymphoma and leave pharmacists to crush the pills for children's use. While this extreme example is not representative of the ethics within the biopharmaceutical industry as a whole, it does highlight the significant disincentives for long-term investment needed to successfully discover and develop a drug for childhood cancers within the current industry environment that emphasizes financial performance and returns.

It has long been recognized by regulators that inducements to the biopharmaceutical industry can be important to the development of pediatric therapeutics for all therapeutic areas, not just in oncology. A variety of regulatory "carrots" and "sticks" have been put into place with varying levels of effectiveness. Pediatric exclusivity and the Rare Pediatric Disease Priority Review Voucher are two of the more successful incentives instituted through the FDA. In 1997, Congress enacted the Food and Drug Administration Modernization Act which included a provision for pediatric exclusivity intended to encourage pharma sponsors through the provision of financial incentives to conduct clinical trials in children. The law provided for 6 months of additional marketing exclusivity to be added to existing patent life for an approved drug. Thus, a pharmaceutical sponsor that performed clinical studies in children in accordance with specific FDA requests could gain a longer period of sales as the entry of generic competition following the expiry of its patent protection would be delayed by one-half year.

The Rare Pediatric Disease Priority Review Voucher was created by FDA in 2012 and is closely modeled off a predecessor voucher program that covered tropical diseases. Importantly, a pediatric voucher obtained by a pharma or biotech sponsor for its candidate drug for a rare childhood disease can then be transferred (sold) to another, usually large pharma, sponsor. The buyer of a pediatric voucher whose drug has nothing to do with pediatric therapeutics can then receive a 6-month priority review by FDA for their NDA or BLA. A priority review by FDA that results in regulatory approval facilitates the drug reaching the market faster to generate greater sales revenues during its patent life. Pharmas quickly recognized the commercial value of these vouchers. The first-ever pediatric voucher was awarded in 2014 and purchased by Sanofi and Regeneron for $67M and used for the approval of Praluent® (alirocumab), a monoclonal antibody for adults with cardiovascular disease. In August 2015, AbbVie paid $350M for a pediatric voucher that it used to accelerate the approval of Rinvoq® (upadacitinib), a Janus kinase inhibitor for adults with rheumatoid arthritis. Since that time, the purchase price for rare pediatric disease vouchers has generally averaged $100M.

Finally, alternative models from within the biopharmaceutical industry have recently emerged that may provide innovative avenues to discover and develop novel drugs for children with cancer. In particular, three start-up biotechs—Day One Biopharmaceuticals, Oncoheroes Biosciences, and M4K Pharma—are deserving of mention. In aggregate these three companies have taken a mix of approaches to building an internal pipeline of drugs aimed at pediatric oncology indications. One focuses on licensing molecules already studied by large pharma in clinical trials for one or more primarily adult tumors and "repurposing" the molecule instead for treatment against a pediatric tumor. Another takes the more traditional path conducting discovery research to identify and optimize molecules created in the laboratory specifically for pediatric cancers of interest. A third is attempting to execute both of these strategies in parallel.

Day One Biopharmaceuticals, based in South San Francisco, launched in 2020 with a $60M

Series A investment. Its first molecule, DAY101, is a brain-penetrant pan-RAF kinase inhibitor from Sunesis Pharma, previously licensed to Takeda Pharmaceutical Company, that Day One is developing as a targeted treatment for children with low-grade gliomas harboring wild-type BRAF fusion proteins. Under Takeda, this molecule had been tested in over 200 adults with melanoma, glioma, and other solid tumors at the time of licensing. In 2021, Day One raised another $130M in a Series B round and licensed pimasertib and MSC2015103B, both allosteric inhibitors of MEK1/2, a key enzyme in the MAPK signaling pathway, from Merck KGaA. Pimasertib had been studied in over ten phase 1 and phase 2 clinical trials in approximately 900 cancer patients by Merck KGaA. Day One has disclosed that it intends to conduct combination development of DAY101 with pimasertib.

Based in Toronto, M4K Pharma is eschewing in-licensing and instead undertaking a robust medicinal chemistry approach to discover its own molecules for children with diffuse intrinsic pontine glioma, a highly lethal and devastating brain tumor of early childhood. Unlike Day One and Oncoheroes, M4K Pharma does not have any VC investment nor does it ever intend to. Instead, M4K which started in 2017 is wholly owned by a charity, the Agora Open Science Trust. M4K is predicated on using the principles of "open science" to revolutionize how affordable new treatments are discovered and developed. In this case, open science for M4K means that it is committed to not restricting access to its research by filing patents, instead freely sharing the scientific knowledge derived from its programs. In fact, M4K records its bimonthly research project team meetings and loads it onto YouTube for anyone with an interest to view in their entirety. M4K's discovery research occurs at academic and government laboratories, such as McGill University, the Institute of Cancer Research in England, Canada's Ontario Institute for Cancer Research, and many others. In addition, CROs like Charles River Laboratories perform research activities for M4K without charge as a charitable in-kind service. By taking this approach and with an initial funding of less than $3M, M4K has been able to identify five potential lead ALK2 inhibitor molecules as it advances through preclinical development.

Oncoheroes Biosciences, started in 2017 and based in Boston and Barcelona, is taking a dual approach of both repurposing existing clinical molecules that it licenses and conducting drug discovery to bring forth its own original molecules. For repurposing, Oncoheroes in 2019 licensed Boehringer Ingelheim's volasertib, a polo-like kinase 1 (PLK1) inhibitor, that had failed to demonstrate sufficient clinical efficacy in combination with low-dose cytarabine in an earlier phase 3 trial in elderly adults with AML (Döhner et al. 2016). However, based on PLK1's involvement in stabilizing PAX3/7-FOXO1, a chimeric oncoprotein implicated in rhabdomyosarcoma, Oncoheroes is pursuing the clinical development of volasertib in children with this soft tissue sarcoma. In 2020, Oncoheroes received Rare Pediatric Disease Designation from the FDA. This would qualify Oncoheroes to receive a priority review voucher should volasertib be approved thus allowing it to further monetize its R&D investment in volasertib by selling the voucher as described above. On the drug discovery front, Oncoheroes is utilizing a synthetic lethality approach in an attempt to identify a preclinical molecule or combination of molecules for high-risk pediatric medulloblastoma with MYC gene amplification.

Day One Biopharmaceuticals, Oncoheroes Biosciences, and M4K Pharma are all too early in their respective gestations as biotechs to have reached the goal that they all seek, namely, the successful clinical development and regulatory approval of a novel medicine for pediatric cancer. The strategy of repurposing molecules for indications other than the one originally intended has occasionally succeeded, e.g., Viagra was first developed for cardiac-related chest pain, but more often than not, this strategy has failed. At the same time, discovering a molecule from scratch is a long, arduous process that in most cases never yields a molecule that even enters into clinical trials. Nevertheless, given the substantial hurdles described above that make pediatric oncology the poor and neglected stepchild of adult malignancies when it comes to attention, investment, and resources from large pharma and biotech, the paths taken by these three innovative biotechs bring hope that atypical avenues may yet be found to stimulate the development of novel and better treatments for children with cancer.

References

Anderson M (2020) Top 10 pharma companies by revenue. Becker's Hospital Review. https://www.beckershospitalreview.com/pharmacy/top-10-pharma-companies-by-revenue.html. Accessed 15 Jan 2021

Daemmrich A, Bowden ME (2005) A rising drug industry. Chem Eng News 83:28–42

Döhner H, Symeonidis A, Sanz MA et al (2016) Phase III randomized trial of volasertib plus low-dose cytarabine (LDAC) versus placebo plus LDAC in patients aged ≥65 years with previously untreated AML, ineligible for intensive therapy. Haematologica 101:abstract S501

GlaxoSmithKline (2005) Annual report

GlaxoSmithKline (2017) Annual report

Harper M (2013) The cost of creating a new drug now $5 billion, pushing big pharma to change. Forbes. https://www.forbes.com/sites/matthewherper/2013/08/11/how-the-staggering-cost-of-inventing-new-drugs-is-shaping-the-future-of-medicine/?sh=2e00f10b13c3. Accessed 16 Jan 2021

Hay M, Thomas DW, Craighead JL et al (2014) Clinical development success rates for investigational drugs. Nat Biotechnol 32:40–51

Hirschfeld S, Ho PTC, Smith M, Pazdur R (2003) Regulatory approvals of pediatric oncology drugs: previous experience and new initiatives. J Clin Oncol 21:1066–1073

Huckman RS, Strick E (2005) GlaxoSmithKline: reorganizing drug discovery (A). Harvard Business School Case 605-074

Merck (2019) Annual report

Mikulic M (2020) Total global spending on pharmaceutical research and development from 2012 to 2026. Statistica. https://www.statista.com/statistics/309466/global-r-and-d-expenditure-for-pharmaceuticals/. Accessed 15 Jan 2021

Mullard A (2013) An audience with... Paul Stoffels. Nat Rev Drug Discov 12:258

Naik G (2003) Glaxo's decentralized discovery pays off. Wall Street Journal, 24 Mar 2003

Novartis (2020) Annual report

Owens PK, Raddad E, Miller JW et al (2015) A decade of innovation in pharmaceutical R&D: the Chorus model. Nat Rev Drug Discov 14:17–28

Pagliarulo N (2017) GSK overhauls R&D, axes 30 programs to regain edge. Biopharma Dive. https://www.biopharmadive.com/news/glaxosmithkline-gsk-rd-pipeline-restructuring-cut-q2-earnings/447924/. Accessed 21 Feb 2021

Paul SM, Mytelka DS, Dunwiddie CT et al (2010) How to improve R&D productivity: the pharmaceutical industry's grand challenge. Nat Rev Drug Discov 9:203–214

Pisano GP (2006) Science business: the promise, the reality, and the future of biotech. Harvard Business School Press, Boston, pp 84–87

Robaczewska J, Vanhaverbeke W, Lorenz A (2019) Applying open innovation strategies in the context of a regional innovation ecosystem: the case of Janssen Pharmaceuticals. Glob Transit 1:120–131

Sallman DA, Asch AS, Al Malki MM et al (2019) The first-in-class anti-CD47 antibody magrolimab (5F9) in combination with azacitidine is effective in MDS and AML patients: ongoing phase 1b results. Blood 134(Supplement 1):569

Schuhmacher A, Gassmann O, Hinder M (2016) Changing R&D models in research-based pharma companies. J Transl Med 14:105–115

Torsoli A (2011) Glaxo scientists 'live or die' with project in research overhaul. Bloomberg News. https://www.bloomberg.com/news/articles/2011-11-30/glaxo-scientists-live-or-die-with-project-in-biggest-research experiment. Accessed 21 Feb 2021

Vallance P (2010) An audience with Patrick Vallance. Nat Rev Drug Discov 9:834. https://doi.org/10.1038/nrd3307. Accessed 12 Feb 2021

Wang SS (2009) J&J's Stoffels says 'Open Innovation' is the R&D answer. Wall Street Journal, 29 Jan 2009

Whalen J (2006) Bureaucracy buster? Glaxo lets scientists choose its new drugs. Wall Street Journal, 27 Mar 2006

Clinical Research Organizations 8

Gregory A. Hale and Jennifer Pullum

Contents

G. A. Hale (✉)
Medpace, Inc., Cincinnati, OH, USA
e-mail: g.hale@medpace.com

J. Pullum
Clinical Trial Management, Medpace, Inc.,
Cincinnati, OH, USA

J. DiMartino et al. (eds.), *Pediatric Cancer Therapeutics Development*, Pediatric Oncology,
https://doi.org/10.1007/978-3-031-06357-2_8

8.1 Introduction

Clinical research organizations (CROs) are independent companies that assist sponsors such as pharmaceutical, biotechnology, medical device companies, as well as universities and research organizations by providing trial management services outsourced by the sponsor under a contractual agreement (Gad et al. 2020a, b; Masri et al. 2012). CROs may also be referred to as contract service organization (CSO) or pharmaceutical development organizations. CROs can be traced back to the 1940s and 1950s with founding of companies such as Charles River Laboratories and Huntingdon Life Sciences that provided animals for testing or conducted the testing themselves (Serota 2020a). However, with the increased regulations for pharmaceutical testing of compounds, CROs began to evolve and now serve as a cornerstone of research, supporting sponsors in full-service offerings in the early stages of development through commercialization through the outsourcing of services from the sponsor to the CRO. While sponsors retain responsibility for the conduct of clinical trials, CROs have the ability to provide the essential support services necessary to conduct the trials.

The outsourcing of trial-related duties is largely driven by the need of sponsors to have access to clinical trial staff, trial sites, their generated data, and efficient processes in conducting clinical trials, thereby reducing costs (Rettig 2000; Landhuis 2018; Rose 2008). Specifically, the International Council for Harmonisation of Technical Requirements for Pharmaceuticals for Human Use defines a CRO as "a person or an organization (commercial, academic, or other) contracted by the sponsor to perform one or more of a sponsor's trial-related duties and functions" (Sfera and Sauber 2019a). This same organization also maintains that although the sponsor may delegate trial-related duties and functions to other entities such as CROs, the sponsor is required to ensure oversight of trial-related duties and functions including those that may be subcontracted to another party by the sponsor's contracted CRO.

Sponsors partner with CROs to further develop a new drug or device from conception to regulatory approval more efficiently than if the sponsor were to conduct the trial activities on their own (Sfera and Sauber 2019a). With the increasing complexity of the regulatory environment governing novel therapeutics such as advanced therapies medicinal products, and cell and gene therapies, CROs play an increasingly important role in helping sponsors develop approval pathways for their drug or device.

Historically, larger pharmaceutical companies conducted these research services internally. However, over time, many of these companies began to outsource these services to CROs who maintain the appropriate trial personnel and overall functionality in order to increase efficiencies and reduce costs of drug or device development (Landhuis 2018). CROs may provide a variety of research services including preclinical research, clinical research, regulatory affairs, clinical trial operations, clinical monitoring, medical monitoring, data management, medical writing, biostatistics, investigational product distribution/tracking, and safety/pharmacovigilance (Gad et al. 2020c; Shih 2015). Larger CROs are likely to be able to provide all these services in a full-service model, while smaller CROs may only provide a few areas, working with vendors to meet the sponsor's other research needs. In fact, there are small CROs that occupy niches in the research field such as specific research functions, serve specific geographic areas, or focus on certain therapeutic areas (Solarin et al. 2020; Gad et al. 2020d).

Some CROs offer additional services such as central imaging review, clinical laboratory, electrocardiogram (ECG) review, biorepositories, and assay development. Centralized evaluation of radiographic images or laboratory assays provides a uniform assessment of these endpoints, minimizing variability introduced by using multiple sites.

CROs may be categorized by geographical coverage, therapeutic area specialization, and size. Some CROs have a global footprint to conduct international trials, while some smaller CROs are limited to a specific country or region of the world. CROs may be specialized in specific disease areas or in healthy volunteers. CROs may be categorized by organization size: large, mid-size, or small (Shih 2015). The size of the CRO is also important not only in its ability to conduct a trial but also in how the CRO is able to relate and meet the needs of the pharmaceutical or biotechnology partner. Academic research organizations (AROs) are similar to CROs in that they fulfill a function in the conduct of clinical trials; however, they are nonprofit entities and more commonly collaborate with other AROs (Reist et al. 2013).

Research and development is a large portion of the corporate budget for the pharmaceutical and biotechnology industry. Recently, sponsors (pharmaceutical and biotechnology companies) have been increasingly contracting with third-party vendors such as CROs to perform certain aspects of their research and development, largely to remain profitable and competitive (Landhuis 2018; Buvailo 2020). This is also the result of decreasing returns on late-stage pipeline products. In 2016, for example, the returns for the top 12 pharmaceutical companies declined from 10.1% in 2010 to 3.7% in 2016. In contrast, there were over 1100 CROs internationally in 2013, with the top 10 CROs controlling 57% of the market by 2018, a 12% increase from 2011 (Buvailo 2020). A 2019 report stated that the global CRO industry grew at 10% compound annual growth rate (CAGR) with a projected increase to 12% by 2022 (Buvailo 2020). This is largely due to the growth in the number of biotechnology companies and the number of research projects in the pharmaceutical arena, combined with the number of drug entities in development nearly doubling from 7737 in 2007 to 15,267 in 2018 (Buvailo 2020). On average, large pharmaceutical companies outsource approximately 45% of their research activities to CROs, while small- and medium-sized organizations outsource up to 70% of their activities with some emerging companies outsourcing 90% (Buvailo 2020).

8.2 Business Development

Sponsors typically will issue to CROs a request for proposal (RFP) when a new clinical trial is to be initiated. The RFP includes a synopsis or complete protocol (a road map for the trial) for the research project and an outline of the specific questions that the sponsor would like the CRO to address in their written response (Gad et al. 2020b). A CRO's response typically includes comments on the research proposal, a description of how the study would be operationalized, criteria for site selection, the timelines for trial initiation and conduct, and an estimated study budget (Burks 2020). The sponsor reviews all CRO responses and selects a small number of CROs for an in-person or "virtual" meeting, which is called a bid defense. During the bid defense, a team of individuals from the CRO, each representing a specific area of specialization or function, "defends" the strategy of how the CRO would execute the sponsor's trial according to the proposed clinical protocol (Rose 2008).

The sponsor may have already selected external vendors, representing functions not provided by the CRO. CRO team members may include a regulatory affairs representative, who provides advice in interactions with regulatory agencies; a regulatory submissions person, who interacts with institutional research boards (IRBs) and ethics committees (EC); a project manager, who oversees the research project; a data manager, who oversees data collection, completeness, and data integrity; a medical monitor, a physician who provides medical advice and safety oversight; a safety manager, who oversees safety parameters in the research project; and a biostatistician, who designs the statistical strategy of the trial (Gad et al. 2020c).

A CROs budget proposal in the RFP response provides the sponsor an estimate of the cost of the research project, which will be important to the sponsor's leadership in prioritizing business aims (Gad et al. 2020e). The trial budget typically includes direct and indirect costs. Direct costs are those required to conduct the trial. Indirect costs are those costs that are passed on from sites and other groups involved in the project to cover expenses costs (e.g., expenses of paying site staff, Institutional Review Board costs, visit procedures, etc.). As the project progresses, it is not uncommon that amendments to the project budget are required. The CRO will address changes to the contract through contract amendments.

Following the bid defense meeting, the sponsor will select a CRO to operationalize their project based on the CRO's experience, proposal and strategy, budget, and alignment with culture/ability to work together with the sponsor (Gad et al. 2020f; CREDEVO 2019). Once the sponsor selects the CRO, the CRO and the sponsor will agree on a final contract and budget for the project, and the CRO generates a scope of work. The scope of work is a document that identifies which tasks of the project will be performed by the CRO, the sponsor, another vendor, or some combination of each. Ultimately, the sponsor is the principal entity responsible for conducting the research project appropriately.

8.2.1 CRO Team Members

A CRO functions as a tcam. Each member is responsible for a component of the trial, always working in close collaboration with the sponsor. These team members include the following project areas: regulatory affairs, study start-up, medical monitoring, project management, clinical monitoring, data management, safety, and biostatistics (we will review each of these areas in the following paragraphs (Gad et al. 2020f). The CRO may be responsible for these positions, or the sponsor may select other vendors to fulfill certain roles, such as biostatistics, data management, or safety. Project managers are individuals who oversee the trial and function as the central point of communication between CRO team members and the sponsor. Clinical research associates (CRAs) are individuals who function as the main communication liaison between the CRO, sponsor, and the trial site. CRAs conduct the site training and are the first line of contact from the site in the event there are questions regarding the protocol. CRAs also conduct monitoring visits of the trial to ensure the data is complete and captured accurately by comparing source documents (e.g., medical records) with the site's database entries (Serota 2020b; Sfera and Sauber 2019b).

8.2.2 Regulatory Affairs

Members of the regulatory affairs group provide guidance and strategy to the sponsor on how to proceed with drug or device development. This advice is particularly important for small-to medium-sized pharmaceutical companies or small biotechnology companies who do not have internal regulatory affairs teams. These team members are able to assist the sponsor in navigating the regulatory environment by designing a strategy for drug or device development, which may include writing the Investigational New Drug (IND) application (or equivalent), responding to regulatory agency (such as the Food and Drug Administration (FDA)) inquiries, or attending meetings with the regulatory agency at the sponsor's request. Their advice is particularly important for global trials, where more than one regulatory agency is involved in trial review and approval (FDA 2021).

8.2.3 Investigational New Drug (IND)/Investigational Device Exemption (IDE) Application

Human testing of a new drug cannot begin until there is evidence that the drug product to be used in humans is reasonably safe. This is called the preclinical phase. The preclinical phase typically takes 1–3 years, and the data collected from this phase will be used to move to the IND phase of the trial. The IND phase of the trial will collect the data needed to support the use of the drug product in humans. This phase can take up to 12 years to complete. If the sponsor wishes to begin testing their drug product in humans, a formal IND application is required. The IMD is a similar application for testing medical devices in humans (Babiarz and Pisano 2008).

8.2.4 FDA Meetings

Meetings with the FDA are conducted to review sponsor protocols and provide proposals, provide answers, and resolve scientific issues that impact the development of a pharmaceutical product. These meetings mark the beginning of determining if this product can move forward to the next stage of investigation. There are several meetings that are important in this process: pre-IND meeting, end of phase 2 meetings, special protocol and ad hoc technical meetings, pre-New Drug Application (NDA) meeting, advisory committee meetings, and labeling meetings. The most important characteristic to remember with all of these meetings with the FDA is that all of these meetings are serious and formal. All discussions are scientific in nature with "scientist to scientist" in many cases (Grignolo and Choe 2008).

8.2.5 Investigator's Brochure (IB)

The Investigator's Brochure (IB) is a compilation of the clinical and nonclinical data on the investigational product(s) that are relevant to the study of the product(s) in human subjects. Its purpose is to provide the investigators and others involved in the trial with the information to facilitate their understanding of the rationale for, and their compliance with, many key features of the protocol, such as the dose, dose frequency/interval, methods of administration, and safety monitoring procedures. The IB also provides insight to support the clinical management of the study subjects during the clinical trial. The information should be presented in a concise, simple, objective, balanced, and nonpromotional form that enables a clinician, or potential investigator, to understand it and make his/her own unbiased risk-benefit assessment of the appropriateness of the proposed trial. For this reason, a medically qualified person should generally participate in the editing of an IB, but the contents of the IB should be approved by the disciplines that generated the described data (Chiodin et al. 2019; Sfera and Sauber 2019c).

8.2.6 Annual Reporting

Under the IND, application sponsors are expected to submit brief reports of the progress of the investigations conducted under their respective IND application within 60 days of the anniversary date that the application went into effect. Such reports are submitted annually (Hamrell 2008).

8.2.7 Protocol Development and Amendments

Some sponsors may provide a general protocol synopsis outlining the study title; subject population; planned number of subjects; background and rationale; investigational product; dosing regimen; duration of the study; eligibility criteria; primary, secondary, and exploratory objectives and their corresponding endpoints; and statistical considerations. These synopses may vary in the amount of detail available. The sponsor may request the CRO to develop the formal clinical trial document (protocol), which is typically a collaboration between medical writers, the medical monitor, operations personnel, and statisticians. The sponsor retains responsibility for the protocol development. Once the protocol is final, the sponsor provides approval. Alternatively, some sponsors may have already developed a protocol and request only that the CRO provides comments on the protocol (Green et al. 2012a).

If at any time the protocol requires changes that impact trial conduction, patient safety, etc., an amendment to the protocol will be required. The same quality control process will be employed in the modification of the protocol to ensure that the rights, safety, and well-being of trial patients are not compromised. If immediate altering of a protocol is required for patient safety, then the sponsor can implement these changes in advance of the protocol amendment (Green et al. 2012a; Brody 2016a).

8.2.8 Feasibility

Feasibility is the process of confirming if a protocol strategy is possible and makes sense. The conduction of a feasibility assessment is usually one of the first steps in conducting the clinical trial for the CRO (Spilker 2009a). The feasibility analysis helps to identify any challenges a trial could encounter and is critical in determining which regions and sites will be considered for trial participation. The CRO will often utilize multiple sources of information when conducting the initial feasibility for a trial. Among these materials is a critical review of the published medical literature for the incidence of the disease being studied as well as any geographic or demographic predisposition. Internal CRO databases can also be important sources of information if the CRO has experience in the disease under investigation by the sponsor. External databases are available by subscription and provide detailed information on prior clinical trials (Rajadhyaksha 2010).

If the sponsor permits, sites can be contacted to speak directly with principal investigators about their opinions on the trial design and eligibility criteria and to assess their interest in participating in the trial. Contacting the PIs provides the advantage to the CRO in the ability to gain an understanding of the standard of care therapies at potential sites, the availability of any specific medications, the number and types of patients treated at the site, competing clinical trials, and the sites' standards of care. These latter issues are important in global trials since there may be significant differences in medication availability and standard of care therapies as well as the quality of medical care available.

Using published, proprietary, and general data, the CRO provides an estimate of the screen failure rate for the subject population targeted by the protocol. This requires an understanding of the specific eligibility criteria regarding subjects being approached for the protocol. Using the screen failure rate, the CRO can provide an estimate of the number of subjects with the disorder being studied who will not be eligible to proceed to the trial intervention. The CRO will identify any pertinent eligibility criteria or trial design factors that contribute to the screen failure rate, allowing the sponsor to consider revisions to the trial design, if appropriate.

Using similar data sources, the CRO will generate an enrollment rate for the trial, reported in patients/site/month; aggregate values are calculated for each site and then for the entire trial.

CROs must have a knowledge about the competitive landscape for the specific patient population. This includes both standard of care options and clinical trials in progress and in development. The public website www.clinicaltrials.gov provides a starting point for this evaluation. These values allow the CRO to provide an estimate for the number of clinical sites and countries that are required to complete the trial in a specific time frame. The CRO is also able to provide various scenarios to a sponsor so that the sponsor can view different scenarios that have different numbers of sites and geographic areas, allowing a comparison of timeline and budget considerations.

The importance of a solid feasibility investigation cannot be underestimated as it will provide the approximate number of patients needed, the number of sites needed to enroll the patients, and the time required to enroll the trial. Timelines are critically important for sponsors, and this can affect their ability to obtain external funding from investors and to adhere to their overall product development budgets.

8.2.9 Study Start-Up

Following the conclusion of the site feasibility assessment, the CRO and sponsor identify potential sites to be contacted for official selection for trial participation. The CRA will contact the potential sites to obtain information about the site's PI, their infrastructure, competitive trials status, potential patient population, and their ability to enroll the trial. In many cases, the CRA will need to conduct an on-site evaluation of the site under consideration for inclusion of the trial to ensure the trial has the right infrastructure in place to conduct the trial (Sfera and Sauber 2019b). For many CROs, if the site is well known with recent study experience with the CRO, this process can be waived and a phone assessment conducted with the site. The CRO will provide the site's particular information to the sponsor for review. Sites who meet all the criteria for trial participation are considered qualified or selected. Per regulations, the sponsor is required to formally approve all trial sites for inclusion in the trial. Once approved by the sponsor, the site will begin the start-up activities.

All sites participating in a clinical trial are required to conduct trial activities according to regulatory documents also known as "critical or essential documents" (Sfera and Sauber 2019c; FDA 2018). These essential documents are required to track and evaluate the ethical and procedural conduct of the trial and are filed in the trial master file (TMF). These essential documents illustrate that the trial site, the sponsor, and the CRO have the proper ethical and regulatory approvals to conduct the trial. The collection and submission of these essential documents can be time-consuming and will affect the time required to enroll the first patient. The site's study budget will cover the time and effort of the PI and the internal research team to collect, submit, and provide the documents to the CRO for review and approval for the site to be "activated" and eligible to enroll patients in the trial.

The Regulatory Authority's permission to start a trial is required. If an IND is required for the trial, the sponsor will need to obtain clearance to proceed from the appropriate regulatory agency. In the United States, this would be the FDA, and in Europe, this would be the Medicines and Healthcare Products Regulatory Agency (MHRA) (Brody 2016b). The FDA will provide clearance to proceed to the sponsor. The sponsor then begins the institutional approval process. In some circumstances, while awaiting "notification to proceed" from the regulatory agency, the sponsor may request the site submit the protocol to their IRB prior to the FDA completing their review. This process is termed "at risk" because if additional changes to the protocol are required, the site may need to resubmit the protocol for another review.

Within the overall process of site approvals, some sites may have internal committees involved in the review process. For example, gene therapy trials require Institutional Biosafety Committee (IBC) review (Eisenman 2019). Oncology trials may require institutional scientific committee review. Additionally, sites will have internal committees review the schedule of assessments to determine which ones are standard of care for their institution; this is important in finalizing the budget as only research activities (those that are not standard of care) for the trial will be covered in the study budget.

8.2.10 Site Activation

In conjunction with the collection of all essential documents, the CRA will conduct a site initiation visit, or site training visit with the site. The CRA will train the site on the clinical protocol and all operational activities required to support the execution of the protocol. Once all regulatory approvals have been obtained, all remaining essential documents collected, and the contract and budget finalized/ executed, the site will be approved and "activated" to begin screening patients into the trial (Sfera and Sauber 2019b). Ongoing training will be provided to the site by the CRO if there are any changes to the protocol or any of the trial processes.

8.2.11 Determining the Impact on Timelines

The CRO will leverage its experience with various clinical sites to determine the timelines (Passot 2020). CROs have an understanding of how each site operates, whether they use a central or local IRB, what internal site committees are required for protocol approval, and the requirements for contract and budget negotiations. Using this knowledge, the CRO can anticipate the length of time required for review at each site; the length of time required will vary between regions of the world as well. The CRO will use this information to generate a timeline for trial enrollment, which will impact the overall timeline of the study from study commencement to trial completion. Sponsors will typically request specific dates for the following: first patient first visit (FPFV), last patient first visit (LPFV), and last patient last visit (LPLV). These dates permit sites to better design their budgets and will be important milestones for the success of the sponsor in conducting the trial.

8.3 Project Management

Each study team is led by a project manager, who serves as the central point of contact for all functional areas involved with the research project, including the CRO, sponsor, and other vendors.

The project manager directs the study team through the life cycle of the clinical trial, initially focusing on feasibility and site identification, moving the study through the start-up and site activation phase, progressing to study enrollment and trial conduct, and concluding with study closeout (Serota 2020b; Sfera and Sauber 2019b). The project manager prioritizes communication between the team members of the CRO and sponsor and any external vendors involved in any of these phases of the clinical trial.

The project manager oversees and manages day-to-day trial operations for all functional area deliverables. The project manager ensures all project milestones are met and functional area deliverables are of the highest quality. The project manager will confirm that all team members are trained on the research project and that the documentation of project-specific training is appropriately filed in the trial master file. Project-specific training provides CRO team members with the background information and clinical trial review in order for them to perform their respective job functions appropriately.

The project manager also oversees the development of the study management tools and operational plans for the conduction of the trial. Examples of these documents include enrollment forms, site initiation visit training slides, monitoring plan, communication plan, deviation plan, safety management plan, and data management plan. The project manager is responsible for organizing regularly scheduled, internal, and external team meetings. Internal team meetings allow the CRO employees involved in the project to discuss the current study status of all functional areas. External team meetings include the CRO, the sponsor, and other vendors involved in the trial.

At most CROs, the project manager will be responsible for the financial management of a clinical trial on behalf of the CRO. It is imperative that the project manager is familiar with the duties agreed upon between the CRO and sponsor and ensures that all functional areas are conducting trial activities according to the scope of work that outlines the CRO responsibilities in the trial. Conducting activities not covered under the contract between the CRO and the sponsor are considered "out of scope" activities and not covered for payment by the sponsor. It is critical for the project manager to consult with the functional areas prior to committing to "out of scope" tasks. If the project manager does identify project activities required that are not covered in the existing scope, it is the responsibility of the project manager to discuss with the sponsor prior to conduction of these activities in order to obtain approval to conduct the activities, which may also require trial budget modification.

8.3.1 Medical Monitoring

Medical monitors are physicians skilled in the conduct of clinical trials (Riddle 2018). These physicians provide medical support for the internal CRO team and work with the sponsor medical director to conduct the trial safely while maintaining the integrity of the trial. The medical monitors answer questions from sites, CRAs, and internal team members regarding eligibility, study conduct, adverse event term coding, and serious adverse event processing and oversee safety of clinical trial participants. Medical monitors typically provide information regarding the investigational medication, concomitant medications, serious adverse event (SAE) reports, stopping rules, safety review triggers, subject withdrawal, and laboratory alerts. Medical monitors may assist in the preparation for Data and Safety Monitoring Committee (DSMC) meetings. Protocol deviations are unavoidable during the conduct of a clinical trial, and most are discovered retrospectively during the monitoring process (Bhatt 2012). However, occasionally site investigators may request the medical monitor to grant a prospective waiver for a protocol-required assessment. As a rule, prospective waivers for eligibility are generally not granted by the medical monitor and are referred to the sponsor for consideration. Most regulatory agencies and review boards do not view prospective protocol deviations favorably as the trial has already undergone a thorough and extensive review by the sponsor, CRO, regulatory agencies, and review boards. These requests are best addressed through a protocol amendment (European Commission n.d.).

8.3.2 Clinical Monitoring

Clinical monitoring is a critical process in the conduct of a clinical trial and is fulfilled primarily by the Clinical Research Associate (CRA). The primary role of the CRA is to act as the liaison between the sponsor, CRO, and the sites where the clinical study is taking place. A successful CRA is detail-oriented, highly educated, and able to communicate clearly with all the individual groups. The CRA must review the source documents, which in most cases includes patient medical records, as well as all site study-related/medical documents that support the data generated from the site trial activities as they reflect the protocol requirements. The review of this data is generally conducted via regular visits—virtually or on-site—to ensure that the site is keeping proper records to support the trial and that all trial data is correctly documented. Sites must be sure to maintain the confidentiality of patient records.

As noted earlier, the CRA plays a critical role in the selection of qualified sites. An experienced CRA is valued for their ability to assess the ability of potential sites to conduct the trial according to the clinical protocol. As a representative of the CRO and sponsor, the CRA must ensure he/she is effectively communicating all requirements needed for the site to function at a high level during the trial.

In an effort to promote efficiency, risk-based monitoring (RBM) has been advocated in some instances. RBM in its simplest form is the use of software, data, and analytics to monitor risk and support the clinical decision-making for the trial (FDA 2019). A risk-based approach to monitoring provides a data-driven approach to identifying and correcting issues as they arise. These measures help to mitigate against unexpected findings by review agencies when the investigational medication undergoes review for regulatory approval.

8.3.3 Safety

The sponsor is charged with assuring and monitoring the safety of research subjects on clinical trials. Pharmacovigilance relates to practices used to identify, assess, comprehend, and prevent adverse events or problems associated with an investigational medication or device (Brody 2009). CROs work with the sponsor to develop a safety monitoring plan outlining how the safety processes will be conducted during the trial, including the definitions and reporting guidelines for adverse events, adverse events of special interest (AESI), and serious adverse events (SAE). AEs are untoward medical occurrences in a clinical trial participant and do not necessarily indicate a causal relationship to the investigational product (FDA 2012). AESIs are serious or non-serious AEs of special interest to the sponsor for which ongoing monitoring and quick communication by the site to the sponsor are required. To be considered serious, the AE must meet one or more of the following criteria: results in death, is life-threatening, leads to hospitalization or prolongation of hospitalization, results in significant disability, or a congenital anomaly/birth defect.

CROs are often the responsible entity for notifying sites of safety concerns, and the sites are typically responsible for notifying their IRB or EC. CROs can also be designated to submit safety reports to regulatory oversight agencies as well. CROs focus on working with sites to facilitate the timely documentation and reporting of adverse events. The reporting timelines are critically important for SAEs. SAEs must be assessed by the PI as related or not related to the study mediation or intervention. The medical monitor will review the SAE narrative, the criteria for seriousness, and the assessments of causality by the PI. The medical monitor will provide an assessment of expectedness of the SAE by reviewing the investigator's brochure (IB) or package insert (Brody 2016c). Expected events are listed in the package insert or are in the reference safety information section of the IB. SAEs that are related and unexpected with respect to the study medication are considered suspected unexpected serious adverse reactions (SUSARs). SUSARs require expedited reporting and have tighter timelines.

CROs frequently oversee the external data monitoring safety board composition and meetings as well as endpoint adjudication committees, if required. As part of their safety oversight responsibilities, CROs will have policies that address tracking of dose limiting toxicities, trial stopping rules, and the implementation of urgent safety measures should a safety issue be identified that needs immediate attention. For global trials, CROs will need to have staff available to provide timely interaction with sites and regulatory oversight entities.

8.3.4 Clinical Data Management (CDM)

CDM is a critical component in clinical research. The function of CDM ensures that the collection and integration of clinical data support the conduct, management, and analysis of the clinical data (Spilker 2009b). The ultimate goal of CDM is that the conclusions of the data support the research that was proposed in the protocol, with particular focus on the primary and secondary endpoints.

Once the protocol is finalized, the protocol-specific data base must be constructed. The method of collecting the trial data that reflects the protocol required information via data entry into trial's case report form, or data collection tool. Most current databases are electronic (electronic data capture, EDC) so that sites can enter source data from the medical record into the database. The database must be secure with password-restricted access and the ability to document the name of individuals making entries as well as the time of the entry. The database must be 21 CFR Part 11 compliant, meaning that electronic records as well as electronic signatures are considered the same as those for paper records and handwritten signatures (FDA 2003). No protected health information is collected in the database, unless specified in the protocol. The entire process of data management is documented in a data management plan. This plan describes the activities to be conducted during data collection and processing.

Data managers, who oversee the function of data management activities, CRAs, and occasionally sponsor representatives have access to the EDC and can issue queries or questions for clarification of data about which they have questions. The site can then address these queries directly. CRO staff work closely with sites to have data entered into the database in a timely manner so that queries can be resolved soon after the data point and that any interim analysis or DSMB meeting can occur.

Data coding is typically overseen by the data management team with assistance by the medical monitor (Babre 2010). Coding is done in compliance with the most recently published version of the MedDRA Term Selection: Points to Consider. The medical monitor may review the coding periodically or at the end of the trial. Final reports are filed in the trial master file, also referred to as the TMF.

8.3.5 Statistics

Biostatisticians provide consultative advice on protocol development, including study design, randomization processes, and questions regarding how clinical trial issues affect statistical analysis (Green et al. 2012b). Biostatisticians take the data collected in the process of clinical data management and use statistical methods to analyze this data. They are responsible for working with the sponsor to generate data sets in the form of tables, figures, and listings to be supplied for interim analyses, trend analyses, safety reviews, regulatory reports, as well as data safety monitoring committees.

When the study is completed, the biostatistician will work with medical writers, the medical monitors, and sponsors to complete the clinical study report (CSR). The CSR is a study document generated at the completion of the trial; the CSR describes the clinical and statistical information required by regulatory authorities in evaluating clinical trial results of an investigational medication or device.

8.3.6 Quality Assurance

CROs conduct their operations to meet the requirements of international regulatory agencies as established by the World Health Organization (WHO),

European Union (EU), US Code of Federal Regulations (CFR), and the International Council for Harmonisation of Technical Requirements for Pharmaceuticals for Human Use (ICH), with emphasis on ICH Good Clinical Practice (GCP). In addition, each site must conduct the trial in an ethical manner in compliance with the protocol and under the approvals of national and institutional regulatory agencies. The sponsor is responsible for the oversight of the trial operations, and quality assurance is a means to ensure this occurs (Green et al. 2012c). It is important that the clinical trial be conducted in compliance with regulatory guidelines so that the conclusions of the trial can be regarded as valid. CROs have internal quality assurance groups that function to oversee these aspects of the trial. When the matter can be addressed by the clinical trial team, the issue may be resolved through discussion with the site to review the issue and to identify ways to prevent it from occurring again. For recurrent issues, a correct action plan may be implemented to formally outline the problem and the corrective actions required. When matters are more serious, the quality assurance team also serves as escalation point should the CRO team members and the sponsor have differences of opinions regarding any matter that could potentially affect the quality of the trial.

8.3.7 Risk Management/Risk Mitigation

Risk mitigation or risk management in clinical research is the process of evaluating opportunities and threats to the execution of a clinical protocol. The primary focus of risk management is to ensure that the rights and well-being of clinical trial patients are protected (Brody 2009). Some of the most egregious issues with failures of clinical trials revolve around the lack of appropriate planning in advance for investigator noncompliance with the clinical protocol. The most recurring issues requiring oversight are in the areas of protocol compliance, incorrect informed consent procedures, inadequate record keeping, and inadequate investigational product accountability. Sporadic issues include problems with screening or enrolling patients on the trial.

Risk mitigation will always be a challenge that needs continual review and time to ensure that patients are supported throughout their participation in the clinical trial. In addition, this process also ensures that the protocol primary and secondary endpoints are protected.

Risk mitigation is an important function of CROs. When the trial begins, the CRO and sponsor will review the protocol and identify risks to the successful conduct of the trial along with prospectively identified mitigation measures. Patient recruitment and retention measures may require modification if the trial fails to meet enrollment goals. Mitigation measures have been particularly important during the COVID-19 pandemic that affected many countries throughout the world, requiring novel methods for clinical monitoring and modifications of timelines due to delays in protocol review by regulatory boards and clinic closures.

8.3.8 Recruitment and Retention

The success of clinical trials hinges on the ability to enroll eligible subjects in a timely manner and to ensure that they can complete the trial to the point that they are evaluable for protocol objectives (Hulley et al. 2007; Spilker 2009c). CROs have expertise in this area based on their experience in the therapeutic area, their data on prior trials in this indication, their usage of social media, and their relationships with sites and patient advocacy groups. Most CROs will have patient recruitment teams that focus on these measures and can develop print- and web-based methodologies. Strategies to improve patient education, increase trial compliance, and enhance patient engagement prove valuable in these efforts. CROs will typically have experience in reviewing clinical trials from a patient perspective so that the trial is written to be minimally cumbersome for patients.

Recently, the FDA has focused on enrolling diverse clinical trial populations where possible (FDA 2020). This diversity allows the sponsor to collect additional data by gender, race, and ethnicity as there may be variations in pharmacokinetic (PK) and pharmacodynamic (PD) assessments. In addition, a recent publication reported that 96.3% of subjects in phase III cancer clinical trials had good performance status (Jaoude et al. 2020). Thus, others have called for enrolling research subjects with lower performance scores to reflect real-world patient populations more accurately. Similarly, given the improved treatments available for HIV and with an increasing number having undetectable viral loads, there has been a focused effort to enroll HIV-positive patients when this diagnosis will not alter patient safety or affect trial endpoints (Dirix et al. 2020). However, sponsors may be hesitant as these subjects with lower performance scores may adversely affect the ability for the trial to assess safety and efficacy.

8.4 Conclusion

CROs are playing an increasingly important role in drug development, collaborating as full-service or partial service partners with pharmaceutical or biotechnology sponsors, to allow the sponsor to conduct their trials expeditiously, safely, in compliance with GCP, and in concordance with pertinent regulatory authorities. What began as a small industry in the 1940s has grown into a significant entity in the clinical research industry with the expectation of a valued section of up to 90 billion by 2026.

References

Babiarz JC, Pisano D (2008) Overview of FDA and drug development. In: FDA regulatory affairs: a guide to prescription drug, medial devices, and biologics, 2nd edn. Informa Healthcare, New York City

Babre D (2010) Perspect Clin Res 1:29–32

Bhatt A (2012) Protocol deviation and violation. Perspect Clin Res 3:117

Brody T (2009) Drug safety. In: Brody T (ed) Guide to drug development: a comprehensive review and assessment, 1st edn. Lippincott Williams & Wilkins, Philadelphia

Brody T (2016a) Clinical trial design: amendments to the clinical study protocol. In: Brody T (ed) Clinical trials, 2nd edn. Elsevier, Amsterdam

Brody T (2016b) Regulatory approval. In: Brody T (ed) Clinical trials, 2nd edn. Elsevier, Amsterdam

Brody T (2016c) Package inserts. In: Brody T (ed) Clinical trials, 2nd edn. Elsevier, Amsterdam

Burks B (2020) Leave no site behind: how sites, sponsors, and CROs can speed clinical research together. Clinical Researcher. https://acrpnet.org/2020/01/14/leave-no-site-behind-how-sites-sponsors-and-cros-can-speed-clinical-research-together/. Accessed 15 Jun 2020

Buvailo A (2020) The evolving pharma R&D outsourcing industry: a bird's eye view. BioPharma Trend. https://www.biopharmatrend.com/post/146-the-evolving-pharma-rd-outsourcing-industry-a-birds-eye-view/. Accessed 1 Nov 2020

Chiodin D, Cox EM, Edmund AV et al (2019) Regulatory affairs 101: introduction to investigational new drug applications and clinical trial applications. Clin Transl Sci 12:334–342

CREDEVO (2019) How to choose a CRO? Small and mid-size pharma companies. http://credevo.com/articles/wp-content/uploads/2020/03/howtochooseaCRO_small_medium_pharma_companies_credevo.png. Accessed 1 Sept 2020

Dirix P, Wyld L, Paluch-Simon S, Poortsmans P (2020) Time for more inclusive cancer trials. J Natl Compr Cancer Netw 18:1431–1434. https://doi.org/10.6004/jnccn.2020.7652

Eisenman D (2019) Established safety profiles allow for a gene therapy boom and streamlining of regulatory oversight. Clinical Researcher, vol 33

European Commission (n.d.) Substantial protocol amendments. https://ec.europa.eu/health/sites/health/files/files/clinicaltrials/docs/pc_rev3_2009-11/list_sa_uk_en.pdf

FDA (2003) Guidance for industry part 11, electronic records; electronic signatures-scope and application. US Dept. Health Human Services

FDA (2012) Guidance for industry and investigators. Safety reporting requirements for INDs and BA/BE studies. US Dept. Health Human Services

FDA (2018) E6 (R2) Good clinical practice: integrated addendum to ICH E6 (R1) Guidance for industry. US Dept. Health Human Services

FDA (2019) A risk-based approach to monitoring of clinical investigations. Questions and answers. Guidance for industry. US Dept. Health Human Services

FDA (2020) Enhancing the diversity of clinical trial populations-eligibility criteria, enrollment practices, and trials designs. Guidance for industry. US Dept. Health Human Services. http://www.fda.gov/drugs/guidance-compliance-regulatory-information/guidances-drugs. Accessed 1 Dec 2020.

FDA (2021) Investigational new drug (IND) application. https://www.fda.gov/drugs/investigational-new-drug-ind-application/ind-application-reporting-annual-reports. Accessed 1 Mar 2021

Gad SC, Spainhour CB, Serota DG (2020a) Introduction. In: Gad SC, Spainhour CB, Serota DG (eds) Contract research and development organizations—their history, selection, and utilization, 1st edn. Springer Nature, Cham

Gad SC, Spainhour CB, Serota DG (2020b) Functions and types of contract support organizations (including CROs, CMDOs, packagers, and contract formulators).

In: Gad SC, Spainhour CB, Serota DG (eds) Contract research and development organizations—their history, selection, and utilization, 1st edn. Springer Nature, Cham

Gad SC, Spainhour CB, Serota DG (2020c) Contract research and development organizations—their history, selection, and utilization, 1st edn. Springer Nature, Cham

Gad SC, Spainhour CB, Serota DG (2020d) CROs in China, India, and elsewhere in the broader world: outsourcing science gone global. In: Gad SC, Spainhour CB, Serota DG (eds) Contract research and development organizations—their history, selection, and utilization, 1st edn. Springer Nature, Cham

Gad SC, Spainhour CB, Serota DG (2020e) Contracting, pricing, and cost or works performed by CROs. In: Gad SC, Spainhour CB, Serota DG (eds) Contract research and development organizations—their history, selection, and utilization, 1st edn. Springer Nature, Cham

Gad SC, Spainhour CB, Serota DG (2020f) Selection of CDROs. In: Gad SC, Spainhour CB, Serota DG (eds) Contract research and development organizations—their history, selection, and utilization, 1st edn. Springer Nature, Cham

Green S, Benedetti J, Smith A, Crowley J (2012a) Clinical trials in oncology, 3rd edn. CRC Press, Boca Raton

Green S, Benedetti J, Smith A, Crowley J (2012b) Reporting of results. In: Green S, Benedetti J, Smith A, Crowley J (eds) Clinical trials in oncology, 3rd edn. CRC Press, Boca Raton

Green S, Benedetti J, Smith A (2012c) Crowley data management and quality control. In: Green S, Benedetti J, Smith A, Crowley J (eds) Clinical trials in oncology, 3rd edn. CRC Press, Boca Raton

Grignolo A, Choe S (2008) Meeting with the FDA. In: Pisano DL, Mantus DS (eds) FDA regulatory affairs: a guide to prescription drug, medical devices, and biologics, 2nd edn. Informa Healthcare, New York City

Hamrell MR (2008) IND. In: Pisano DL, Mantus DS (eds) FDA regulatory affairs: a guide of prescription drug, medical devices, and biologics, 2nd edn. Informa Healthcare, New York City, p 20

Hulley SB, Newman TB, Cummings SR (2007) Choosing the study subjects: specification, sampling, and recruitment. In: Hulley SB, Cummings SR, Browner WS, Grady DG, Newman TB (eds) Designing clinical research, 3rd edn. Lippincott Williams & Wilkins, Philadelphia

Jaoude JA, Kouzy R, Mainwaring W et al (2020) Performance status restriction in phase III cancer clinical trials. J Natl Compr Cancer Netw 18:1322–1326. https://doi.org/10.6004/jnccn.2020.7578

Landhuis E (2018) Careers: the rise of outsourcing. Nature 556:263–265

Masri MD, Ramirez B, Popescu C, Reggie EM (2012) Contract research organizations: an industry analysis. Int J Pharm Healthc Mark 6:336–350. https://doi.org/10.1108/17506121211283226

Passot C (2020) Trend of longer trial timelines is likely to continue. CenterWatch

Rajadhyaksha V (2010) Conducting feasibility in clinical trials: an investment to ensure a good study. Perspect Clin Res 3:106–109

Reist CJ, Rorick TL, Berdan LG, Lopes RD (2013) The role of academic research organization in clinical research. In: Lopes RD, Harrington RA (eds) Understanding clinical research, 1st edn. McGraw-Hill Medical, New York City

Rettig RA (2000) The industrialization of clinical research. Health Aff 19:129–146

Riddle WM (2018) Medical monitoring 101: providing medical expertise for clinical trials. C3isolutions.com/blog/meical-monitoring-101. Accessed 12 Jul 2020

Rose L (2008) Pharmafile. http://www.pharmafile.com/news/stop-micro-managing-cros. Accessed 18 Aug 2020

Serota DG (2020a) The history of CROs: including CRO snapshots. In: Gad SC, Spainhour CB, Serota DG (eds) Contract research and development organizations—their history, selection, and utilization, 1st edn. Springer Nature, Cham

Serota DG (2020b) Study and project monitoring. In: Gad SC, Spainhour CB, Serota DG (eds) Contract research and development organizations—their history, selection, and utilization, 1st edn. Springer Nature, Cham

Sfera D, Sauber C (2019a) Regulations. In: Sfera D, Sauber C (eds) The comprehensive guide to clinical research. A practical handbook for gaining insight into the clinical research industry, 1st edn. Sweat Equity & Investments, LLC, East San Bernardino

Sfera D, Sauber C (2019b) Monitoring. In: Sfera D, Sauber C (eds) The comprehensive guide to clinical research. A practical handbook for gaining insight into the clinical research industry, 1st edn. Sweat Equity & Investments, LLC, East San Bernardino

Sfera D, Sauber C (2019c) Site level dynamics. In: Sfera D, Sauber C (eds) The comprehensive guide to clinical research. A practical handbook for gaining insight into the clinical research industry, 1st edn. Sweat Equity & Investments, LLC, East San Bernardino

Shih M (2015) Roles of contract research organizations in translational medicine. J Orthop Trans 3:85–88

Solarin O, Mohammed SI, Ndlovu N et al (2020) Partnerships and collaborations: the right alliances for clinical trials in Africa. JCO Glob Oncol 6:954–958. https://doi.org/10.1200/JGO.1900194

Spilker B (2009a) Feasibility of multinational trials. In: Spilker B (ed) Guide to drug development: a comprehensive review and assessment, 1st edn. Lippincott Williams & Wilkins, Philadelphia

Spilker B (2009b) Data management. In: Spilker B (ed) Guide to drug development: a comprehensive review and assessment, 1st edn. Lippincott Williams & Wilkins, Philadelphia

Spilker B (2009c) Project management: balancing line function and matrix approaches. In: Spilker B (ed) Guide to drug development, 1st edn. Lippincott Williams & Wilkins, Philadelphia

9 Role of Patients and Advocates in Cancer Therapeutics Development

Donna Ludwinski, Nicole Scobie, and Leona Knox

Contents

This chapter is dedicated to the children and young people who participate in clinical research and their families. Their bravery and contribution to advancing research are recognized and valued.

D. Ludwinski (✉) · L. Knox
Solving Kids' Cancer UK, London, UK
e-mail: donna@solvingkidscancer.org

N. Scobie
Zoé4life, Sullens, Switzerland

J. DiMartino et al. (eds.), *Pediatric Cancer Therapeutics Development*, Pediatric Oncology,
https://doi.org/10.1007/978-3-031-06357-2_9

9.1 Introduction and Landscape Perspective

In the past 50 years, 5-year survival rates for most childhood cancers have vastly improved in high-income countries (GBD 2017 Childhood Cancer Collaborators 2019), giving the impression that the challenge of childhood cancer has largely been solved. But, some childhood cancers still have no effective treatments, have treatments with limited success, or have unacceptable toxicities. In addition, children in low-income and middle-income nations continue to suffer very low survival rates. This 5-year survival rate statistic does not account for those who develop secondary cancers, children who have recurrent or progressive disease or die because of their cancer beyond this 5-year mark, and those who experience chronic life-threatening health conditions caused by their cancer treatments.

For patients and advocates focused on addressing these significant unmet needs, there is a great sense of frustration that more is not being done to alleviate the suffering of children and young people that is disguised in the data.

Despite significant cumulative investment in direct basic and translational research and thousands of clinical trials in childhood cancer, few drugs were approved for pediatric malignancies in the past 40 years, particularly in the frontline setting, relative to adult oncology drugs. Today, children are commonly treated with the same toxic chemotherapies off-label, developed and tested in adults, dose-adjusted for body weight or surface area (Adamson et al. 2016). Although these therapies may continue to have a role to play in debulking disease, they were never designed for young children going through developmental growth (Hudson et al. 2013). Over 40% of survivors live with debilitating acute and long-term side effects due to the toxicity of their treatments (Pearson et al. 2020a).

Patients and advocates not only champion specific areas of significant unmet need, but they also bring lived experience, ideas, resources, in-depth knowledge of the disease landscape, and a passion for finding solutions that are crucial to accelerating progress. Advocates are catalysts for innovation and policy change—fostering and facilitating collaboration and enabling new initiatives otherwise deemed impossible or not worth pursuing. They seek regulatory alignment, streamlined efforts to reduce duplication and the consequences of silo working, and find new ways to incentivize investment in drug development. Advocates who bring direct access or influence over philanthropic funding for academic research and initiatives to improve clinical care can be powerful enablers and drivers of innovation.

The objective of patients and advocates is always clear and unambiguous—to improve the lives of patients and to remain steadfast in that pursuit. Advocates can hold others accountable and bring stakeholders together in a way that may not otherwise be achievable, something that is a potential force in medicines research and development (R&D). Despite natural tensions because of differing and competing pressures among stakeholders, all share a single goal (as shown in Fig. 9.1)—to maximize the reach of evidence-based, more effective, and less toxic treatments for children and young people with cancer.

Therefore, addressing the challenges and maximizing the potential of multi-stakeholders work will bring benefits for all—most importantly for children and young people with cancer.

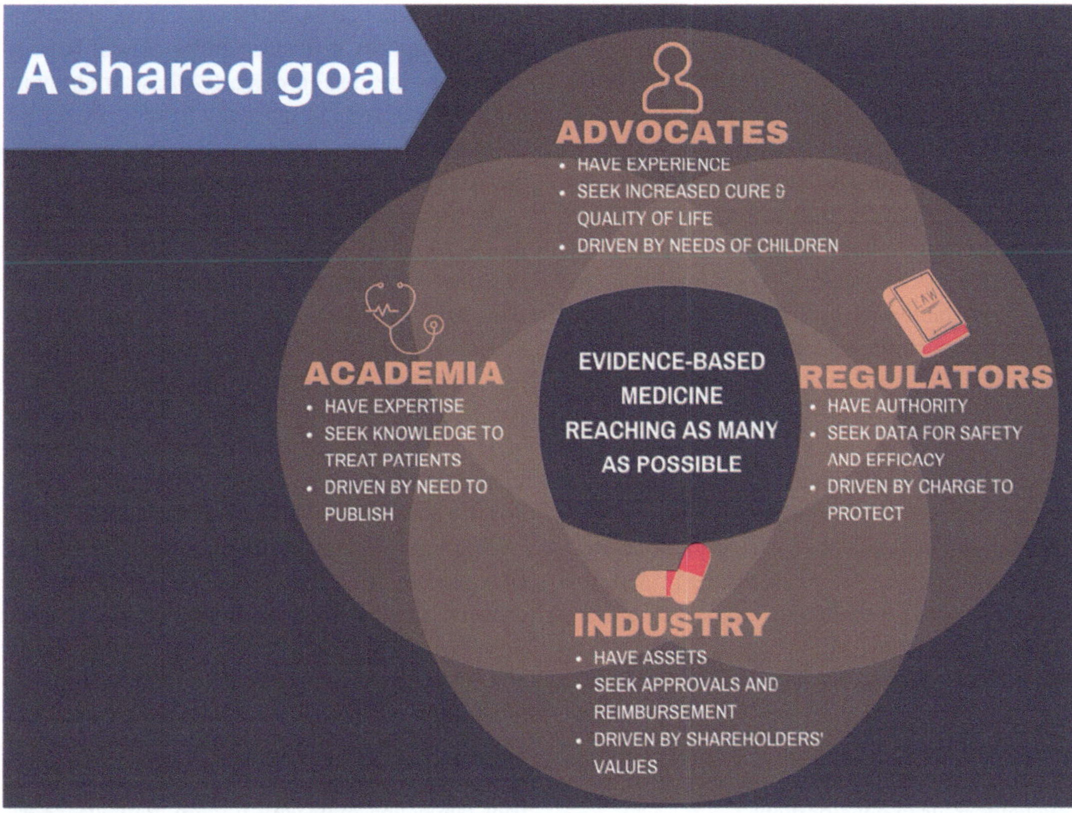
A shared goal
ADVOCATES
• HAVE EXPERIENCE
• SEEK INCREASED CURE & QUALITY OF LIFE
• DRIVEN BY NEEDS OF CHILDREN
ACADEMIA
• HAVE EXPERTISE
• SEEK KNOWLEDGE TO TREAT PATIENTS
• DRIVEN BY NEED TO PUBLISH
EVIDENCE-BASED MEDICINE REACHING AS MANY AS POSSIBLE
REGULATORS
• HAVE AUTHORITY
• SEEK DATA FOR SAFETY AND EFFICACY
• DRIVEN BY CHARGE TO PROTECT
INDUSTRY
• HAVE ASSETS
• SEEK APPROVALS AND REIMBURSEMENT
• DRIVEN BY SHAREHOLDERS' VALUES

Fig. 9.1 Stakeholders have different perspectives but a shared goal in cancer therapeutics development

9.2 A Brief History and the Rise of Advocate Involvement

Over the past four decades, engaging the patient community in all aspects of the research and development of medicines has significantly evolved. In the 1980s, HIV advocates changed the way the scientific community viewed patient involvement. In contrast to the ACT UP grassroots efforts to raise public awareness through demonstrations and civil disobedience, scientific-minded HIV advocates insisted on "nothing for us without us" and worked directly with scientists at the National Institutes of Health (NIH) to give input to drug testing, clinical trial design, and research priorities—with the important ability to bring money and patients needed to conduct the clinical research (De Cock et al. 2011).

Other disease groups have also been able to successfully influence the research priorities and conduct, bringing the patient voice to the scientists and clinicians. Notable examples of these efforts are well recognized in breast cancer, multiple myeloma, Parkinson's, and Alzheimer's. In the pediatric community affected by ultra-rare diseases, advocacy roles are critical. Challenges to effective advocacy can be compounded by the rarity of the conditions (Pearson et al. 2020a).

In the past decade, greater interconnectedness via the digital world played a key role in the rare disease patient community. Caregivers are more accessible to each other and share experiences, most notably through social media. This has facilitated a better organization and coalescing of initiatives within advocacy groups. Advocates with deep knowledge in specific disease areas are respected as trusted and influential thought leaders by other patients and families. At the same time, they provide critical insight for academia and industry because they are embedded in the patient community. Valued by all stakeholders, it is important to note that advocates' ethical obligations are first to the patient community they represent.

Incorporating the patient perspective throughout the drug development pathway has led to a growing trend to involve advocates in academic study teams and grant reviews for various phases of drug testing. Furthermore, industry, Health Technology Assessment (HTA) agencies, and payers are increasingly consulting with advocates post-approval, which provides opportunities to ensure patient needs are met in the "real world."

The evolution of the role of advocates from endorsement through consultation, to genuine engagement and involvement, is clear and irreversible. Including advocates early on in drug development processes can result in tangible impact. Even so, challenges remain including tokenism, low expectations of advocates, and outdated views of the risks of involving advocates. Significant efforts are underway to address these challenges and provide best practices for the effective and impactful role of patients and advocates in drug development.

9.3 Defining the Roles of Patients and Advocates

Within drug development, patients are most often *participants* in clinical research. Families seek access to novel agents and investigational therapies in the hope that they will benefit the child, specifically in the relapse and refractory setting. This is true even in early phase trials. However, the median life expectancy of children after enrollment in pediatric oncology Phase 1 trials is 3.6–6.4 months (Bautista et al. 2015; Kim et al. 2008; Morgenstern et al. 2014). Consequently, children with cancer enrolled in Phase 1 trials spend the limited time remaining being treated in a trial that is not focused on directly benefiting them (Crane et al. 2018). This raises ethical concerns, especially where children rely on their parents or guardians as proxy decision-makers. It is important to recognize and respect the hope, courage, and desperation of these families. Minimal upheaval for the family should be considered in the design of early-phase trials, with less discomfort and time away from home for the children, including required to travel to specialized treatment centers being important priorities.

Patient advocates are generally defined by those who advocate for an individual's care. Patients have personal experience with a disease and its treatment and bring an important firsthand account of the full range of emotional, social, psychological, and physical impacts of therapy. Adolescent and teen survivors bring important insight into experiencing the rigors of cancer treatment. In poor prognosis cancers, there may not be many survivors to bring the patient's voice.

The voice of the young child is, by necessity, conveyed by the parents or caregivers. Although parents do not undergo treatment themselves, they bring important perspectives as caregivers and decision-makers, and how treatment affects the family dynamic. Parents advocate for their child throughout cancer treatment and beyond. Knowledge of the disease, research, and clinical trial landscape may vary widely. Patient experts distinguish those advocates who are best suited to contribute meaningfully to identify unmet needs, prioritize research focus, provide input on drug development plans and clinical trial design, and serve on regulatory advisories and comment on HTA appraisals.

While the scientific community increasingly recognizes the importance of including advocates in the effort to create and test new drugs for children with cancer, specific advocacy roles reflect increasing specialization just as with other disciplines. Terms to describe and define these roles are not universal and differ significantly between countries and continents.

Pediatric cancer advocate roles in the past have been blurred, meaning any advocate was assumed to fulfill any role—whether focused on individual patient care, public awareness, government funding, and policy or patient-centric research. Advocacy in medicine is no longer a singular homogeneous role. For efficient and meaningful exchanges with academia, industry,

Table 9.1 Distinguishing advocate roles and activities

Advocate role	Description of activity
Patient	Personal experience of living with a disease, contribute with their subjective disease and treatment experience
Caregivers/parents	Supporting individual patients such as family members
Patient advocates	Insight and experience in engaging and representing a larger population of patients living with a specific disease
Patient organization representatives	Mandated to represent and express the collective views of a patient organization on a specific issue or disease area
Policy experts	Knowledge of legislative and policy opportunities to impact the regulatory environment to enhance and speed drug development
Patient experts	In addition to disease-specific expertise, have technical knowledge on the full spectrum of medicines R&D, subject matter experts

and government agencies, careful consideration should be given to identifying the right advocates for a specific activity, as outlined in Table 9.1.

Pediatric cancers include various tumor types with corresponding treatment paths that may vary significantly in intensities and modalities, resulting in a wide range of toxicities and outcomes. Therefore, effective patient experts must be well versed in specific tumor types, including their clinical research history. There is a great need for patient experts with an existing scientific aptitude and thorough training or experience to network within the pediatric cancer funding and research communities to drive priorities and accelerate drug development so that all tumor types are well represented.

Many agencies and regulatory bodies have established advocacy programs embedded, such as the National Cancer Institute (NCI) and the US Food and Drug Administration (FDA), and use terms such as patient representatives, research advocates, patient experts, and consumers. In 2017, the European Patients' Academy on Therapeutic Innovation (EUPATI) developed one of the most evolved frameworks for defining, training, and engaging patients and patient representatives to meaningfully contribute to the key points in the full range of the drug development life cycle. To date, EUPATI published four guidance documents covering patient involvement in pharmaceutical industry-led medicines R&D (Warner et al. 2018), ethics committees (Klingmann et al. 2018), regulatory processes (Haerry et al. 2018), and health technology assessments (Hunter et al. 2018). A guidance document for advocate involvement in academic-sponsored research would be a helpful addition to this series.

These are distinct activities in terms of training or experience required and differ widely in the appropriate settings for engagement. This presents an emerging challenge to academic researchers, industry teams, and government and regulatory agencies to identify advocates with the relevant knowledge and experience needed to provide meaningful input in the drug development enterprise. Distinguishing these elements of expertise and applying the right advocate to the right situation will result in more impactful engagement.

9.4 Policy and Regulatory Issues

9.4.1 United States

The pediatric cancer advocacy movement is becoming more organized and unified to benefit children with cancer. A well-informed movement of hundreds of organizations with impressive records for achieving change, including patient advocacy groups such as Kids V Cancer (KVC), Coalition Against Childhood Cancer (CAC2), and Childhood Cancer International (CCI), works on regulatory issues nationally and internationally. In recent years, advocates had a significant impact on legislative and regulatory policy driving the enactment of two federal laws directly affecting childhood cancer drug development—moving from identifying a problem to proposing a solution.

The Creating Hope Act (CHA) was enacted in 2012 to address the lack of industry interest in developing new treatments for rare pediatric diseases. As a financial incentive, the CHA established a program of Priority Review Vouchers awarded upon FDA approval of a drug for a rare pediatric disease. The voucher grants the right for FDA priority review of any other product, shortening the regulatory review time from the standard 10 months to 6 months. The voucher can also be sold; to date, pricing for sold vouchers has ranged from $67 to $350 million, and as of 2020, the total value of sales is over $1.3 billion.

The full impact of this program will be better understood in the coming years. However, early indications show a significant growth in the development of drugs for children: 28 new drugs for rare pediatric diseases made it to market in the past 8 years, including three new oncology drugs developed specifically for children. Since the passage of the CHA, there has been a tenfold increase in the number of applications to the FDA for a rare pediatric disease drug designation. In 2020, 25% of rare pediatric disease drugs under this program were approved (Kids V Cancer 2018).

Another concern identified by advocates is the adult vs. pediatric innovation gap in oncology drug development. While there are over 900 oncology drugs for adults in the pipeline, only a handful of treatments are being developed specifically for children. Historically, studies in children have lagged trials in adults by over 6 years (Neel et al. 2019). KVC proposed an update to the Pediatric Research Equity Act, resulting in the 2017 Research to Accelerate Cures and Equity for Children Act (RACE Act) which went into effect in 2020. Formerly, PREA gave the FDA the authority to require pediatric studies of certain therapies, but in practice, there have been no studies of cancer drugs for children under PREA.

The RACE Act authorizes the FDA to require drug developers to initiate pediatric studies if a molecular target of an agent is "substantially relevant to the growth and progression" of any childhood cancers. The FDA created and published a list of molecular targets and exceptions, as well as guidance documents for the industry on how to comply with the RACE Act requirements (Reaman 2018; FDA 2019). This effectively closed the regulatory loophole in PREA that waived the requirement for drugmakers to conduct pediatric studies of orphan cancer drugs.

Both laws address the critical unmet needs of children with cancer, driven by advocacy, resulting in increased optimism in the field (Rinde 2021).

9.4.2 Europe

Instrumental in shaping policy and making the voice of pediatric oncology heard throughout Europe, advocates from Childhood Cancer International (CCI) and other charity leaders have become increasingly recognized for promoting better European Union policies for children with cancer. Advocates have collaborated with academic scientists and clinicians and liaised with the key stakeholders in the childhood cancer field, organizing awareness-raising events, producing communication documents, explaining legislation backed by the childhood cancer community, and identifying policies and legislation of the European Medicines Agency (EMA) that should be changed and why.

In 2016, a group of parents, researchers, and health professionals succeeded in lobbying the EU Parliament to adopt a resolution on the Regulation on Pediatric Medicines. A goal of the resolution was to eliminate a waiver used to skirt the obligation to investigate a drug in children if the adult cancer for which the drug was originally developed does not occur in children. However, numerous drugs being waived could still be potentially used to treat common childhood cancer types (European Parliament 2016).

The European Commission (EC) published its report on 10 years of the EU Pediatric Regulation in 2017. In response, advocates called for a targeted revision since children with cancer do not benefit from the Orphan Drug Regulation. By contrast, the RACE for Children Act had just been passed in the United States, allowing the FDA to require pediatric studies of new cancer drugs that addressed a relevant target. It is not yet clear how this legislation will affect European children with cancer (Daue 2017).

In 2019, advocates joined forces with the European Society for Paediatric Oncology (SIOPE) to present a manifesto for the European elections. This manifesto outlined the vision "Beating childhood cancer: Cure more and cure better – Towards zero deaths and zero late effects." The same year, the EC began its comprehensive evaluation of the legislation for medicines for rare diseases and children by assessing the strengths and weaknesses of the Orphan and Pediatric Medicine Regulation and released the results of the evaluation in 2020. Advocates argued that regulation neither served the needs of children and adolescents with cancer nor addressed long-term side effects caused by older medicines. Furthermore, it was clear that inequalities persist in access to new and essential medicines across Europe. Advocates at CCI along with academia partners at SIOPE responded with key recommendations including aligning the regulations with science and unmet needs of children, ensuring child-specific and first-in-child innovation, implementing multi-stakeholder cooperation and prioritization as a standard recommendation, allocating public investment in medicine development for children, and ensuring equal access to essential and novel anticancer medicines and to supportive care medicines (Cardoen 2020; SIOPE 2016, 2019).

An impact assessment on the revision of the Pediatric and Orphan Regulations was begun by the EC in 2020, taking into account input from all stakeholders. The major point in the assessment was that a revision of both regulations should define and address unmet medical needs and develop a system to prioritize compounds for childhood cancers. The topic was discussed in depth at a breakout session during the ACCELERATE meeting in February 2021, which resulted in the decision to write a joint statement on the definition of unmet needs from the childhood cancer community (European Commission 2021).

Most recently in 2020/2021, advocates have been involved in Europe's Beating Cancer Plan (BECA) Commission. They successfully called for pediatric cancers to be included among the priorities of BECA and are advocating for better access to cancer drugs for all children in the EU. A BECA initiative entitled "Helping Children with Cancer" aims to ensure that children have access to rapid and optimal detection, diagnosis, treatment, and care. This initiative will facilitate access to early diagnosis and quality treatment through the network of centers of excellence, the European Reference Network on Paediatric Cancer (ERN PaedCan). The initiative will also support training and enable the sharing of best practices and standards of care for children with cancer, complementing the actions implemented within the European Reference Networks (SIOPE 2021).

9.4.3 Canada

The Advocacy for Canadian Childhood Oncology Research Network (Ac2orn) was founded in 2014 by parents and patients to help the pediatric oncology research community break down barriers and build bridges when conducting research in hopes of finding better treatments for children, adolescents, and young adults with cancer. Ac2orn has been instrumental in reducing the administrative burden when using off-label non-investigational drugs in clinical trials, providing patient input for the approval of drugs in the pan-Canadian Oncology Drug Review (pCODR) process, creating pathways and resources for patients who must travel out of province and out of the country for treatment, advocating for specific therapies (e.g., CAR T-cell, proton beam radiation), and working as patient partners for a variety of child health initiatives (e.g., cross-Canada pediatric research ethics board). Ac2orn has joined forces with childhood health advocacy groups across Canada and internationally to strengthen the collective voice in fighting for world-class care for children (SIOPE 2021; Meyers et al. 2021; de Claro et al. 2020).

9.4.4 Low- and Middle-Income Countries

CCI, founded in 1994, is the largest patient support organization for childhood cancer. It is a global, parent-driven nonprofit that represents more than 170 organizations, in over 90 countries, across 5 continents. An important focus of CCI is in advocating for improvements in treatments and socioeconomic conditions for children in low- and middle-income (LMIC) countries. To this end, CCI has partnered with the World Health Organization (WHO) to work at improving conditions in specific target countries. In 2018 CCI was officially recognized as a non-state actor in official relations with the WHO. In September 2018, WHO announced a new effort—the WHO Global Initiative for Childhood Cancer—with the aim of reaching at least a 60% survival rate for children with cancer by 2030, thereby saving an additional 1 million lives. This new target represents a doubling of the global cure rate for children with cancer.

The Initiative has two goals: to increase prioritization of childhood cancer through awareness raising at global and national levels and to expand the capacity of countries to deliver best practice in childhood cancer care. Concretely, WHO will support governments to assess current capacities in cancer diagnosis and treatment including the availability of medicines and technologies; set and cost priority cancer diagnosis and treatment programs; and integrate childhood cancer into national strategies, health benefits packages, and social insurance schemes (WHO 2021).

9.5 Support and Learning for Patient Experts

Opportunities for training patient experts are rapidly expanding and can be modeled after successful and well-organized efforts in many other disease areas, such as breast cancer. The National Breast Cancer Coalition trained hundreds of research advocates and created a network to support and enhance the role of these advocates in the research enterprise (NBCC 2019).

Active advocates have a deep disease knowledge with a wide lens perspective; they constantly seek information about the status of the field including basic science, new targets, and clinical developments. This broad-based information is an extremely valuable resource for academic and industry-driven research in pediatric cancer drug development.

To be effective, patient experts must be scientifically grounded, immersed in the patient community, comprehensive in their familiarity with the tumor biology research and trials landscape, and attuned to breakthroughs in the adult oncology arena. They must be well-versed in the drug development life cycle and understand regulatory requirements. Participating in various training opportunities to address knowledge gaps and keeping up with the steady stream of relevant journal articles builds a robust knowledge base. Attending key scientific meetings is a necessary component and an important way for advocates to become immersed in the pediatric cancer research community. Understanding all the stakeholder roles and perspectives is also required for patient experts to engage meaningfully with academia, industry, regulatory agencies, HTAs, as well as the opportunity to collaborate with other advocates and charity leaders. Most importantly, an advocate who specializes in a single tumor type can bring significant knowledge to the research community. These patient experts have the bandwidth to develop deep expertise in the cumulative tumor-specific research history which brings valuable insight to other stakeholders in the drug development continuum.

While the depth of scientific and technological knowledge of patient experts will most often have limitations, the breadth of understanding of the research environment coupled with a thirst for continuous knowledge acquisition can enable the patient expert to play a critical role in helping to drive forward progress.

An example of this unique expertise is demonstrated by a patient expert who presented on history, current research, and development of anti-GD2 antibodies at the ACCELERATE platform meeting in 2019. To date, no exploration has been so thorough on this important topic in the treatment of neuroblastoma (Bird 2021).

9.6 Involving Patient Experts in the Drug Development Life Cycle

The full spectrum of advocate involvement in medicines' R&D, including policy and legislative changes (Fig. 9.2), seeks faster and increased

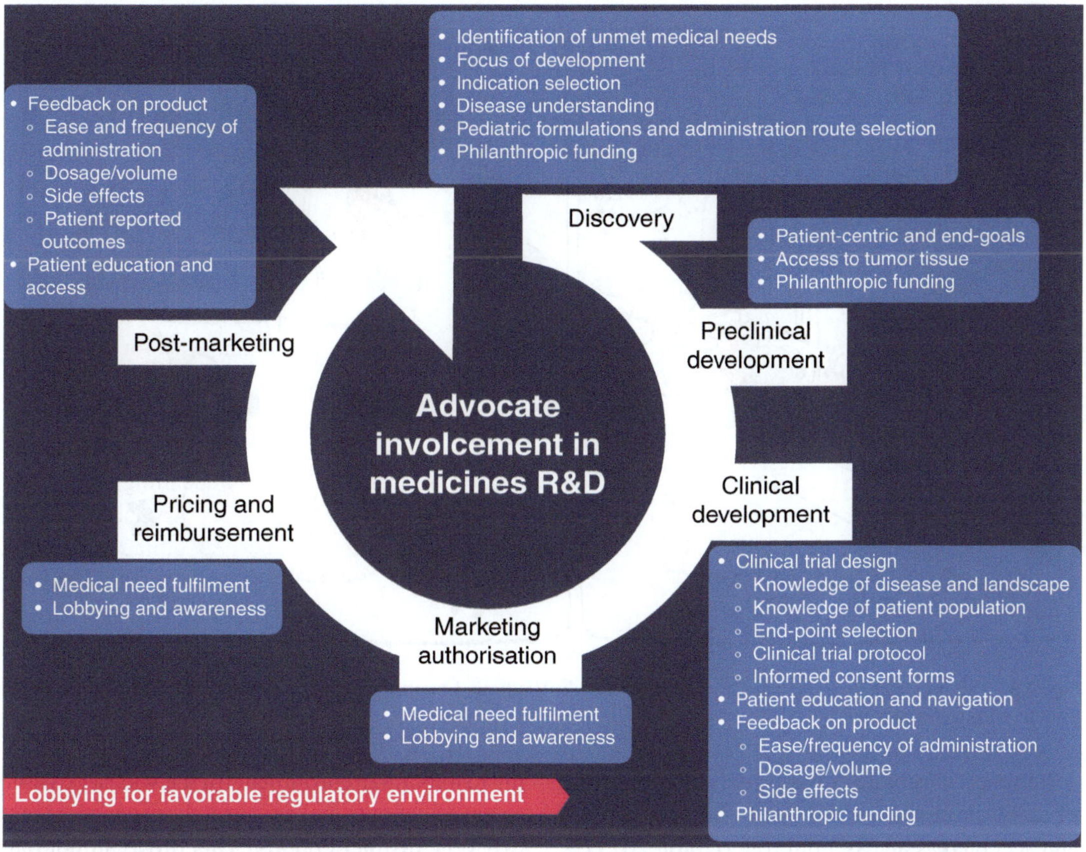

Fig. 9.2 Advocate involvement in medicines R&D

access to innovative therapies for children and young people.

Engaging advocates is the most common practice—where information is shared and exchanged. However, *involving* advocates more fully throughout the drug development process is more effective (Hoos et al. 2015; Lowe et al. 2016).

Successful product development in any industry starts with understanding the "user perspective" as illustrated in Fig. 9.3.

Industry engagement of advocates presents unique opportunities to hear patient-centric views early in development and give input on post-approval informational materials for patients and families.

The goal of drug development is to bring a new compound with proven therapeutic effect to the market. Of every 5000 cancer molecules identified in the laboratory, about 250 will enter preclinical testing. Of these 250, fewer than 10 are tested in clinical trials, and on average, only 1 will be approved by regulatory authorities (Akhondzadeh 2016). Patient experts add intrinsic value—they can provide important input at key points in the drug development life cycle. This specialist expertise helps shape outcomes more relevant to patients and more likely to be supported by regulatory agencies and payers.

Advocates create an important bridge between the scientific and patient communities, helping to raise awareness, tackle sensitive issues, disseminate information between both groups, and serve to always keep the needs of patients at the forefront of everyone's mind.

The industry has recently shown an increasing interest in incorporating patient engagement through adding positions on staff such as a "patient advocacy officer." Their duties are to learn about the patient communities and develop relationships with patient organizations. But while some are more advanced than others in embracing and optimizing patient advocacy

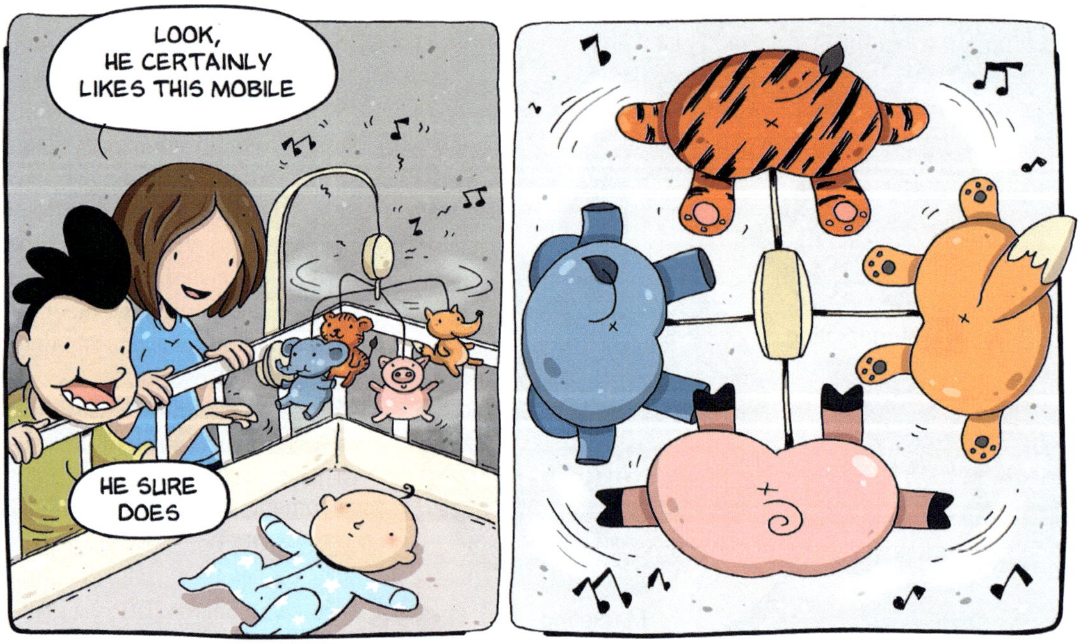

Fig. 9.3 The importance of the user perspective. (Credit Vladimir Lopatin, used with permission: https://www.instagram.com/piterskii_punk/)

within their corporate cultures, the function is still in early development and yet to be standardized and accepted as an essential role (Upton 2019).

9.6.1 Setting Research Priorities and Catalyzing New Ideas

Research advocates who keep abreast of the research landscape, note advances in adult oncology research, and track pediatric clinical trials can identify specific gaps and unmet needs. Open dialogue with scientists and clinicians can spark new research questions and influence the research agenda, but advocates must be in the "right room" (Bird 2021; Pearson et al. 2020b).

When advocates collaborate with nonprofit research funders, making grant calls to address specific unmet needs can stimulate the research community to respond to the challenge and accelerate bold and innovative research. For example, clinical trials testing new agents in pediatric tumors almost always include refractory chemoresistant tumors together with relapsed disease, so the need for novel approaches in refractory neuroblastoma was identified as a priority. While seeking to maximize enrollment for the widest possible group of patients makes sense, these can represent two very distinct cohorts. This drove an international collaboration of charities to initiate a grant call that specifically sought to focus on chemoresistant primary refractory neuroblastoma, which succeeded in stimulating scientifically robust proposals, resulting in funding support for multiple approaches (Solving Kid's Cancer 2021a).

Another example is the Canadian "100% Fund," fully funded by charities, with 100% of the funds going to the winning research proposals. The charities collaboratively select the area(s) of research focus and are part of the decision-making committee who score and discuss all of the research applications to the funding competition (C17 Council Blog 2021).

9.6.2 Basic and Translational Research

Many patient organizations and nonprofits support basic and translational research with the end goal to create more effective and less toxic therapies for children—not to simply contribute more scientific knowledge about the tumor. Advocates ask, "What does this knowledge mean for the patient?" Asking pertinent questions can help shape and steer the nature of the work and its direction, with more focus on patient-centric outcomes. Often, advocates ask the obvious question that proves to be extremely pertinent.

Advocates in the United States and EU called for transatlantic collaboration and coordination in the preclinical testing arena, to avoid duplication and share data. The advocates serving on the Pediatric Cancer Working Group (PCWG) Steering Committee proposed this focus for the PCWG, and AACR held a special joint session on the US and EU preclinical testing platforms in 2018, which was followed by the first joint meeting of the Innovative Therapies for Children with Cancer Pediatric Preclinical Proof-of-Concept Platform (ITCC-P4) and the National Cancer Institute's Pediatric Preclinical Testing Consortium (NCI PPTC). By invitation-only, industry, academic researchers, regulatory experts, and advocates attended and discussed the state-of-the-art preclinical testing models in the United States and EU. This workshop resulted in an international consensus on minimum preclinical testing requirements before studying an agent in children and adolescents with cancer (Solving Kid's Cancer 2021b; Powell 2018; Vassal et al. 2021).

9.6.3 Tumor Tissue for Preclinical Testing

An important area of translational research that patients and advocates provide critical support to is the creation of orthotopic patient-derived xenografts (PDX) animal models and other tumor-derived models. With increased understanding of the importance of biopsies and altruistic donations of tumor for research purposes, major knowledge gaps can be filled, and more realistic models can be created potentially leading to more indicative results when testing new molecules.

A particularly sensitive issue for both the scientific community and families is the need for access to postmortem tumor tissue. Analyzing the tumor and immune environment at the point where the disease causes death is another vital piece of the puzzle in increased understanding leading to more effective therapies. This is particularly true in diseases where biopsies throughout the course of treatment are very difficult, such as brainstem tumors. Although some families graciously offer to support research in this way to help future children, there is still a need for greater awareness in this area, and advocates are best placed to help. For example, Swifty Foundation and KVC among other charities collaborated to create a navigation pathway with specific help for both families and physicians to reduce the practical and emotional burden for everyone (Kids V Cancer 2021).

9.6.4 Philanthropic Funding of Early Drug Development

Government and philanthropic funding for drug development are important to de-risk industry investment. Models show poor rates of returns for private drug development in pediatric cancers and suggest hybrid business models are needed to successfully develop and market new agents:

> The purely private-sector portfolio exhibited expected returns ranging from −24.2% to 10.2%, depending on the model variables assumed. This finding suggests significant financial disincentives for pursuing pediatric oncology therapeutics and implies that financial support from the public and philanthropic sectors is essential (Das et al. 2018).

When an academic-held drug is ready for translation to a clinical-grade product before there is an interested industry partner, applying for highly competitive government funding may be unsuccessful or result in long delays. Advocate involvement can stimulate charity funding for this gap to launch the work quickly. A recent example of this is the SN22 nanoparticle formulation at Children's Hospital of Philadelphia that was rapidly completed as a result of support from several charities (The Children's Hospital of Philadelphia 2021). Charity funding launched in 2007 sped the development and testing of a humanized antibody for neuroblastoma, with a company licensing the agent in 2015, resulting in FDA approval in 2020 (Band of Parents 2021; Center for Drug Evaluation, Research 2021).

Other advocates go a step further and create their own for-profit or nonprofit drug companies. Notable examples of this are pediatric cancer parents who founded Y-mAbs Therapeutics, Oncoheroes, and Kids Cure Pharmaceuticals. Additionally, others are pediatric oncologists who start companies like Day One Biotherapeutics (The Boston Globe and Baker 2021; Y-mAbs Therapeutics 2019; Oncoheroes 2021; Day One Biotherapeutics 2021).

Without these advocate-led efforts, a major gap would exist in the drug development continuum, slowing progress that could benefit children and young people with cancer.

9.6.5 Clinical Trial Design and Ethics Review

Involving trained advocates in trial design can effectively address key elements such as best target population, endpoints, benefit/risk considerations, and inclusion/exclusion criteria and provide insight on issues that may impact accrual. Understanding firsthand what the patient journey involves alongside continued engagement in the patient community, research advocates can pinpoint reasons trials without patient-centric input are at risk of slow or no accrual and trial abandonment. These may include the opportunity cost due to more compelling competing trials and off-the-shelf therapies, burdensome travel, time in hospital or clinic, toxicities, quality of life, and negative reports of personal experiences in patient group social media forums. Additional factors advocates can help explore are equitable access and what international sites should be considered to broaden availability to patients for enrollment (Crocker et al. 2018).

Most pediatric clinical trials are conducted within academic-run study groups or consortia such as the Children's Oncology Group (COG), Pediatric Early Phase Clinical Trials Network (PEP-CTN), New Approaches to Neuroblastoma Therapy (NANT), Pediatric Brain Tumor Consortium (PBTC), the European Society for Paediatric Oncology (SIOP Europe), Innovative Therapies for Children with Cancer in Europe (ITCC), and many more. Some, but not all, formally include advocates on advisory boards for ongoing input and review of proposed trials. To improve patient and advocate involvement in the trial design and review, initial and continuing education should be embedded in the advocate advisory structure. Communicating accurate trial information in the disease forums is another way advocates serve their communities. Advocates who closely monitor the clinical trials landscape can offer valuable and objective assistance in navigating clinical trials and support in the difficult area of decision-making.

When a drug company has an asset they want to consider developing for a pediatric cancer indication, early engagement with knowledgeable advocates is invaluable to understand the entire treatment path and potential market. Determining the shortest path to regulatory approval versus considering the optimal application of a particular agent in the treatment path may create very different development plans when planning early phase and registration trials. Another highly important topic is the production of suitable pediatric formulations, especially where very young patient populations are concerned. If a child is unable to swallow medicine or is reluctant to take the required dose because of taste or volume, this raises important questions around trial adherence and dosing.

Industry-sponsored focus groups and advisory committees with clinicians and advocates are ideal for industry sponsors to formulate the pediatric drug development plan. In addition, FDA hosts the Pediatric Subcommittee of the Oncologic Drugs Advisory Committee which requires a Patient Representative (Advocate) position.

Once a clinical trial protocol is written, advocates on research ethics boards, or institutional review boards (IRBs), have an opportunity to examine the risks and benefits to children with regard to ethics in human research regulations.

Advocates review language contained in recruiting pamphlets, consent, and assent forms to assure purpose, rationale, risks, and benefits are accurately and objectively presented in lay language. Advocates have important input on ethical concerns such as biopsies for research purposes only, among other interventions or tests required with no prospect of clinical benefit.

9.6.6 Regulatory Approval and Reimbursement

9.6.6.1 FDA

In the 1960s, scientists and other public health experts believed that instituting public advisory committees at the FDA would allow for more effective consumer protection. In 1972, the Congress established the formal use of advisory committees throughout the federal government with the passage of the Federal Advisory Committee Act. The FDA includes consumer representatives and patient advocates in advisory committees alongside academic and industry experts in related disciplines. The advocates present "real-world" concerns of the patient who is to be the potential recipient of the new medical product (Center for Drug Evaluation, Research 2018).

9.6.6.2 EMA

EMA engages individuals and patient organizations at all points in the regulatory life cycle of a medicine. Patient experts are involved in protocol development, orphan designation, and ad hoc expert groups and advisories (European Medicines Agency 2021).

9.6.6.3 HTAs

Health Technology Assessment (HTA) bodies and payer organizations are increasingly recognizing patient advocates as important stakeholders, but the level of involvement remains low, and critical attention to increase involvement is needed. Some countries engage with patients during reimbursement decisions for payer decision-making, as outlined in *Partnering With Patients in the Development and Lifecycle of Medicines: A Call For Action* (Hoos et al. 2015) (Table 9.2).

Table 9.2 Countries engaging with patients during reimbursement decisions for payer decision-making

Australia	Pharmaceutical Benefits Advisory Committee
Canada	Canadian Agency for Drugs and Technologies in Health (CADTH) in the pan-Canadian Oncology Drug Review (pCODR)
England and Wales	National Institute for Health and Care Excellence
France	French National Authority for Health
Germany	Institute for Quality and Efficiency in Healthcare as well as Federal Joint Committee
New Zealand	Pharmaceutical Management Agency
Scotland	Scottish Medicines Consortium
Sweden	Dental and Pharmaceutical Benefits Agency
The Netherlands	National Health Care Institute (formerly College voor Zorgverzekeringen, Healthcare Insurance Board)
United States	Patient-Centered Outcomes Research Institute

Patients and advocates play a crucial role in helping payers evaluate the social impact and "cost-effectiveness" of medicines in ultra-rare diseases such as childhood cancers, and their contribution as part of this process can have far-reaching effects. For example, in 2016 after the United Kingdom's National Institute for Health and Care Excellence (NICE) published a negative recommendation for dinutuximab, an anti-GD2 antibody approved by the FDA in 2015 for neuroblastoma, advocates lodged an appeal of the decision, and the appeal was subsequently upheld (NICE 2015). Several issues were raised including the methods of assessment: single technology assessment (STA) versus highly specialized technology (HST) and lack of fit for purpose of applying the same end-of-life criteria to toddlers and elderly patients, claiming "...there was no evidence in the committee papers that the Committee had considered the special position of children, or treated their best interests as a primary concern." This action led to a favorable recommendation in 2018 for dinutuximab-beta (NICE 2018).

Advocates emphasize that drug approval is not the end goal; it is access for children everywhere.

9.7 Collaboration Among Stakeholders to "ACCELERATE"

ACCELERATE, a collaborative platform of international stakeholders, was jointly created in 2015 by SIOPE, Innovative Therapies for Children with Cancer in Europe (ITCC), and Cancer Drug Development Forum (CDDF) within the European Network for Cancer Research in Children and Adolescents (ENCCA). The primary aim is to accelerate innovation in drug development for children and adolescents with cancer (Vassal et al. 2015).

The platform with equal representation of academic scientists and clinicians, advocates, industry representatives, regulators, and HTA authorities provides a transparent forum to discuss and address overarching issues in the development of innovative anticancer medicines for children and adolescents with cancer. It assembles all stakeholders in pediatric oncology drug development as equal partners to identify key problems and work together to address them by developing comprehensive strategies.

In 2018, ACCELERATE was reorganized to strengthen international cooperation in order to improve the global development of new pediatric oncology drugs. This strategic decision to strengthen international cooperation turned ACCELERATE into an organization spanning Europe, North America, and beyond. The ACCELERATE platform explores the current drug development landscape, identifies bottlenecks and hurdles, and makes proposals to improve the development of anticancer drugs in the pediatric and adolescent population.

The ACCELERATE Annual Conference is the occasion when progress is monitored, proposals are implemented, and new areas of focus are identified. A working plan is established each year at the conference to be executed during the following year. Progress is monitored and reported from the previous year's working plan. The plan is implemented by the working groups. Working groups are systematically composed of members from the four stakeholder groups. Representatives from other stakeholders can be invited to join on an ad hoc basis.

Working groups are composed of representatives of the four stakeholders (patient experts, academia, pharmaceutical companies, and regulatory bodies) and any other stakeholder on an ad hoc basis.

Current and previous working groups looked at new incentives and strategies for specific pediatric drug development and drug repositioning, business models for financing, implementation of long-term follow-up measures of children and adolescents receiving new anticancer drugs, developing best principles on how the design and deliver a trial with a dataset that can be included in a package for filing as well as Fostering Age Inclusive Research (FAIR) Trials for Adolescents & Young Adults.

Lastly, ACCELERATE has begun a series of relevant educational webinars specifically for stakeholders involved in drug development, with the most recent one held in March 2021 (ACCELERATE 2021).

9.7.1 Pediatric Strategy Forums

One of the important outputs of the ACCELERATE platform is their Paediatric Strategy Forums, which are entering their fifth year in 2021.

Timely and successful drug development for rare cancer populations, such as pediatric oncology, requires consolidated efforts in the spirit of shared responsibility. In order to advance tailored development efforts, the concept of multi-stakeholder strategy forums involving industry, academia, patient organizations, and regulators has been developed. The goals of these forums are to evaluate the current state of the science, facilitate dialogue, and provide an opportunity for constructive discussions between relevant stakeholders on specific topics to assure the development of medicines in the best interests of children and adolescents with cancer is prioritized. The objective of these meetings is to share information and to facilitate the development of innovative medicines and ultimately their introduction into the standard of care of children with malignancies. Advocates have been instrumental in the planning, organizing, and participating in the forums and have contributed to publications that resulted (Pearson et al. 2019, 2020b, c, d).

9.8 Challenges and Opportunities

Being identified as an advocate, or engaging in an "advocate" activity, comes with many challenges. The same is perhaps even more so for patients who are advocates, who often bear the physical and psychological scars of the disease. Other stakeholders have a very important role to play in prioritizing the involvement of advocates while respecting the cumulative cost to the advocate and his/her family.

Advocates and patients can be seen as having a very one-dimensional role, available to provide insight on what it is like to live with a disease or to *remind people of what is important*. For even within the best-intentioned groups, advocate involvement can be seen as an add-on activity, or worse still, something to check the box of Patient and Public Involvement (PPI). This can be distressing for people who genuinely want to support in a co-production role, providing an understanding not only of the condition but also of the disease landscape and potential challenges and opportunities within.

For the most part, advocates have direct experience of the disease, having lived through the devastation of diagnosis, grueling treatment, and setbacks, cared for an extremely ill child or young person, and often suffered bereavement. Advocates are embedded in the patient community, carrying significant personal and collective trauma and pressure to ensure they do what is right for those they represent. Where advocates are engaged at any stage of the drug development pathway, it is extremely important to not add to the emotional cost of their involvement. It is critical to make the processes and role clear, ensure they have the tools and support they need to fulfill the role, and respect them as equals. Without this, advocates can feel exploited, helpless, and guilty, or it can exacerbate post-traumatic stress.

Compensating advocates for their time and knowledge exchange is a nuanced topic. To achieve maximum inclusion, it is important to ensure no individual is excluded simply because they cannot afford to participate. Advocates often self-fund their travel to meetings, hotel stays, and associated costs and spend time away from paid work. Full compensation should be offered for these costs. Additional compensation to recognize the value of the knowledge exchange to the company or organization may be gratefully received, but many advocates do not accept payment for their time to minimize potential conflicts of interest and maintain their independence. Advocates should disclose industry advisory and consulting roles, as medical professionals are required (Richards et al. 2018).

Aside from covering costs, another way to help promote diversity and inclusion is to ensure patients and advocates have access to relevant and timely information. If clear and effective two-way communication is not promoted by industry, academia, and regulatory bodies, then advocates with higher socioeconomic status and increased health literacy will dominate the landscape, and important views and perspectives are likely to be lost from the conversation. At present, knowledge of the drug development process is acquired by patients and advocates through self-directed learning. Opportunities for learning need to be increased, with consideration for those less likely to have access to digital technology.

Where advocates are engaged in discussions with commercial sensitivities, it is important to ensure there is a clear understanding of the nature of these discussions and any steps the company needs to take to protect its interests. However, making this process onerous, involving extensive unfamiliar legalese will only add to the burden for advocates and further alienate potentially marginalized groups. Equally, advocates need to be made aware—in advance—of how any information they share will be held and used by the company.

9.9 Recommendations for Academic, Industry, and Regulatory Bodies

1. View patients and advocates as important and equal partners and bring patient experts into the development process early.
2. Be clear in your expectations and rules of engagement and the role of the patient expert, foster honest two-way dialogue, and provide regular feedback.
3. Increase opportunities for learning in the drug development process, with consideration for those less likely to have access to digital technology.
4. Maximize inclusion and diversity to ensure full perspective while engaging the right people in the right roles. Advocates active in the patient community provide insight from current and emerging issues, as well as from their own experience.
5. Make industry contractual obligations as simple and straightforward as possible.
6. Appreciate the personal investment of advocates, which includes time, money, and emotion.
7. Evaluate and credit advocate input and impact (Richards et al. 2020).

9.10 Summary and What's Next?

Patients and advocates bring intrinsic value to the drug development process, and recognition of this has vastly increased in recent decades. The scientific and drug industry communities are engaging with advocates more deeply and more extensively.

Highly motivated advocates who are active and knowledgeable about the childhood cancer landscape play an important role in the process of drug development. Their input and impact are increasingly recognized by all stakeholders.

Things are moving in the right direction; however, more work is needed to strengthen this collaboration and its impact and to achieve true partnership for the benefit of children.

The field of cancer therapeutics development for children and young people has many scientific, ethical, logistical, and regulatory issues to solve. To drive progress in this critical disease area, a partnership of equals is required within the multi-stakeholder approach.

Identifying the challenges and opportunities in this multi-stakeholder process is essential to accelerate access to innovative therapies for the children and young people who desperately need them. To achieve the full impact of combining scientific knowledge with in-depth horizon scanning, lived experience, and global drug development, advocates need support and better-defined roles. The seven recommendations in this chapter outline a way forward: from bringing advocates into the drug development process earlier and helping educate them in this field to increasing inclusion and recognition of both advocates and the patients themselves in participating in clinical research. Only by working together as a team will all stakeholders succeed in the common goal to rapidly bring new and better treatments to children with cancer everywhere.

Acknowledgments The authors gratefully acknowledge contributions and review by Elena Gerasimov of Kids V Cancer, Nick Bird of Solving Kids' Cancer UK, Antonia Palmer of Kindred Foundation, Pia Rhiner and Kristi McKay of Solving Kids' Cancer, and Garrett Robinson.

References

ACCELERATE (2021) ACCELERATE Educational Webinar on drug development in paediatric oncology (30 Mar)—Accelerate platform. Accelerate--platform.org [cited 2021 Jun 16]. Available from: https://www.accelerate-platform.org/2021/02/23/accelerate-educational-webinar/

Adamson P et al (2016) Translating discovery into cures for children with cancer. https://www.cancer.org/content/dam/cancer-org/research/translating-discovery-into-cures-for-children-with-cancer-landscape-report.pdf

Akhondzadeh S (2016) The importance of clinical trials in drug development. Avicenna J Med Biotechnol 8(4):151

Band of Parents (2021) Major Initiatives. Bandofparents.org [cited 2021 Jun 16]. Available from: https://www.bandofparents.org/our-impact/major-initiatives/

Bautista F, Di Giannatale A, Dias-Gastellier N, Fahd M, Valteau-Couanet D, Couanet D et al (2015) Patients in pediatric phase I and early phase II clinical oncology trials at Gustave Roussy: a 13-year center experience: a 13-year center experience. J Pediatr Hematol Oncol 37(2):e102–e110

Bird N (2021) Dinutuximab: a newly approved immunotherapy for the treatment of neuroblastoma. Accelerate-platform.org [cited 2021 Jun 15]. Available from: https://www.accelerate-platform.org/wp-content/uploads/sites/4/2019/03/3.-Nick-Bird.pdf

C17 Council Blog (2021) The 100% Fund—C17 Council Blog. Wordpress.com [cited 2021 Jun 16]. Available from: https://c17blog.wordpress.com/category/the-100-fund/

Cardoen G (2020) Evaluation of the medicines for rare diseases and children legislation. Europa.eu [cited 2021 Jun 16]. Available from: https://ec.europa.eu/health/human-use/paediatric-medicines/evaluation_en

Center for Drug Evaluation, Research (2018) Advisory committees: critical to the FDA's product review process. Fda.gov [cited 2021 Jun 16]. Available from: https://www.fda.gov/drugs/information-consumers-and-patients-drugs/advisory-committees-critical-fdas-product-review-process

Center for Drug Evaluation, Research (2021) FDA grants accelerated approval to naxitamab for high-risk neuroblasto. Fda.gov [cited 2021 Jun 16]. Available from: https://www.fda.gov/drugs/resources-information-approved-drugs/fda-grants-accelerated-approval-naxitamab-high-risk-neuroblastoma-bone-or-bone-marrow

Crane S, Haase JE, Hickman SE (2018) Well-being of child and family participants in phase 1 pediatric oncology clinical trials. Oncol Nurs Forum 45(5):E67–E97

Crocker JC, Ricci-Cabello I, Parker A, Hirst JA, Chant A, Petit-Zeman S et al (2018) Impact of patient and public involvement on enrolment and retention in clinical trials: systematic review and meta-analysis. BMJ 363:k4738

Das S, Rousseau R, Adamson PC, Lo AW (2018) New business models to accelerate innovation in pediatric oncology therapeutics: a review. JAMA Oncol 4(9):1274–1280

Daue R (2017) The 2017 commission report on the paediatric regulation. Europa.eu [cited 2021 Jun 16]. Available from: https://ec.europa.eu/health/human-use/paediatric-medicines/developments/2016_pc_report_2017_en

Day One Biotherapeutics (2021) About—DayOne. Dayonebio.com [cited 2021 Jun 16]. Available from: https://dayonebio.com/about/

de Claro RA, Spillman D, Hotaki LT, Shum M, Mouawad LS, Santos GML et al (2020) Project Orbis: global collaborative review program. Clin Cancer Res 26(24):6412–6416

De Cock KM, Jaffe HW, Curran JW (2011) Reflections on 30 years of AIDS. Emerg Infect Dis 17(6):1044–1048

European Commission (2021) Medicines for children & rare diseases—updated rules. https://ec.europa.eu/info/law/better-regulation/have-your-say/initiatives/12767-Medicines-for-children-&-rare-diseases-updated-rules_en

European Medicines Agency (2021) Getting involved: patients, consumers and carers are involved in a wide range of European Medicines Agency (EMA) activities. Europa.eu [cited 2021 Jun 16]. Available from: https://www.ema.europa.eu/en/partners-networks/patients-consumers/getting-involved

European Parliament (2016) Texts adopted—Paediatric medicines—Thursday, 15 Dec 2016. Europa.eu [cited 2021 Jun 16]. Available from: https://www.europarl.europa.eu/doceo/document/TA-8-2016-0511_EN.html

FDA (2019) FDARA implementation guidance for pediatric studies of molecularly targeted oncology drugs: amendments to sec. 505B of the FD&C act guidance for industry. Fda.gov [cited 2021 Jun 15]. Available from: https://www.fda.gov/media/133440/download

GBD 2017 Childhood Cancer Collaborators (2019) The global burden of childhood and adolescent cancer in 2017: an analysis of the Global Burden of Disease Study 2017. Lancet Oncol 20(9):1211–1225

Haerry D, Landgraf C, Warner K, Hunter A, Klingmann I, May M et al (2018) EUPATI and patients in medicines research and development: guidance for patient involvement in regulatory processes. Front Med (Lausanne) 5:230

Hoos A, Anderson J, Boutin M, Dewulf L, Geissler J, Johnston G et al (2015) Partnering with patients in the development and lifecycle of medicines: a call for action: a call for action. Ther Innov Regul Sci 49(6):929–939

Hudson MM, Ness KK, Gurney JG, Mulrooney DA, Chemaitilly W, Krull KR et al (2013) Clinical ascertainment of health outcomes among adults treated for childhood cancer. JAMA 309(22):2371–2381

Hunter A, Facey K, Thomas V, Haerry D, Warner K, Klingmann I et al (2018) EUPATI guidance for patient involvement in medicines research and development: health technology assessment. Front Med (Lausanne) 5:231

Kids V Cancer (2018) Priority Review Vouchers for rare pediatric diseases, issued and sold 2012–present. Kidsvcancer.org [cited 2021 Jun 15]. Available from: https://www.kidsvcancer.org/priority-review-vouchers/

Kids V Cancer (2021) Post-mortem tissue donation. Kidsvcancer.org [cited 2021 Jun 16]. Available from: https://www.kidsvcancer.org/tissue-donation/

Kim A, Fox E, Warren K, Blaney SM, Berg SL, Adamson PC et al (2008) Characteristics and outcome of pedi-

atric patients enrolled in phase I oncology trials. Oncologist 13(6):679–689
Klingmann I, Heckenberg A, Warner K, Haerry D, Hunter A, May M et al (2018) EUPATI and patients in medicines research and development: guidance for patient involvement in ethical review of clinical trials. Front Med (Lausanne) 5:251
Lowe MM, Blaser DA, Cone L, Arcona S, Ko J, Sasane R et al (2016) Increasing patient involvement in drug development. Value Health 19(6):869–878
Meyers DE, Jenei K, Chisamore TM, Gyawali B (2021) Evaluation of the clinical benefit of cancer drugs submitted for reimbursement recommendation decisions in Canada. JAMA Intern Med 181(4):499–508
Morgenstern DA, Hargrave D, Marshall LV, Gatz SA, Barone G, Crowe T et al (2014) Toxicity and outcome of children and adolescents participating in phase I/II trials of novel anticancer drugs: the Royal Marsden experience: the royal Marsden experience. J Pediatr Hematol Oncol 36(3):218–223
NBCC (2019) Project LEAD. Stopbreastcancer.org [cited 2021 Jun 16]. Available from: https://www.stopbreastcancer.org/what-we-do/education/project-lead/
Neel DV, Shulman DS, DuBois SG (2019) Timing of first-in-child trials of FDA-approved oncology drugs. Eur J Cancer 112:49–56
NICE (2015) National Institute for Health and Care Excellence single technology appraisal appeal hearing. Dinutuximab for treating high-risk neuroblastoma [ID799]. Org.uk [cited 2021 Jun 15]. Available from: https://www.nice.org.uk/guidance/gid-tag507/documents/appeal-decision
NICE (2018) Overview | Dinutuximab beta for treating neuroblastoma | Guidance | NICE [cited 2021 Jun 15]. Available from: https://www.nice.org.uk/guidance/ta538
Oncoheroes (2021) Founders—Oncoheroes Biosciences. Oncoheroes.com [cited 2021 Jun 16]. Available from: https://oncoheroes.com/founders
Pearson ADJ, Scobie N, Norga K, Ligas F, Chiodin D, Burke A et al (2019) ACCELERATE and European Medicine Agency Paediatric Strategy Forum for medicinal product development for mature B-cell malignancies in children. Eur J Cancer 110:74–85
Pearson ADJ, Karres D, Reaman G, DuBois SG, Knox L, Scobie N et al (2020a) The RACE to accelerate drug development for children with cancer. Lancet Child Adolesc Health 4(10):714–716
Pearson ADJ, Zwaan CM, Kolb EA, Karres D, Guillot J, Kim SY et al (2020b) Paediatric Strategy Forum for medicinal product development for acute myeloid leukaemia in children and adolescents: ACCELERATE in collaboration with the European Medicines Agency. Eur J Cancer 136:116–129
Pearson AD, Stegmaier K, Bourdeaut F, Reaman G, Heenen D, Meyers ML et al (2020c) Paediatric Strategy Forum for medicinal product development of epigenetic modifiers for children: ACCELERATE in collaboration with the European Medicines Agency with participation of the Food and Drug Administration. Eur J Cancer 139:135–148
Pearson ADJ, Rossig C, Lesa G, Diede SJ, Weiner S, Anderson J et al (2020d) ACCELERATE and European Medicines Agency Paediatric Strategy Forum for medicinal product development of checkpoint inhibitors for use in combination therapy in paediatric patients. Eur J Cancer 127:52–66
Powell M (2018) Highlighting pediatric preclinical drug testing at the annual meeting 2018. Aacr.org [cited 2021 Jun 16]. Available from: https://www.aacr.org/blog/2018/04/12/highlighting-pediatric-preclinical-drug-testing-at-the-annual-meeting-2018/
Reaman GH (2018) Oncology Products. Relevant molecular targets for cancer drug development for children. Fda.gov [cited 2021 Jun 15]. Available from: https://www.fda.gov/media/128614/download
Richards DP, Jordan I, Strain K, Press Z (2018) Patient partner compensation in research and health care: the patient perspective on why and how. Patient Exp J 5(3):6–12
Richards DP, Birnie KA, Eubanks K, Lane T, Linkiewich D, Singer L et al (2020) Guidance on authorship with and acknowledgement of patient partners in patient-oriented research. Res Invol Engag 6(1):38
Rinde M (2021) Surge of new drugs fuels optimism in pediatric oncology. OncLive [cited 2021 Jun 15]. Available from: https://www.onclive.com/view/surge-of-new-drugs-fuels-optimism-in-pediatric-oncology
SIOPE (2016) European Childhood Cancer Organisations' Recommendations following the European Commission's evaluation of the legislation for medicines for rare diseases and children and the launch of the pharmaceutical strategy for Europe. Siope.eu [cited 2021 Jun 16]. Available from: https://siope.eu/media/documents/recommendations-for-paediatric-cancer-following-launch-of-the-pharmaceutical-strategy-for-europe.pdf
SIOPE (2019) European elections 2019 manifesto for childhood cancer. Siope.eu [cited 2021 Jun 16]. Available from: https://siope.eu/news/european-elections-2019-manifesto-paediatric-oncology-haematology-communit/
SIOPE (2021) Childhood cancer is under the spotlight in Europe's Beating Cancer Plan :: SIOP Europe. Siope.eu [cited 2021 Jun 16]. Available from: https://siope.eu/news/childhood-cancer-under-spotlight-eu-cancer-plan/
Solving Kid's Cancer (2021a) Landmark transatlantic trial for children with high-risk neuroblastoma funded by parent-led charities. Org.uk [cited 2021 Jun 16]. Available from: https://www.solvingkidscancer.org.uk/landmark-trans-atlantic-trial-for-children-with-high-risk-neuroblastoma
Solving Kid's Cancer (2021b) PTPP—ITCC-P4 Collaboration. Org.uk [cited 2021 Jun 16]. Available from: https://www.solvingkidscancer.org.uk/ptpp-itcc-p4
The Boston Globe, Baker B (2021) The Power of Will. Bostonglobe.com [cited 2021 Jun 16]. Available from: https://apps.bostonglobe.com/metro/graphics/2016/12/will/?p1=Lacey_Short_URL

The Children's Hospital of Philadelphia (2021) New treatment shows success in high-risk solid tumors. Chop.edu [cited 2021 Jun 16]. Available from: https://www.chop.edu/news/new-treatment-shows-success-high-risk-solid-tumors

Upton J (2019) Patient advocacy: the corporate mandate. PharmExec [cited 2021 Jun 16]. Available from: https://www.pharmexec.com/view/patient-advocacy-corporate-mandate

Vassal G, Rousseau R, Blanc P, Moreno L, Bode G, Schwoch S et al (2015) Creating a unique, multi-stakeholder Paediatric Oncology Platform to improve drug development for children and adolescents with cancer. Eur J Cancer 51(2):218–224

Vassal G, Houghton PJ, Pfister SM, Smith MA, Caron HN, Li X-N et al (2021) International consensus on minimum preclinical testing requirements for the development of innovative therapies for children and adolescents with cancer. Mol Cancer Ther 20:1462–1468

Warner K, See W, Haerry D, Klingmann I, Hunter A, May M (2018) EUPATI guidance for patient involvement in medicines research and development (R&D); guidance for pharmaceutical industry-led medicines R&D. Front Med (Lausanne) 5:270

WHO (2021) WHO launches new tools to help countries build effective childhood cancer programmes. Who.int [cited 2021 Jun 16]. Available from: https://www.who.int/news/item/15-02-2021-who-launches-new-tools-to-help-countries-build-effective-childhood-cancer-programmes

Y-mAbs Therapeutics (2019) Overview. Ymabs.com. [cited 2021 Jun 16]. Available from: https://ymabs.com/company/overview/

The Role of Regulatory Agencies in Pediatric Cancer Drug Development

10

Martha Donoghue, Lori Ehrlich, Margret Merino, Sonia Singh, Dominik Karres, Franca Ligas, Giovanni Lesa, and Gregory Reaman

Contents

M. Donoghue (✉)
Division of Oncology 2, Office of Oncologic Diseases, Center for Drug Evaluation and Research, U.S. Food and Drug Administration, Silver Spring, MD, USA

Pediatric Oncology Program, Oncology Center for Excellence, U.S. Food and Drug Administration, Silver Spring, MD, USA
e-mail: martha.donoghue@fda.hhs.gov

L. Ehrlich · M. Merino · S. Singh · G. Reaman
U.S. Food and Drug Administration, Silver Spring, MD, USA

D. Karres · F. Ligas · G. Lesa
Paediatric Medicines Office, Scientific Evidence Generation Department, Human Medicines Division, European Medicines Agency (EMA), Amsterdam, The Netherlands

J. DiMartino et al. (eds.), *Pediatric Cancer Therapeutics Development*, Pediatric Oncology, https://doi.org/10.1007/978-3-031-06357-2_10

10.1 Introduction and History of Legislation Affecting Pediatric Drug Development

Drug development for children operates within a highly regulated environment that has evolved over the past 120 years to address the provision of safe and effective drugs to treat pediatric patients (Table 10.1). The laws which dictate the approval and licensing of safe and effective drugs in general in the United States largely originated as a result of catastrophic events that occurred in children. These include deaths due to tetanus from contaminated typhoid vaccines leading to the Biologics Control Act of 1902, deaths from unknown drug substances in patent medicines prompting enactment of the Pure Food and Drug Act of 1906, and deaths in children due to diethylene glycol poisoning from elixir of sulfanilamide culminating in the Food, Drug, and Cosmetic (FD&C) Act of 1938 which authorized the Food and Drug Administration (FDA) to review and control the safety profile of new drugs (Ballentine 1981; Hirschfeld and Ward 2013; Institute of Medicine 2008). More than two decades later, yet another tragic event affecting newborn infants, phocomelia and other limb abnormalities due to maternal use of thalidomide during pregnancy, resulted in the 1962 Kefauver-Harris amendment to the FD&C Act, which imposed specific guidelines leading to drug approval based on proven measures of effectiveness in addition to safety (Kim and Scialli 2011).

Although the policies derived from these landmark pieces of legislation did not specifically address participation of children in clinical trials, the tragedies which predominated in children leading to their passage were of such a magnitude that the absence of specific requirements for pediatric studies unfortunately led to their exclusion from clinical trials evaluating effectiveness and safety of new drugs. This led to the description of children as "therapeutic orphans" by Dr. Harry Shirkey in a Journal of Pediatrics editorial in 1968 noting the obvious disparity of children included in clinical trials despite the incidence of adverse events in children due to use of new drugs in the absence of adequate dosing and safety information directing their use (Shirkey 1968; Wilson 1999). Despite the incorporation of a pediatric use section in product labeling by the FDA and passage of the final labeling rule requiring sponsors of approved products to review existing data to potentially support expansion of pediatric labeling provisions (U.S. Food and Drug Administration 1994), there was little improvement in substantive pediatric use information.

Pediatric Regulations in the United States Years of professional advocacy and voluntary efforts on the part of clinical investigators and pharmaceutical sponsors culminated in a formal program to economically incentivize sponsors to conduct pediatric studies of new drugs with the passage in 1997 of the Food and Drug Administration Modernization Act (FDAMA) (U.S. Congress 1997) that included Sec 505A of the FD&C Act granting 6 months of marketing exclusivity to manufacturers who voluntarily conducted studies in children under a written request issued by the FDA. The following year, a companion law, the Pediatric Rule, was introduced that required pharmaceutical sponsors to conduct studies in children to support pediatric use of the product for the approved indication (U.S. Federal Register 1997). The Pediatric Rule and the exclusivity provision (Sec 505A) were envisioned to work together to foster pediatric drug development by driving appropriate investigations of new drugs in children. However, the Pediatric Rule was struck down in 2002 by the Federal Court of the District of Columbia on the grounds that it exceeded the statutory authority of the FDA to require expansion of the indication of an approved product (U.S. District Court for the District of Columbia 2002). Later that year, the Best Pharmaceuticals for Children Act (BPCA) was enacted, reauthorizing the exclusivity provision of Sec 505A and creating a process for pediatric studies of off-patent drugs by the National Institutes of Health (U.S. Congress 2002). In 2003, the Pediatric Research Equity Act (PREA) was passed by the US Congress, which incorporated most of the provisions of the Pediatric Rule; however, it exempted products for orphan-

Table 10.1 US legislation affecting pediatric drug development

Year	Legislation	Pediatric regulatory implications
1902	Biologics Control Act	Required annual licensure by the Public Health Service for sale or exchange of biologic products such as vaccines or antitoxins
1906	Pure Food and Drug Act	Prohibited sale of misbranded or adulterated food and drugs
1938	Food, Drug, and Cosmetic (FD&C) Act	Gave the FDA authority to oversee the safety of food, drugs, and cosmetics
1962	Kefauver-Harris Amendment	Safety and effectiveness required for FDA approval of new drug applications
1979	Pediatric Information Requirements	FDA required product labeling to include information regarding whether safety and effectiveness have been established in pediatric patients
1994	Pediatric Drug Labeling	Regulation required manufacturers of marketed drugs to provide information summarizing available information to determine whether there was sufficient information to include information on pediatric use in drug labeling
1997	Food and Drug Administration Modernization Act (FDAMA)	Incorporated Sec 505A into the FD&C Act, creating incentives (including a 6-month extension of patent protection and marketing exclusivity) for companies to voluntarily study drugs in pediatric patients and submit data from these studies in response to a written request for pediatric studies issued by the FDA
1998	Pediatric Rule	Required drug manufacturers to submit results of studies of their drug in New Drug Application (NDA) if there is potential use in children. Overturned by Federal Court (2002)
2002	Best Pharmaceuticals for Children Act (BPCA)	Reauthorized the exclusivity provision of Sec 505A through 2007 and created process for pediatric evaluation of off-patent drugs by the National Institutes of Health
2003	Pediatric Research Equity Act (PREA)	Amended the FD&C Act to authorize the FDA to require pediatric studies of drugs or biologics that are likely to be used in a substantial number of pediatric patients or would provide a meaningful benefit to children over existing treatments. Also restored aspects of the Pediatric Rule. Requirement for pediatric studies linked to indication sought in adults; orphan-designated products exempt
2007	FDA Amendments Act (FDAAA)	Congress renewed and extended BPCA and PREA and enacted the Pediatric Medical Device Safety and Improvement Act (PMDSIA) to facilitate development of pediatric medical devices. National Institutes of Health was given authority to propose pediatric study of off-patent drugs
2010	Biologics Price Competition and Innovation Act	Pediatric exclusivity provisions under BPCA extended to biological products
2012	Title V of the Food and Drug Administration Safety and Innovation Act (FDASIA)	Permanently authorized BPCA and PREA Authorized FDA to require earlier pediatric study plan submission (iPSP) for drugs subject to PREA Under Section 529, provided additional incentive for development of new drugs for rare pediatric diseases (Pediatric Rare Disease Priority Review Voucher, extended in December 2020 for four additional years)
2017	Title V of the FDA Reauthorization Act (FDARA)	Amended Sec 505B of the FD&C Act to require pediatric investigations of certain targeted cancer drugs with new active ingredients based on molecular mechanism of action rather than clinical indication. Applied to original applications submitted on or after August 18, 2020 for new drugs intended for treatment of an adult cancer and directed at a molecular target substantially relevant to growth or progression of one or more pediatric cancers, irrespective of orphan designation

designated indications from the requirement for pediatric studies and did not require submission of a proposed timeline and plan for the submission of pediatric studies during the investigational new drug application (IND) phase of drug development (U.S. Congress 2003). In 2007, the FDA Amendments Act (FDAAA) modified BPCA to allow the National Institutes of Health to propose pediatric study requests that the FDA could issue as a written request to a commercial sponsor (U.S. Congress 2007). In 2010, the pediatric exclusivity provision was also extended to biologics under the Biologics Price Competition and Innovation Act (U.S. Congress 2010). In 2012, PREA was amended under the FDA Safety and Innovation Act (FDASIA) to require pharmaceutical sponsors to submit an initial Pediatric Study Plan (iPSP) early (60 days after an end-of-phase 2 meeting) in development and reach agreement with the FDA on the iPSP prior to the submission of a new drug application (NDA) or a biologics licensing application (BLA) (U.S. Congress 2012). This was done in an attempt to require consideration of pediatric development earlier in a product's development timeline, thereby facilitating responsible and timely access of safe and effective drugs to children. Both PREA and BPCA had sunset provisions requiring reauthorization; they were reauthorized under the Food and Drug Administration Amendments Act (FDAAA) in 2007 and permanently reauthorized under FDASIA in 2012.

Together, PREA and BPCA provided complementary opportunities to foster pediatric drug development through a combination of mandates to and incentives for the pharmaceutical industry. However, because cancers that occur in adults rarely occur in pediatric patients and the requirement for pediatric assessments under PREA was tied to the adult indication under development, the FDA granted full waivers of the requirement for pediatric assessments to marketing applications in oncology, if the indication was not already exempt from PREA requirements due to orphan drug designation. Therefore, PREA did not facilitate pediatric oncology drug development. However, in 2017, Title V of the FDA Reauthorization Act (FDARA) amended Section 505B of the FD&C Act to require pediatric investigations of certain targeted cancer drugs with new active ingredients based on molecular mechanism of action rather than clinical indication (U.S. Congress 2017). The provisions under FDARA apply to original applications submitted on or after August 18, 2020 for new drugs intended for treatment of an adult cancer and directed at a molecular target considered substantially relevant to the growth or progression of one or more pediatric cancers, irrespective of orphan designation (United States Food and Drug Administration 2021a).

Pediatric Regulations in the European Union In 1997, a committee convened by the European Commission determined that existing legislation in the European Union (EU) should be strengthened to facilitate the development of pediatric medicines. Additional discussion resulted in the July 2002 International Conference on Harmonization (ICH) Guideline E11, providing guidance on clinical investigation of medicinal products in pediatric patients. A series of subsequent legislative initiatives incorporating a system of obligatory and voluntary provisions resulted in the European Commission's regulation 1901/2006 (the Paediatric Regulation). The Paediatric Regulation came into effect in January 2007, governing the development and authorization for pediatric use of drugs by the European Medicines Agency (EMA). The Paediatric Regulation requires drug companies seeking marketing authorization for a new drug, new indication, new drug product formulation, or new route of administration for adults to submit a plan for pediatric development, called a Paediatric

Investigation Plan (PIP), to the EMA by the time of completion of first-in-human trials in adults; this time frame was established to provide for early consideration of pediatric development and sufficient time for review and formulation of an opinion by the Paediatric Committee regarding the necessity for and appropriateness of a pediatric development plan. Products for rare diseases or orphan-designated drugs products are not exempt from this requirement. Fulfillment of the requirement for conduct of studies under a PIP qualifies the product for the incentive component of the law, providing a 6-month extension of their supplementary protection certificate (SPC) or an additional 2 years of market exclusivity for orphan medicines. An additional voluntary program for pediatric studies of off-patent drugs, incentivized by data protection for a drug product's innovator from use by a competitor leading to a Paediatric Use Marketing Authorisation, was included in the Paediatric Regulation (European Parliament and the Council of the European Union 2006a, b). The Paediatric Regulation included a provision for class waivers based on the drug class or medical condition; recognizing the need for a mechanism of action-based approach to pediatric drug development in oncology, the EU revised the list of class waivers to reduce the number of drugs that would qualify for an automatic exclusion from the requirement for pediatric development in 2015 (Reaman et al. 2020).

Pediatric Regulations in Other Countries Canada and Switzerland enacted pediatric drug regulations following their institution in the United States and EU. In 2011, the Canadian government amended Part C of its Food and Drug Regulations to provide a 6-month extension of data protection based on results of trials designed to demonstrate safety and efficacy of approved drugs in children leading to a supplemental filing for pediatric use when completed within 5 years of the initial approval for the adult indication. Revision and refinement of this regulatory initiative are underway to more actively support pediatric drug development (The Council of Canadian Academies 2014). An even more far-reaching incentive program with obligatory components, the Therapeutics Products Law, was passed by the Swiss Parliament in 2016 authorizing its regulatory agency, Swissmedic, to encourage companies to submit pediatric use data (Bucci-Rechtweg 2017).

Most countries do not currently have specific regulations to facilitate pediatric drug development. For example, there are currently no specific regulations that extend special authority to the Pharmaceuticals and Medical Devices Agency (PMDA) in Japan and the Therapeutic Goods Administration (TGA) in Australia to facilitate pediatric drug development, other than the potential to extend the reexamination of an approved drug in Japan upon submission of pediatric use survey and clinical study data (Bucci-Rechtweg 2017).

10.1.1 US Regulatory Programs to Expedite Development of Drugs and Biologics

In an effort to facilitate and expedite drug development for serious conditions and to address an unmet need, starting in 1997, health authorities began to offer programs to facilitate and expedite development and regulatory review of products that meet qualifying criteria. Although not unique to oncology or pediatrics, a large percentage of drug development in oncology is conducted under these programs. Table 10.2 provides a summary of the FDA expedited programs for drugs and biologics intended to treat serious conditions, including cancer (United States Food and Drug Administration 2014a). Most drug development programs resulting in approval in pediatric patients have leveraged one or more of these expedited programs.

Table 10.2 Summary of FDA expedited programs for serious conditions—drugs and biologics (United States Food and Drug Administration 2014a)

	Priority review	Accelerated approval	Fast-track designation	Breakthrough therapy designation
Year initiated	1992	1992	1997	2012
Qualifying criteria	– An application (original or efficacy supplement) for a drug that treats a serious condition AND, if approved, would provide a significant improvement in safety or effectiveness OR – Any supplement that proposes a labeling change pursuant to a report on a pediatric study under 505A OR – Any application or supplement for a drug submitted with a priority review voucher	A drug that treats a serious condition and generally provides a meaningful advantage over available therapies and demonstrates an effect on a surrogate endpoint that is reasonably likely to predict clinical benefit or on a clinical endpoint that can be measured earlier than irreversible morbidity or mortality (IMM) that is reasonably likely to predict an effect on IMM or other clinical benefit (i.e., an intermediate clinical endpoint)	A drug that is intended to treat a serious condition AND nonclinical or clinical data demonstrate the potential to address unmet medical need	A drug that is intended to treat a serious condition AND preliminary clinical evidence indicates that the drug may demonstrate substantial improvement on a clinically significant endpoint over available therapies
Timing of submission	With original BLA, NDA, or efficacy supplement	The sponsor should discuss the possibility of accelerated approval with the review division during development	With IND or after, ideally no later than the pre-BLA or pre-NDA meeting	With IND or after but ideally no later than the end-of-phase 2 meeting
Features	Shortens the review clock by 4 months	Approval based on an effect on a surrogate endpoint or intermediate clinical endpoint that is reasonably likely to predict a drug's clinical benefit	Actions to expedite development and review Frequent interactions with the review team during development Rolling review	Intensive guidance on efficient drug development Organizational commitment Rolling review Other actions to expedite review

Source: United States Food and Drug Administration 2014a

10.1.2 European Regulatory Programs to Expedite Development of Drugs and Biologics

In Europe, EMA expedited programs include accelerated assessment, conditional marketing authorization, and Priority Medicines (PRIME) designation (European Medicines Agency 2018) (Table 10.3).

As in the United States, these programs are not unique to oncology but have had a significant impact in the development of oncology drugs for adult indications and are also utilized in development programs for drugs intended to treat pediatric cancers.

10.1.3 US Orphan Drug Program

In order to encourage and facilitate development of new treatments for rare diseases or conditions including pediatric cancers, the Orphan Drug Act (ODA), established in 1983, authorized the FDA to grant special status referred to as "orphan designation" to certain drugs and biological products intended to treat a rare disease or condition, upon the request of a sponsor. In order to qualify for orphan designation, the drug and the disease or condition need to meet certain criteria outlined in FDA regulations (21 CFR Part 316). Applications for orphan designation typically

Table 10.3 EMA expedited programs

	Accelerated assessment	Conditional marketing authorization	PRIME designation
Year initiated	2005	2006	2016
Qualifying criteria	Major public health interest, particularly from the point of view of therapeutic innovation	Benefit to public health by treating, preventing, or diagnosing seriously debilitating or life-threatening diseases, with immediate availability to patients greater than the risk inherent in the fact that additional data are still required	Nonclinical and exploratory clinical data support a potential major public health interest prior to the initiation of confirmatory clinical studies
Features	Shorter EMA review time (150 days instead of standard 210 days)	Less comprehensive evidence at time of initial authorization compared with normal requirement	Support tailored to the stage of development, scientific advice, early Committee for Medicinal Products for Human Use (CHMP) Rapporteur appointment, eligible for accelerated assessment

Source: European Medicines Agency (1995–2021a, b); European Medicines Agency (1995–2022)

include documentation to show that the disease or condition for which the drug is intended affects less than 200,000 persons in the United States, or more than 200,000 persons, but for which there is no reasonable expectation that the cost of developing and making available in the United States a product for such disease or condition will be recovered from the sale in the United States. This status is potentially applicable to all pediatric cancers given their rarity.

Orphan designation qualifies the sponsor of the product for various development benefits including tax credits, research grants for clinical testing expenses, waiver of the marketing application user free, and FDA protocol assistance. Further, orphan designation attracts industry interest through a 7-year period of market exclusivity for a product approved to treat an orphan disease (United States Food and Drug Administration 2020a).

10.2 Regulatory Standards for Approval of Drugs and Biologics

In the United States and EU, the regulatory standards for approval of a new drug or biologic product intended for use in pediatric patients are the same as those for products intended for adults. The FDA must conclude that a drug or biologic is safe and effective and provides benefits that outweigh its known and potential risks for the intended patient population.

In 1962, the US Congress required for the first time that drugs be shown to be not only safe but also effective. A drug's effectiveness must be established by "substantial evidence," which is defined as:

> evidence consisting of adequate and well-controlled investigations, including clinical investigations, by experts qualified by scientific training and experience to evaluate the effectiveness of the drug involved, on the basis of which it could fairly and responsibly be concluded by such experts that the drug will have the effect it purports or is represented to have under the conditions of use prescribed, recommended, or suggested in the labeling or proposed labeling thereof. (The FD&C Act Section 505(d) (21 U.S.C. § 355(d))

Under Section 351 of the Public Health Service (PHS) Act (42 U.S.C. § 262), marketing licenses (BLA or sBLA) can be issued only when products are demonstrated to be "safe, pure, and potent" (United States Government Publishing Office 2010a, b). The FDA interprets potency to include effectiveness and has also generally considered "substantial evidence" of effectiveness to be necessary to support licensure of a biological product under Section 351 of the PHS Act (United States Food and Drug Administration 2019c).

Historically, the FDA has interpreted the law as generally requiring at least two adequate and well-controlled clinical investigations to establish effectiveness (21 CFR 314.126) (United

States Code of Federal Regulations 2020), but the FDA is authorized to rely on a single adequate and well-controlled investigation when it is deemed appropriate. Additionally, the FDA may also rely on a previous finding of effectiveness of an approved drug when scientifically justified and legally permissible (United States Food and Drug Administration 2019c).

The approaches to providing substantial evidence to support the safe and effective use of drugs in pediatric populations can vary depending upon the pediatric indication sought, the extent of knowledge about the drug in adult patients, and the extent to which the course of the disease and effects of the drug in adult and pediatric patients are similar. The traditional approach would rely on evidence from one or more adequate and well-controlled trials in pediatric patients to support a pediatric indication, which would generally require a full pediatric development program. In the 1994 Final Regulation on Pediatric Labeling, the FDA finalized a set of rules permitting extrapolation of efficacy to the pediatric patient population, concluding that "a pediatric use statement may also be based on adequate and well-controlled studies in adults, provided that the agency concludes that the course of the disease and the drug's effects are sufficiently similar in the pediatric and adult populations to permit extrapolation from the adult efficacy data to pediatric patients (U.S. Food and Drug Administration 1994). Where needed, pharmacokinetic data to allow determination of the appropriate pediatric dosage and additional pediatric safety information must also be submitted" to support a pediatric indication (United States Food and Drug Administration 2014b). Extrapolation of efficacy can be based on "full extrapolation" in cases where there is a similar progression of disease, similar response to treatment, and similar exposure-response relationship in adult and pediatric patients and when the drug or its active metabolite concentration is measurable and predictive of response; with full extrapolation, if there is insufficient PK information to support pediatric dosing, then a PK study would be needed to identify the pediatric dose that would provide similar exposure to adults. "Partial extrapolation" of adult efficacy data supplemented by pharmacokinetic and pharmacodynamic information from studies in pediatric patients may be warranted in cases where the exposure-response relationship in pediatric patients is not adequately defined or thought not to be sufficiently similar to that in adults. In general, extrapolation from adult studies is not sufficient to establish the safety of a drug in pediatric patients; the extent of pediatric safety studies needed depends on multiple factors including prior clinical experience with similar drugs in pediatric populations, the safety profile observed in adult or pediatric patients, unique safety considerations based on the drug's mechanism of action, potential concerns identified by toxicology studies, and feasibility of conducting studies in pediatric patients (United States Food and Drug Administration 2014b).

As with products intended for use in adult patients, the process for review and approval (or arriving at a decision not to approve) of a new drug application (NDA) or biologics license application (sBLA) or associated supplemental applications is multidisciplinary and occurs within a structured framework; this framework includes analysis of the condition and available treatments and assessment of the benefits and risks associated with the drug based on clinical data, as well as strategies for managing these risks. Risk-benefit assessments are not always straightforward, and therefore decisions made by regulatory authorities do not always align.

10.3 Implementation of Pediatric Regulations (Before FDARA)

10.3.1 Implementation of Pediatric Regulations in the United States

The passage of FDAMA in 1997 and the subsequent publication of the Pediatric Rule followed by the passage of PREA in 2003 were intended to provide a two-pronged approach to foster pediatric drug development: a mandate for pediatric studies under PREA and an incentive program under BPCA to encourage pediatric drug development that is not required under PREA. Although these programs resulted in some progress in pediatric drug development, PREA did not result in timely pediatric cancer drug development, and no approvals for pediatric oncology indications occurred as a result of PREA due to provisions for waivers and exemptions to PREA that were not addressed until the 2017 passage of FDARA. The following sections outline the implementation of pediatric regulations prior to the implementation of the provisions enacted under FDARA.

10.3.2 Legislative Requirements for Pediatric Studies

10.3.2.1 United States

Under PREA, a manufacturer must submit a pediatric assessment when submitting a new drug application (NDA), biologics licensing applications (BLA), or supplement to an application to market a new active ingredient, new indication, new dosage form, new dosing regimen, or new route of administration, unless a waiver or deferral has been obtained. PREA also authorized FDA to require holders of applications for previously approved marketed drugs and biological products to submit a pediatric assessment under certain circumstances. Prior to FDARA, requirements for pediatric assessments under PREA were linked to the adult indication under study, and applications that received orphan designation were exempt from PREA requirements.

The original PREA legislation did not specify a timing requirement for the submission of a pediatric study plan; however, in an effort to shorten the timeline for initiation of pediatric studies in 2012 under FDASIA, PREA was amended to require submission of an initial Pediatric Study Plan (iPSP) outlining the plan for conduct of an assessment of the drug or biologic no later than 60 calendar days from the date of the end-of-phase 2 (EOP2) meeting. In the absence of an EOP2 meeting, iPSPs should be submitted as early as possible and at a time agreed upon by the FDA and sponsor. The iPSP should be submitted prior the initiation of phase 3 studies and no later than 210 days prior to the submission of a marketing application.

Under PREA, the iPSP can include a plan for requesting a deferral of pediatric assessments if the marketing application seeking an indication in adults is ready for submission prior to completion of pediatric studies, or if additional safety or efficacy data are warranted prior to conducting pediatric studies. The iPSP can also include a plan for a waiver of the requirement to conduct pediatric assessments for all pediatric age groups (full waiver) or a subset of the pediatric population (partial waiver) if one or more of the following criteria are met:

- Necessary studies are impossible or highly impracticable.
- Evidence strongly suggests the drug/biologic would be ineffective or unsafe.
- Drug/biologic does not represent a meaningful therapeutic benefit over existing therapies for pediatric patients and is not likely to be used by a substantial number of pediatric patients.
- Reasonable attempts to produce a pediatric formulation necessary for a pediatric age group have failed (partial waiver only).

In July 2020, the FDA issued a final guidance document outlining the content and process for submitting iPSPs and modifications to iPSPs (United States Food and Drug Administration 2020b).

Figure 10.1 provides an overview and timeline associated with the iPSP submission and agreement process. The FDA review of iPSPs occurs in consultation with the FDA Oncology Center of Excellence (OCE) subcommittee of the Pediatric Review Committee (PeRC), and the total length of time for FDA review of an iPSP should not generally exceed 210 days. Sponsors should not submit an original or supplemental marketing application until the FDA issues a letter confirming agreement with the agreed iPSP; FDA may refuse to file an application that does not include an agreed iPSP if the application is subject to PREA.

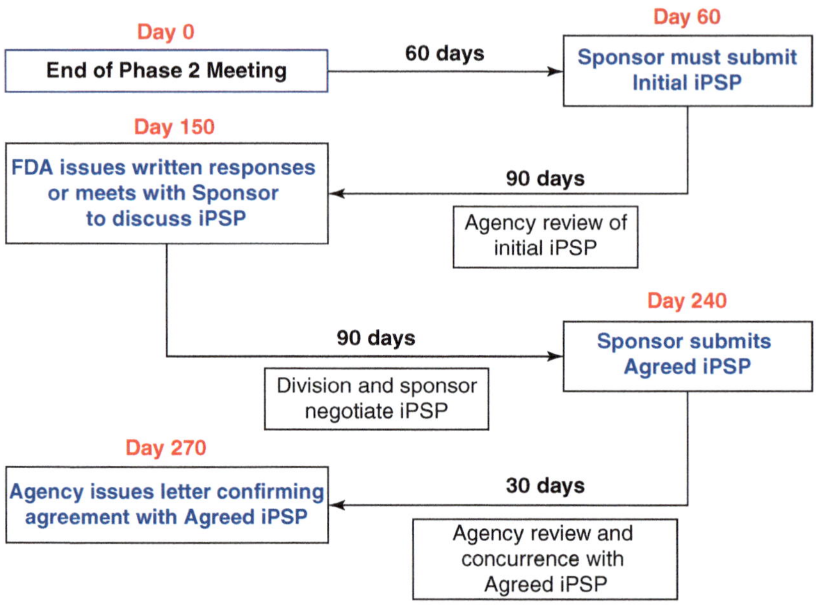

Fig. 10.1 FDA pediatric study plan submission and review process

10.3.2.2 European Union

The European Union's Paediatric Regulation (European Parliament and the Council of the European Union 2006a, b), which came into effect in January 2007, has objectives similar to US legislation but a different system of implementation. The Regulation requires all applications for marketing authorization for a new product, new indication, new pharmaceutical formulation, or new route of administration to establish a pediatric development program known as a Paediatric Investigation Plan (PIP), unless a product-specific or class waiver is granted. The PIP must be agreed to by the European Medicines Agency (EMA) Paediatric Committee (PDCO) and is a mandatory step to gain marketing authorization for adults for most on-patent products.

The PIP is intended to ensure that the necessary data to support the authorization of a product for children are obtained through studies in children. Unlike in the United States where pediatric exclusivity and requirement programs are delineated in distinct legislations (voluntary BPCA and mandated PREA, respectively) with different legal frameworks, in the EU, the exclusivity incentive and requirement for pediatric study are unified under the Regulation.

The PIP details administrative and product information including age-appropriate formulations, the disease to be treated and therapeutic benefit, whether juvenile nonclinical studies are needed, and a description of clinical studies that will generate data to support a pediatric approval. It should also include application for a product-specific waiver or deferral, if relevant. The PIP is submitted early in product development and should be submitted at the end of phase 1. Due to this early timeline, studies are often deferred until there are sufficient data to demonstrate the efficacy and safety of the product in adults.

Similar to the FDA, the PDCO may grant PIP deferrals and waivers as appropriate. Deferrals are justified on one of the following grounds: scientific and technical basis; reasons related to public health; studies should be conducted in adults prior to initiating studies in the pediatric population; and when pediatric studies will take longer to conduct than studies in adults. Waivers may be granted for reasons such as the disease does not occur in children, the product is likely to be ineffective or unsafe, or the product does not represent a significant therapeutic benefit over existing treatments. Products for rare diseases or orphan-designated products are not exempt; however, as in the United States under PREA prior to institution of the FDARA provisions, pediatric development of anticancer drugs is often waived because a therapy is being developed for an adult disease that is rare or does not occur in children.

The EMA maintains a list of class waivers for products that are not required to submit a PIP as part of a marketing authorization application. The EMA provided an updated list of classes of products in July 2015 (European Medicines Agency 2015); in this list, 80% of the class-waived conditions were malignancies. In October 2017, the European Commission published a 10-year scientific and medico-economic report of the EU Paediatric Regulation which showed that it had considerable impact on the development of pediatric products, particularly in therapeutic areas such as rheumatology and infectious disease, but insufficient progress was made for children with cancer (European Medicines Agency 2017). Due to the issue of class waivers in oncology and the EMA's acknowledgment of the need for a mechanism of action-driven approach to pediatric drug development, in July 2018, the EMA launched the revised class waiver list which was intended to result in increased discussions with the PDCO on the ability of a product to address unmet medical needs for children with cancer and consequently reductions in the number of malignant conditions for which a waiver would be granted.

After assessment of an application for a PIP, deferral, waiver, or modification, the PDCO adopts an opinion, and the applicant is notified about it within 10 days from its adoption. The applicant then has an opportunity to request a reexamination of the opinion within a certain period, if desired. Once the PDCO issues its final opinion, the EMA then adopts a decision and makes it publicly available (European Medicines Agency 1995–2021a). The pharmaceutical company must strictly follow the agreed PIP but can modify the PIP at any time, as evidence emerges requiring changes to the plan. Once completed, the EMA confirms that the applicant has complied with all measures through a compliance check which has to be requested by the sponsor or at the validation of a regulatory application, if no prior request to the PDCO has been made by the sponsor. The company can then submit the data generated as part of a PIP for assessment at the Committee for Medicinal Products for Human Use (CHMP). Once a PIP is completed and the data are reflected in the summary of product characteristics (SmPC), the product is eligible for 6 months of supplementary protection certificate (SPC) or patent extension (European Parliament and the Council of the European Union 2006a, b), which differs from the 6-month extension of market protection on the active moiety afforded by BPCA. For orphan-designated medicinal products in the EU, the 10-year period of market exclusivity is extended to 12 years.

10.3.3 Voluntary Incentive Pediatric Development Programs

10.3.3.1 United States

Under BPCA, a written request can be issued by the FDA independently or in response to a request from the sponsor. A sponsor may request the FDA to issue a written request by submitting a Proposed Pediatric Study Request (PPSR). A PPSR contains the rationale for the studies and design, a detailed study design, and a plan for the development of appropriate formulations for each age group. If the terms of the written request have been met and studies were conducted as agreed upon by the agency, the company may be awarded an additional 6 months of patent exclusivity. The studies need not have positive results in order to qualify for exclusivity but must provide clinically meaningful information to be incorporated in product labeling. The FDA may grant a written request for conditions that are different from the adult indication for which the agent may have originally been developed, an important distinction from PREA requirements.

A written request may be amended based on new or evolving data. Amendments to a written request may include addition or removal of studies in the written request or other modifications to the original plan and must be issued by the FDA. The amendment can be issued in response to a request by the sponsor or at the FDA's initiative.

A sponsor is not obligated to conduct studies in response to a written request nor penalized for failure to fulfill the terms of a written request. In addition, trials conducted under a written request do not have to demonstrate efficacy in order to for the written request to be considered fulfilled (United States Food and Drug Administration 2022).

Under FDASIA, an additional program, the Rare Pediatric Disease Priority Review Voucher, under the Creating Hope Act, was added which provides for awarding of priority review vouchers to sponsors of certain pediatric disease product applications (United States Food and Drug Administration 2019a). A priority review voucher entitles the holder to designate a single drug application as qualifying for priority review, which shortens the PDUFA-mandated time frames for review by 4 months. This program was designed to encourage development in disease spaces that otherwise may not see development and to provide an incentive that may offset some of the cost incurred by a company to develop a drug for a rare disorder where clinical studies may be challenging. A rare pediatric disease is a rare disease or condition that is serious or life-threatening in which the serious or life-threatening manifestations primarily affect individuals aged from birth to 18 years, including neonates, infants, children, and adolescents. These criteria qualify all pediatric cancers as rare diseases. Typically, a sponsor submits a request for rare pediatric disease designation prior to submitting a new drug application. The sponsor then may request a voucher at the time of the submission of the application. The FDA must approve the marketing application and the voucher request. Upon approval, the FDA issues a voucher to the company. The priority review voucher is transferable and can be used for any future application irrespective of the indication being sought. The rare pediatric disease voucher program was reauthorized in 2020 and requires reauthorization in 2024 (United States Food and Drug Administration 2017).

As of 2021, the following four rare pediatric disease priority review vouchers have been issued as a result of the approval of an agent for a pediatric oncology or oncology-relevant indication: Unituxin (for neuroblastoma), Kymriah (for B-cell precursor acute lymphoblastic leukemia), Gamifant (for primary hemophagocytic lymphohistiocytosis), and Danyelza (for neuroblastoma).

10.3.3.2 European Union

Similar to BPCA in the United States, the financial incentive stipulated by the EU Paediatric Regulation can be obtained regardless of whether the pediatric studies conducted lead to granting of a new pediatric indication or failed to demonstrate efficacy. Importantly, it is required that the results of these studies are reflected in product labeling, and as such, "negative" studies, which indicate when a product should not be used in children, are also of interest to the FDA and EMA.

Another type of marketing authorization in the EU is the Paediatric Use Marketing Authorisation (PUMA) which was established to incentivize pediatric development of authorized products that are no longer under patent protection. PUMAs are intended to stimulate research of existing medicines to provide better treatments for children or to help transform a known off-label use into an authorized use that is safer and better framed through the marketing authorization. A PUMA granted for a product developed exclusively for use in pediatric patients in compliance with an agreed PIP benefits from 10 years of market protection. So far, only a very limited number of PUMAs have been granted (European Commission 2017).

10.4 Impact of US Pediatric Regulations Prior to FDARA on Pediatric Drug Development

Prior to FDARA, PREA requirements for pediatric studies resulted in meaningful accumulation of data to inform pediatric use for many non-oncologic drugs but did not result in any drug approvals for a pediatric oncologic disease. The lack of approvals is largely because oncology drug development primarily occurs for adult oncologic conditions which are not prevalent in the pediatric population and because many oncol-

Table 10.4 Drugs approved for pediatric oncology indication using data submitted to fulfill a pediatric written request

Agent	Year of pediatric approval	Indication
Imatinib	2003	Ph+ ALL and Ph+ CML
Clofarabine	2004	Relapsed and Refractory ALL
Blinatumomab	2016	ALL
Dasatinib	2017	Ph+ CML in chronic phase
Ipilimumab	2017	Unresectable or metastatic melanoma
Tisagenlecleucel	2017	R/R ALL
Larotrectinib	2018	Metastatic or refractory tumors with NTRK gene fusion
Nilotinib	2018	Ph+ CML R/R Ph+ ALL
Daunorubicin and Cytarabine	2021	t-AML or AML-MRC ages 1 and older

Source: US Food and Drug Administration. Drugs@FDA: FDA-Approved Drugs

ogy drugs under development qualify for orphan drug designation; for these reasons, the vast majority of marketing applications for oncology drugs qualified for full waivers based on the disease or, in the cases of relevant diseases, an exemption from PREA requirements due to orphan designation. Therefore, prior to FDARA, the impact of regulatory provisions to pediatric oncologic drug development in the United States was solely driven by incentivized programs under BPCA provisions.

As of the end of 2020, 40 written requests have been issued for oncologic agents for pediatric indications (Akalu et al. 2021). From the time of the initiation of the BPCA through 2021, nine drugs or biologic products were approved for a pediatric oncologic indication based on a study included in a written request issued by the FDA (Table 10.4).

10.5 Evolving Regulatory Landscape

10.5.1 PREA and the RACE for Children Act

The necessary change in focus of legislative initiatives to protect children through responsible research to ensure their access to safe and effective drugs has resulted in meaningful advances in the development of drugs for many non-oncologic diseases occurring in children but has had a limited impact on improving the treatment of childhood cancers.

Historically, manufacturers have been reluctant to study products in children due to economic, ethical, and perceived legal concerns, among other obstacles. This is particularly true for children with cancer, a vulnerable population with rare and ultra-rare diseases that comprise a small financial market for commercial sponsors developing cancer therapies. Accordingly, approval of a new cancer drug for a pediatric cancer indication without prior approval for an adult cancer indication occurs rarely, and there is an urgent unmet need for new and less toxic treatments for pediatric malignancies.

As discussed in the previous sections, PREA had no impact in oncology because orphan drug designation rendered drug applications exempt from PREA requirements and waivers from the requirement for pediatric assessments were permitted for drugs intended to treat an adult cancer (e.g., breast cancer and prostate cancer) that either does not occur in children or occurs so rarely that the necessary pediatric studies would be impossible or highly impracticable to conduct.

To address this unintended loophole, the Research to Accelerate Cures and Equity (RACE) for Children Act was signed into law on August 18, 2017, as Title V of the 2017 FDA Reauthorization Act (FDARA) to amend PREA, Sec 505B of the FD&C Act, to require, for original applications submitted on or after August 18,

2020, pediatric investigations of certain targeted cancer drugs with new active ingredients, based on molecular mechanism of action rather than clinical indication. FDARA thereby created a mechanism to require evaluation of certain novel agents that may potentially address an unmet medical need in the pediatric population (i.e., children ages 0–2 years, 2–11 years, and adolescents ages 12–<17 years). Specifically, if an initial NDA or BLA (excluding supplemental applications) is for a new active ingredient, and the product that is the subject of the application is intended for treatment of an adult cancer and directed at a molecular target FDA determines to be substantially relevant to the growth or progression of a pediatric cancer, reports on the molecularly targeted pediatric cancer investigation required under Section 505B(a)(3) of the FD&C Act must be submitted with the marketing application, unless the required investigations are waived or deferred (United States Food and Drug Administration 2021a).

FDA, in consultation with the National Cancer Institute, and members of the internal committee established under section 505C of the FD&C Act, the Pediatric Oncology Subcommittee of the Oncologic Drugs Advisory Committee, maintains a publicly accessible list of molecular targets that are considered to be substantially relevant to the growth or progression of a pediatric cancer and that may trigger the requirements for pediatric investigations. Of note, a molecular target to which a specific drug is directed is not required to be on the "The Relevant Molecular Target List" to require a clinical evaluation of the drug in the pediatric population. There is also a separate list of molecular targets that are considered "not substantially relevant" to the growth or progression of pediatric cancers and that could warrant a waiver of pediatric study requirements.

The RACE for Children Act requires affected applications to have an agreed iPSP describing a plan for pediatric clinical investigation(s) designed to yield meaningful data regarding dosing, safety, and preliminary efficacy to inform pediatric labeling, regardless of orphan designation, or a plan to request a waiver or deferral with appropriate justification. The iPSP must be agreed upon by the FDA. The iPSP must include information on the cancer(s) in the pediatric population for which the drug warrants early evaluation, planned pediatric studies, sample size, age-appropriate formulations, statistical analysis plan, timeline of the pediatric development plan, and agreements for pediatric studies with other regulatory agencies.

The RACE for Children Act effectively eliminates orphan exemption for pediatric studies for cancer drugs directed at molecular targets relevant to pediatric cancers. As such, it reinforces FDA's authority to require pediatric studies of oncology products and has the potential to substantially decrease the time frame between characterization of the antitumor activity and safety of novel targeted anticancer drugs in adults and the initial assessment of activity, dosing, and tolerability in children with cancers that have the potential to respond to these drugs.

To facilitate compliance with amended PREA requirements, sponsors can request Early Advice (Type F) meetings, which are held within 30 days of submission of the request, to engage with the Oncology Center of Excellence's Pediatric Oncology Program. The FDA encourages sponsors to consider requesting a meeting during the early stages of formulation of an iPSP to discuss the relevance of a specific target and expectations for early assessment in pediatric populations, unless justification for waiver or deferral can be provided. In pediatric patients with a rare cancer, sponsors are advised to consider innovative study design and seek feedback from FDA regarding planned clinical trials for investigational agents with a specific molecular target. In the first several months following enactment of the FDARA provisions, a significant number of Type F meetings have been requested by industry, and discussions during these meetings have contributed to formulation of agreed iPSPs earlier in the development timeline and resulted in a greater number of agreed iPSPs that contain descriptions of planned pediatric studies. Additionally, there have been more frequent discussions, including Pediatric Cluster Calls and Common Commentaries, among global regulatory health agencies regarding oncology products.

Pediatric legislation in the United States and EU has been successful in increasing the number of clinical studies in children in recent years and providing opportunities for timely initial investigations of potentially safe and effective novel therapies. Although benefits have been delayed in children with cancer, the implementation of the RACE for Children Act in the United States and reduction in class waivers in the EU provide opportunities to further accelerate early pediatric evaluation and development of new anticancer agents for children.

10.6 Responding to the Changing Cancer Drug Development Paradigm

10.6.1 Evolving Cancer Drug Development

The emergence of precision medicine represents a paradigm shift in drug discovery and development. Genomic profiling of cancers has enabled the identification of actionable variants and led to development of targeted agents, changing the landscape of oncology products. Sequencing efforts have found that molecular drivers of certain adult cancers are also implicated in malignancies occurring in children and adolescents across histologies. Up to 50% of pediatric cancers have been reported to harbor a potentially druggable target that may be addressed by a drug already approved for use in adults (Gröbner et al. 2018). Accordingly, novel targeted oncology products may prove effective in the treatment of children with cancer, even if the adult cancer indication does not occur in the pediatric population.

Regulatory agencies acknowledge that conventionally designed pediatric trials may be inefficient and difficult to conduct in children with cancer due to rarity of the disease and pressing unmet need, and as such, flexibility in trial design may be both warranted and necessary. Additionally, due to the inherently different types of cancers that occur in adults and children, limited opportunities exist for extrapolation of efficacy from adult cancer indications to children. As a result, innovative study designs must be also be considered.

Bayesian designs present a more modern clinical trial approach, and pediatric cancer studies are particularly well suited to benefit from these methods. Bayesian approaches account for uncertainty in prior knowledge and incorporate prior knowledge from external data while basing decision-making on posterior probability of efficacy or continuous monitoring as data accrue. Sequential monitoring for efficacy with Bayesian analysis can be a valuable tool that may minimize risk to children by potentially stopping a trial early when warranted based on lack of antitumor activity and preventing further exposure to an ineffective agent (Ye et al. 2020). This reduces risk of unnecessary toxicity and allows patients to pursue other investigational products that may provide greater clinical benefit.

Use of real-world data (RWD) to generate real-world evidence (RWE), including design of external and historical controls, natural history studies, and expanded access data, is being actively explored by commercial sponsors to support clinical drug development and regulatory submissions. The incorporation of such alternative data sources gained momentum through the passage of the twenty-first Century Cures Act in 2016, which tasked the FDA with creating a framework for evaluating RWE for the approval of a medical product. RWD is increasingly relevant in pediatric oncology due to challenges such as disease rarity, vulnerability of patients, poor prognosis including relapsed/refractory tumors, and lack of effective therapies or standard of care which limit the options for a reasonable control in certain diseases. If trials utilizing RWD are well designed and the RWD are fit for purpose, among other criteria, use of RWD has the potential to provide evidence supporting the effectiveness or safety of a new product or in support of labeling changes (e.g., expanded indications) or post-market study requirements for an approved product (United States Food and Drug Administration 2018). Although there is limited experience with use of RWD to support the establishment of efficacy for oncology drugs, the FDA is actively engaging in complex and typically iterative discussions with sponsors interested in pursuing pediatric oncology drug development programs that incorporate use of RWD.

Industry may also consider a variety of strategies to pursue early pediatric assessment of novel therapeutics in the context of adult studies. A pediatric cohort can be included in the expansion phase of an adult clinical trial investigating a target that also occurs in a specific pediatric tumor(s), thereby enabling earlier development in children without having to initiate a dedicated pediatric trial. Adolescent patients may be included at even earlier time points in clinical studies. In general, the FDA strongly encourages broadening eligibility criteria to permit enrollment of adolescent patients in adult oncology trials at all relevant stages of development when the histology and biologic behavior of the cancer is the same in, or the molecular target of the drug is relevant to, cancers in both adult and adolescent patients (United States Food and Drug Administration 2019b). As systemic exposure and clearance of a product are generally similar in adults and adolescents after accounting for the effect of body size on pharmacokinetics, it is often feasible to lower the age requirement of an adult trial to 12 years.

When evaluating a product for a target that is rare in the pediatric population, embedding a pediatric trial within an ongoing adult trial can be an attractive option as it can leverage resources of existing global studies at multiple clinical sites, enhancing enrollment and utilizing infrastructure that is already in place.

Similarly, tissue-agnostic drug development, which typically encompasses tumor types that occur in both pediatric and adult patients, has the potential to provide pediatric patients more timely access to safe and effective targeted therapies that are effective against an oncogenic driver that is essential to the growth of multiple cancers of varying histologies. Investigation of targeted agents in diverse cancers that share a genetic aberration (e.g., neurotrophic receptor tyrosine kinase (NTRK) fusion-positive tumors) or inclusion of pediatric cohorts in adult trials that share a molecular target with pediatric cancers allows for simultaneous study and potential approval of an agent across tumor histologies, resulting in a more widespread impact on patients, particularly those with rare tumor types. In 2017, the FDA granted its first tissue-agnostic approval to pembrolizumab for adult and pediatric patients with unresectable or metastatic, microsatellite instability-high (MSI-H) or mismatch repair deficient (dMMR) solid tumors that have progressed following prior treatment and who have no satisfactory alternative treatment options. Efficacy for pediatric patients with these cancers was extrapolated from the respective adult populations because based on the mechanism of action of pembrolizumab, it would not be expected that response would differ in pediatric patients with MSI-H/dMMR tumors; therefore, the FDA considered it reasonable to extrapolate the effects of pembrolizumab from adults to children. The second product to receive tissue-agnostic FDA approval for the treatment of cancer was larotrectinib, specifically for the treatment of adult and pediatric patients with advanced solid tumors with an NTRK gene fusion without a known acquired resistance mutation who have no satisfactory alternative treatments. Efficacy was established based on data from 55 patients with unresectable or metastatic solid tumors harboring an NTRK gene fusion who were enrolled across three trials. Of these 55 patients, 12 were less than 18 years of age and had rare tumor types including infantile fibrosarcoma, soft tissue sarcoma, and thyroid cancer (U.S. Food and Drugs Administration 2021).

In hand with tissue-agnostic development, master protocols, in the form of basket, umbrella, and platform trials, are being utilized more often in pediatric cancer drug development. Such pediatric precision oncology trials are generally designed to permit streamlined and potentially adaptive biomarker-driven clinical trials while saving time, cost, and other resources. One example of a pediatric master protocol is the Pediatric MATCH (Molecular Analysis for Therapy Choice) trial (NCT03155620), led by the National Cancer Institute and Children's Oncology Group. This US study enrolls patients 1–21 years of age with relapsed or refractory solid tumors, non-Hodgkin lymphoma, and histiocytosis. A sample of the patient's recurrent tumor is submitted for sequencing (over 160 cancer-related genes are tested) and analyzed to determine whether an actionable mutation of interest is present. As of 2021, there are 11 treatment arms with distinct molecular targets using agents that have been tested in or approved for adults. Early reports of this trial have found that 24% of pediatric patients with advanced cancer who had their tumors tested were eligible to receive one of the targeted agents being studied (Parsons et al. 2019).

10.7 International Multi-Stakeholder Collaboration

Because of the limited number of patients diagnosed with pediatric malignancies who may be eligible to be enrolled in clinical trials, particularly with the subdivision of pediatric cancers into smaller subsets based on tumor molecular characteristics, international multi-stakeholder collaboration to facilitate the conduct of global pediatric clinical trials is vital.

Although there are many similarities between the EU and US pediatric laws and regulations, which both aim to facilitate the development of drugs to treat pediatric patients, there are key differences as outlined below (Penkov et al. 2017).

- In the EU, the incentives and requirements for pediatric studies are unified under the Pediatric Regulation, whereas in the United States, pediatric requirements and incentives are provided under separate legal frameworks and therefore have different requirements, processes, and timelines. Thus, fulfillment of the requirement to conduct a pediatric study under PREA in the United States does not confer exclusivity, whereas in the EU, fulfillment of requirements under the pediatric regulation confers exclusivity.
- The scope of EU and US pediatric legislative requirements differs. The EU applies the term "condition" broadly when determining whether pediatric studies are required. In contrast, for US applications submitted prior to the implementation of FDARA, the scope of the requirement for conduct of studies under PREA applied only to the adult indication under development. Under FDARA, the requirement for certain new molecularly targeted cancer drugs and biologics submitted on or after August 18, 2020 to include pediatric investigations in relevant pediatric cancers will facilitate efforts to bring the EU and US requirements in closer alignment.
- The timing of submissions of initial pediatric study plans in the United States (no later than 60 days after an end-of-phase 2 meeting) and pediatric investigational plans (no later than the end of initial tolerability studies) differs.
- After FDASIA, biosimilar products are covered by both PREA requirements and BPCA incentives under US legislation but are exempt from EU requirements.
- In the United States, a mandatory pediatric-focused public safety assessment must be conducted by the Pediatric Advisory Committee 18 months following incorporation of information from pediatric studies conducted under BPCA or PREA into product labeling.

The differences in regulatory requirements and incentives across regulatory bodies and the timing of iPSP and PIP review (see Table 10.5) make communication between agencies crucial to ensure that regulatory milestones are met. The FDA require-

Table 10.5 Comparison of PIP and PSP timelines for review and resubmission

PIP review (EU)	iPSP review (US)
Start of procedure after EMA validation to first PDCO discussion 30 days	Comments to sponsor after initial submission: 90 days
PDCO issuing a request for modification: 30 days	Sponsor to respond: comments or agreement—30 days
Clock stop	Agreed
Restart of procedure to third PDCO discussion: 30 days	Non-agreed: 90 days
Opinion: 30 days	Sponsor response: 30 days
Total length: 120 days (excluding clock stop)	Total length: 210 days

Source: Reaman et al. (2020), U.S. Food and Drug Administration and European Medicines Agency (2021)

ments under the FDARA amendment to PREA require early evaluations of pharmacokinetics, safety, and preliminary efficacy, with further safety and efficacy studies encouraged under the BPCA program. These programs provide overlap with the EMA process under the PIP, allowing opportunity for alignment, when feasible. Programs are in place to foster global interaction between agencies as well as multi-stakeholder engagement.

Transparency by industry sponsors regarding their pediatric development plans to satisfy US and EU requirements, as well as scientific discourse between agencies, can facilitate timely initiation of early-phase studies and a synchronized approach to later-phase development. The main avenue for communication between agencies occurs through Pediatric Cluster Calls. These teleconferences occur regularly between pediatric oncology experts at the FDA and EMA and can also include representatives from Health Canada, Pharmaceuticals and Medical Devices Agency (PMDA) in Japan, and the Therapeutic Goods Administration (TGA) in Australia. Under a confidentiality agreement, the agencies are able to discuss pediatric development plans for new drugs, share scientific insights, and discuss the regulatory decision-making of each entity. Every attempt is made to reach alignment on the design of the pediatric development program for each new drug. After discussion at a Pediatric Cluster Call, the agencies may issue a Common Commentary. Common Commentaries provide a high-level summary of the Pediatric Cluster Call discussion to the commercial sponsors to indicate where alignment was reached, whether additional information may be needed to reach alignment, or where differences in regulatory requirements or clinical management may preclude agreement. The Common Commentary is non-binding but can guide commercial sponsors on their approach to developing the new drug in the pediatric population. Commercial sponsors may request a common commentary for a specific iPSP or PIP. By engaging with regulatory agencies in parallel, commercial sponsors can foster the coordination that is integral to advancing development of drugs to treat pediatric cancers.

The Parallel Scientific Advice (PSA) program provides a more formal mechanism for concurrent dialogue between FDA, EMA, and commercial sponsors. This interaction can be initiated by the commercial sponsor to present their overall product development with both agencies concurrently and is not limited to the pediatric program for that drug. Through the PSA program, a joint meeting is held between all parties for scientific exchange. The PSA is typically limited to a single occurrence for a product, usually early in the lifecycle, so while it can provide an overview of the approach for development of a new drug in the pediatric space, it can have limited utility for ongoing development as new evidence of safety or efficacy develops in a specific pediatric malignancy.

The development of international pediatric clinical trials is challenging due to not only differences in regulatory requirements but also regional differences in clinical management and the overall conduct of clinical trials. Development of an international program requires input of multiple stakeholders including regulatory agencies, commercial sponsors, clinical investigators, parents, patients, and advocacy groups. The ACCELERATE platform was developed by the European Society for Paediatric Oncology (SIOP Europe), the EMA, and ITCC (Innovative Therapies for Children with Cancer in Europe) to bring together all stakeholders in pediatric drug development, including regulatory agencies. The ACCELERATE platform, now international in scope, with active participation by the FDA, has multiple working groups and hosts focused strategy forums to promote international collaboration and multi-stakeholder engagement regarding relevance of a drug to pediatric malignancies, prioritization of agents within disease areas, and development of international pediatric clinical trial programs. The discussions during the strategy forums are published and can provide valuable insight into the approach to drug development for a particular disease area or drug class.

Another venue to provide engagement between the FDA, commercial sponsors, and clinical investigators is the meeting of the Pediatric Oncology Subcommittee of the Oncologic Drugs Advisory Committee. Topics for discussion at the pediatric oncology subcommittee of ODAC can be directed at a particular topic relevant to pediatric drug development or can be focused on a particular drug of interest to the pediatric oncology community to discuss avenues for developing robust clinical trials in anticipation of a written request. These meetings are organized by the FDA with presentations by the commercial sponsors and discussion with the investigator community. Other regulatory agencies are invited to observe these public meetings. The FDA also engages in regular interactions with disease-specific subcommittees of the Children's Oncology Group to increase communication on the prioritization and design of pediatric oncology clinical trials and hosts minisymposia with external constituents often including international regulators to discuss disease-specific research strategies.

Development of novel targeted agents in increasingly small subsets of target-specific pediatric malignancies requires global drug development and discussion between all relevant stakeholders. The multiple venues for scientific exchange allow alignment of pediatric development plans and advancing investigations of potential new agents for the treatment of children with cancer.

10.8 Prospects for Future Advances

The recent FDARA amendment to PREA authorizing the FDA to require pediatric investigation of drugs under development for adult cancers that target a gene or pathway that is substantially relevant to one or more pediatric cancers, in concert with EMA regulations providing incentive and requirements for pediatric drug development and multi-stakeholder initiatives fostering global collaboration, has the potential to transform the landscape of pediatric cancer drug development. This will result in earlier and more complete pediatric assessments for new anticancer drugs. Because appropriate new agents are required to undergo early pediatric evaluations, this will assist the clinical investigators and the patient community to guide new drug development for pediatric malignancies. The BPCA incentive program can then support the conduct of additional pediatric clinical trials, if warranted, based on results of the initial required pediatric investigation, designed to fully characterize the safety and effectiveness of targeted drugs in one or more pediatric cancers that are capable of supporting approval of a marketing application. These two FDA programs allow broad alignment with the EMA PIP and therefore support international pediatric drug development, which is needed for drug development in rare pediatric malignancies.

The combined efforts of the FDA, EMA, and global stakeholder community will result in support for a greater number of new drugs to be investigated in children. This will ultimately shorten the lag time between development of novel agents for adult diseases and initiation of pediatric investigations. While not all drugs under development for adult cancer will be effective in treating pediatric malignancies, it is clear that timely evaluation of appropriate novel agents in pediatric patients will result in an increase in pediatric formulations, dosing and safety information, and demonstration of effectiveness in some pediatric cancers for drugs that may otherwise not have been evaluated. Forward-thinking regulatory flexibility and initiatives are required to facilitate development and approval of agents specifically intended to treat the cancers of childhood.

References

Akalu A et al (2021) A review of the experience with pediatric written requests issued for oncology drug products. Pediatr Blood Cancer 68(2):e28828. https://doi.org/10.1002/pbc.28828

Ballentine C (1981) Taste of raspberries, taste of death: the 1937 elixir sulfanilamide incident. FDA Consumer Magazine. https://www.fda.gov/about-fda/histories-product-regulation/sulfanilamide-disaster. Accessed 28 Aug 2021

Bucci-Rechtweg C (2017) Enhancing the pediatric drug development framework to deliver better pediatric therapies tomorrow. Clin Ther 39(10):1920–1932. https://doi.org/10.1016/j.clinthera.2017.07.043. Epub 2017 Aug 14

European Commission (2017) State of paediatric medicines in the EU: 10 years of the EU Paediatric Regulation. https://ec.europa.eu/health/sites/default/files/files/paediatrics/docs/2017_childrensmedicines_report_en.pdf

European Medicines Agency (1995–2022) Conditional marketing authorisation. https://www.ema.europa.eu/en/humanregulatory/marketing-authorisation/conditional-marketing-authorisation. Accessed 17 July 2022

European Medicines Agency (1995–2021a) Accelerated assessment [online]. Human regulatory, marketing authorisation. https://www.ema.europa.eu/en/human-regulatory/marketing-authorisation/accelerated-assessment. Accessed 30 Aug 2021

European Medicines Agency (1995–2021b) Prime: priority medicines [online]. Human regulatory, research and development. https://www.ema.europa.eu/en/human-regulatory/research-development/prime-priority-medicines. Accessed 30 Aug 2021

European Medicines Agency (2015) European Medicines Agency decision: CW/0001/2015. https://www.ema.europa.eu/en/documents/other/european-medicines-agency-decision-cw-0001-2015-23-july-2015-class-waivers-accordance-regulation-ec_en.pdf. Accessed 30 Aug 2021

European Medicines Agency (2017) 10-year report to the European Commission. https://ec.europa.eu/health/sites/default/files/files/paediatrics/docs/paediatrics_10_years_ema_technical_report.pdf. Accessed 31 Aug 2021

European Medicines Agency (2018) Enhanced early dialogue to facilitate accelerated assessment of PRIority Medicines (PRIME). https://www.ema.europa.eu/en/documents/regulatory-procedural-guideline/enhanced-early-dialogue-facilitate-accelerated-assessment-priority-medicines-prime_en.pdf. Accessed 28 Aug 2021

European Parliament and the Council of the European Union (2006a) Regulation (EC) No. 1902/2006 on medicinal products for pediatric use. https://eur-lex.europa.eu/legal-content/EN/TXT/PDF/?uri=CELEX:32006R1902&from=EN

European Parliament and the Council of the European Union (2006b) Regulation (EC) No. 1901/2006 on medicinal products for pediatric use. https://eur-lex.europa.eu/legal-content/EN/TXT/PDF/?uri=CELEX:32006R1901&from=EN. Accessed 28 Aug 2021

Gröbner S et al (2018) The landscape of genomic alterations across childhood cancers. Nature 555:321–327. https://doi.org/10.1038/nature.25480

Hirschfeld S, Ward RM (2013) History of children and the development of regulations at the FDA. In: Mulberg AE, Murphy D, Dunne J, Mathis L (eds) Pediatric drug development, 2nd edn. Wiley, Hoboken, NJ, pp 6–15

Institute of Medicine (2008) Addressing the barriers to pediatric drug development: workshop summary. The National Academies Press, Washington, DC. http://www.nap.edu/catalog/11911.html. Accessed 28 Aug 2021

Kim J, Scialli A (2011) Thalidomide: the tragedy of birth defects and the effective treatment of disease. Toxicol Sci 122:1–6

Parsons DW et al (2019) Identification of targetable molecular alterations in the NCI-COG pediatric MATCH trial [abstract 10011]. J Clin Oncol 37(15). https://doi.org/10.1200/jco.2019.37.15_suppl.10011

Penkov D, Tomasi P, Eichler I, Murphy D, Yao LP, Temeck J (2017) Pediatric medicine development: an overview and comparison of regulatory processes in the European Union and United States. Ther Innov Regul Sci 51(3):360–371

Reaman G et al (2020) Accelerating the global development of pediatric cancer drugs: a call to coordinate the submissions of pediatric investigation plans and pediatric study plans to the European Medicines Agency and US Food and Drug Administration. J Clin Oncol 38(36):4227–4230. https://doi.org/10.1200/JCO.20.02152

Shirkey H (1968) Editorial commentary: therapeutic orphans. J Pediatr 1968(72):119–120

The Council of Canadian Academies (2014) Improving medicines for children in Canada: the expert panel on therapeutic products for infants, children, and youth. https://cca-reports.ca/wp-content/uploads/2018/10/therapeutics_fullreporten.pdf. Accessed 28 Aug 2021

U.S. Congress (1997) Food and Drug Administration Modernization Act (Public Law 105-115). https://www.govinfo.gov/content/pkg/PLAW-105publ115/pdf/PLAW-105publ115.pdf. Accessed 28 Aug 2021

U.S. Congress (2002) Best Pharmaceuticals for Children Act Amending Section 505A of the Federal Food, Drug & Cosmetic Act (Public Law 107-109). https://www.congress.gov/107/plaws/publ109/PLAW-107publ109.pdf. Accessed 28 Aug 2021

U.S. Congress (2003) Pediatric Research Equity Act Amending Section 505B of the Federal Food, Drug & Cosmetic Act (Public Law 108-155). https://www.congress.gov/108/plaws/publ155/PLAW-108publ155.pdf. Accessed 28 Aug 2021

U.S. Congress (2007) Food and Drug Administration Amendments Act of 2007 (Public Law 110-85). https://www.congress.gov/110/plaws/publ85/PLAW-110publ85.pdf. Accessed 28 Aug 2021

U.S. Congress (2010) Biologics Price and Competition Innovations Act of 2009: Title VII of the Patient Protection and Affordable Care Act (Public Law 111-148). https://www.congress.gov/111/plaws/publ148/PLAW-111publ148.pdf. Accessed 28 Aug 2021

U.S. Congress (2012) Food and Drug Administration Safety and Innovation Act amending Sections 505A, 505B, and 510 of the Federal Food, Drug & Cosmetic Act (Public Law 112-144). https://www.congress.gov/112/plaws/publ144/PLAW-112publ144.pdf. Accessed 28 Aug 2021

U.S. Congress (2017) FDA Reauthorization Act of 2017 (Public Law 115-52). https://www.congress.gov/115/plaws/publ52/PLAW-115publ52.pdf. Accessed 28 Aug 2021

U.S. District Court for the District of Columbia (2002) FDA does not have the authority to require pediatric testing of drugs—Association of American Physicians and Surgeons, Inc. v. U.S. Food and Drug Admin., 226 F.Supp.2d 204 (D.D.C. Oct 17, 2002). Versuslaw. https://biotech.law.lsu.edu/cases/fda/aaps_v_fda.htm. Accessed 28 Aug 2021

U.S. Federal Register (1997) Pediatric patients; regulations requiring manufacturers to assess the safety and effectiveness of new drugs and biological products; proposed rule. https://www.govinfo.gov/content/pkg/FR-1997-08-15/pdf/97-21646.pdf. Accessed 28 Aug 2021

U.S. Food and Drugs Administration (2021) Drugs@FDA: FDA-approved drugs. https://www.accessdata.fda.gov/scripts/cder/daf/index.cfm. Accessed 28 Aug 2021

United States Code of Federal Regulations (2020) Title 21, Volume 5. https://www.accessdata.fda.gov/scripts/cdrh/cfdocs/cfcfr/cfrsearch.cfm?fr=314.126. Accessed 28 Aug 2021

United States Food and Drug Administration (1994) FDA specific requirements on content and format of labeling for human prescription drugs; revision of "pediatric use" subsection in the labeling; Final Rule (21 CFR Part 201). https://www.govinfo.gov/content/pkg/FR-1994-12-13/html/94-30238.htm. Accessed 28 Aug 2021

United States Food and Drug Administration (2014a) Guidance for industry: expedited programs for serious conditions—drugs and biologics. https://www.fda.gov/media/86377/download. Accessed 28 Aug 2021

United States Food and Drug Administration (2014b) Guidance for industry (draft): general clinical pharmacology considerations for pediatric studies for drugs and biological products. https://www.fda.gov/media/90358/download. Accessed 28 Aug 2021

United States Food and Drug Administration (2017) Rare pediatric disease (RPD) designation and voucher programs. https://www.fda.gov/industry/developing-products-rare-diseases-conditions/rare-pediatric-disease-rpd-designation-and-voucher-programs. Accessed 28 Aug 2021

United States Food and Drug Administration (2018) Framework for the FDA's real world evidence program. https://www.fda.gov/media/120060/download. Accessed 28 Aug 2021

United States Food and Drug Administration (2019a) Guidance for industry (draft): rare pediatric disease priority review vouchers. https://www.fda.gov/media/90014/download. Accessed 28 Aug 2021

United States Food and Drug Administration (2019b) Guidance for industry: considerations for the inclusion of adolescent patients in adult oncology clinical trials. https://www.fda.gov/media/113499/download. Accessed 28 Aug 2021

United States Food and Drug Administration (2019c) Guidance for industry (draft): demonstrating substantial evidence of effectiveness for human drug and biological products. https://www.fda.gov/media/133660/download. Accessed 28 Aug 2021

United States Food and Drug Administration (2020a) Designating an orphan product: drugs and biological products. https://www.fda.gov/industry/developing-products-rare-diseases-conditions/designating-orphan-product-drugs-and-biological-products. Accessed 28 Aug 2021

United States Food and Drug Administration (2020b) Guidance for industry: pediatric study plans: content and process for submitting initial pediatric study plans and amended initial pediatric study plans. https://www.fda.gov/media/86340/download. Accessed 28 Aug 2021

United States Food and Drug Administration (2021a) Guidance for industry: FDARA implementation guidance for pediatric studies of molecularly targeted oncology drugs: amendments to Sec. 505B of the FD&C Act. https://www.fda.gov/media/133440/download. Accessed 29 Aug 2021

United States Food and Drug Administration (2022) Qualifying for pediatric exclusivity under Section 505A of the Federal Food, Drug, and Cosmetic Act: frequently asked questions on pediatric exclusivity (505A). https://www.fda.gov/drugs/developmentresources/qualifying-pediatric-exclusivity-under-section-505a-federal-food-drug-and-cosmetic-act-frequently. Accessed July 17 2022

United States Food and Drug Administration and European Medicines Agency (2021) Common Commentary EMA/FDA—common issues requested for discussion by the respective agency (EMA/PDCO and FDA) concerning paediatric oncology development plans (Paediatric Investigation Plans [PIPs] and initial Pediatric Study Plans ([iPSPs]). https://www.ema.europa.eu/en/documents/other/common-commentary-ema/fda-common-issues-requested-discussion-respective-agency-ema/pdco-fda-concerning-paediatric-oncology-development-plans-paediatric-investigation-plans-pips_en.pdf. Accessed 30 June 2021

United States Government Publishing Office (2010a) United States Code, 2006 Edition, Supplement 4, Title 42-The public health and welfare. https://

www.govinfo.gov/content/pkg/USCODE-2010-title42/pdf/USCODE-2010-title42-chap6A-subchapII-partF-subpart1-sec262.pdf. Accessed 28 Aug 2021

United States Government Publishing Office (2010b) United States Code, 2006 Edition, Supplement 4, Title 21-Food and drugs. https://www.govinfo.gov/content/pkg/USCODE-2010-title21/pdf/USCODE-2010-title21-chap9-subchapV-partA-sec355.pdf. Accessed 28 Aug 2021

Wilson J (1999) An update on the therapeutic orphan. Pediatrics 104:585–590

Ye JY et al (2020) A Bayesian approach in design and analysis of pediatric cancer clinical trials. Pharm Stat 19(6):814–826. https://doi.org/10.1002/pst.2039

Ethical Considerations in Pediatric Cancer Therapeutics Development

11

Melanie E. Bhatnagar and Donna L. Snyder

Contents

11.1 Introduction

Significant progress in the treatment of childhood cancer has occurred over the last several decades, attributed largely to medical advances resulting from research and high participation rates for pediatric oncology clinical trials (Adamson 2015). The moral imperative to conduct scientifically and ethically sound research in pediatric oncology is clear—clinical investigation of pediatric cancer therapeutics is necessary to ensure children with cancer have access to safe and effective treatments. Despite this imperative,

M. E. Bhatnagar · D. L. Snyder (✉)
Office of Pediatric Therapeutics, Office of the Commissioner, Food and Drug Administration, Silver Spring, MD, USA
e-mail: Melanie.Bhatnagar@fda.hhs.gov; Donna.Snyder@fda.hhs.gov

J. DiMartino et al. (eds.), *Pediatric Cancer Therapeutics Development*, Pediatric Oncology,
https://doi.org/10.1007/978-3-031-06357-2_11

pediatric oncology research is steeped in moral dilemmas that stem from the necessity of exposing children to research risks despite their inability to provide informed consent, the conflict of the dual role of clinician and investigator, and the struggle to balance hope and realism for families facing a life-threatening condition (Kodish 2003; de Vries et al. 2011). Herein, the ethical principles that guide the conduct of research in children and that underlie US regulatory protections for children involved in clinical investigations will be described with an emphasis on implementing the principles and regulatory requirements in pediatric cancer therapeutics development.

The historical evolution of policies surrounding human research ethics and US human subject protection regulations provide perspective to understand the current paradigm for the ethical conduct of research in children. Implementation of policies in human research ethics largely postdates the Second World War with adoption of the Nuremberg Code in 1947 in response to the atrocities of medical experimentation performed by Nazi physicians (Institute of Medicine 2004). Explicitly interpreted, the Nuremberg Code does not allow for research in children who lack autonomy and decision-making capacity to legally consent to research participation (U.S. Government Printing Office 1949). Children are vulnerable to exploitation because they are subject to the authority of others and may not be able to fully protect their own interests (Roth-Cline and Nelson 2015). Historical examples lay bare the reality of the vulnerabilities of children, the most prominent example being the experiments at New York's Willowbrook State School from 1956 to 1972 wherein researchers intentionally infected healthy institutionalized children with hepatitis to study the natural history of the disease (Institute of Medicine 2004). Henry Beecher described unethical research practices in this study and others in his often-cited 1966 article published in the New England Journal of Medicine. Beecher's article contributed to public debate and controversy over the ethics of human subject research (Beecher 1966). Societal outcry was further spurred in the 1970s after revelations of the Tuskegee Study of the natural history of syphilis were publicized. In this study, researchers had followed black men diagnosed with syphilis without informing them of their condition nor treating them (Institute of Medicine 2004).

In response to these human research abuses, Congress passed the National Research Act in 1974 which established institutional review board (IRB) oversight of human subject research and created a National Commission for the Protection of Human Subjects of Biomedical and Behavioral Research ("National Commission") which was tasked with defining the underlying principles by which to abide when conducting human subject research, including research in children (Institute of Medicine 2004). Aware of deliberations over the ensuing decades since the Nuremberg Code, including concerns that children had become "therapeutic orphans" (quoted from pediatrician and clinical pharmacologist Harry Shirkey in 1968), the National Commission keenly understood that without involvement in clinical trials, children may not fully benefit from the rapid progress in medicine that is driven by scientific research. This imperative to conduct research in children was further evidenced by later legislative efforts such as the Pediatric Rule of 1994, the Best Pharmaceuticals for Children Act (BPCA) of 2002, and the Pediatric Research Equity Act (PREA) of 2003 which either encourage or require pharmaceutical industry sponsors to study drug and biological products in children.

Industry sponsors for oncology products often have received waivers of PREA requirements because the adult cancer indication does not occur or occurs rarely in children or because the product has received an exemption based on orphan designation. With passage of the Research to Accelerate Cures and Equity (RACE) for Children Act in 2017, the principles underlying the legislative mandates of PREA are applied to pediatric cancer research when the molecular target of the product is relevant to the growth or progression of a pediatric cancer (Food and Drug Administration 2019a). In this context, the evolution of clinical research in pediatric cancer continues—as does the importance of maintaining ethical standards to protect children involved in research.

11.2 Ethical Principles Defined by the National Commission and Regulatory Framework for Safeguarding Children Involved in Clinical Investigations

The National Commission's most prominent manuscript, the *Belmont Report*, outlined three basic principles to guide ethical research involving humans: respect for persons, beneficence, and justice (National Commission 1979). Embedded in respect for persons is the principle of autonomy—with an emphasis on the provision of voluntary, informed consent for participation in research—and added protections for those with diminished autonomy. An important element of respect for persons is ensuring that research participants are not asked to expose themselves to risks in studies that are not properly designed to answer an important scientific question. The importance of the knowledge to be gained from research must be given utmost consideration. In clinical research, this requires an understanding of the disease and the landscape of therapeutic development to clearly delineate information gaps and therapeutic needs, ensure research equipoise (i.e., genuine uncertainty regarding whether the study intervention or control is better), and prioritize patient enrollment in studies for promising therapeutics. When establishing a clinical trial protocol, consideration must be given to whether completion of the study is feasible (e.g., enough patients exist to meet the target enrollment) and whether the study design and statistical analysis will be adequate to confidently answer the research questions. Beneficence refers to the researcher's obligation to care for an individual's well-being first by doing no harm (nonmaleficence) and second by maximizing potential benefits and minimizing potential harms in research. In the research context, the concept of justice involves ensuring the burden and potential harms and benefits of research are distributed fairly (Institute of Medicine 2004).

Injustice can range from exploitation of vulnerable groups or groups who are unlikely to benefit from any knowledge gained in the research to the converse extreme of failure to include groups who could benefit from the scientific knowledge. When establishing recommendations for its report on *Research Involving Children*, the National Commission considered the vulnerabilities of children that raise questions about the ethical acceptability of involving them in research. The National Commission also considered the need to conduct clinical research in children to ensure that children have therapies available with evidence to support their safe and effective use in children (i.e., as a matter of justice) (National Commission 1978). One concept described by the National Commission that is grounded in considerations of social justice has been coined the "principle of scientific necessity." This principle maintains that children should not be enrolled in a clinical trial unless necessary to answer an important scientific and/or public health question about the health and welfare of children that cannot be answered by enrolling consenting adults (Roth-Cline and Nelson 2014; Roth-Cline et al. 2011). In addition to this core principle, the National Commission described three other pillars which together serve as the ethical framework for research in children, namely, that (1) absent a prospect of direct clinical benefit, the risks to which children are exposed must be low, (2) children should not be placed at a disadvantage by being enrolled in a clinical trial, and (3) children should have a suitable proxy to provide permission for them to enroll in a clinical trial. The National Commission's report was used as the basis for establishing the additional safeguards for children involved in research that are codified into US regulations under Subpart D of 45 CFR 46 for federally supported or conducted research and Subpart D of 21 CFR 50 for research regulated by the Food and Drug Administration (FDA).

11.2.1 Additional Safeguards for Children Involved in Clinical Investigations (21 CFR 50, Subpart D)

Children involved in research are afforded additional protections under FDA regulations (21 CFR 50, Subpart D) (Food and Drug Administration 2001, 2013). These regulations specify that children should not be enrolled in research that exceeds a defined level of risk unless the risks are justified by the prospect of direct benefit to the child and the balance of risks and benefits is at least as favorable as that of the available alternatives. In this context, the term "children" applies to neonates, infants, children, and adolescents who have not reached the legal age to consent to treatments or procedures in clinical trials (21 CFR 50.3(o)). Under these regulations, IRBs can approve research involving children only if the research falls into one of the following categories:

1. Clinical investigations not involving greater than minimal risk (21 CFR 50.51).
2. Clinical investigations involving greater than minimal risk but presenting the prospect of direct benefit to individual subjects (21 CFR 50.52).
3. Clinical investigations involving greater than minimal risk and no prospect of direct benefit to individual subjects but likely to yield generalizable knowledge about the subjects' disorder or condition (note: the level of risk allowed in this category is capped at a "minor increase over minimal risk") (21 CFR 50.53).

For clinical investigations that are not approvable under any of these categories but present an opportunity to understand, prevent, or alleviate a serious problem affecting the health and welfare of children, an IRB may refer the proposed investigation to the FDA Commissioner for review in consultation with a panel of experts and an opportunity for public comment (21 CFR 50.54). For all clinical investigations involving children, adequate provisions must be in place for obtaining parental permission and, when appropriate, child assent (21 CFR 50.55).

11.3 Interpreting and Applying the Ethical Principles and Regulatory Framework in Pediatric Cancer Therapeutics Development

11.3.1 Scientific Necessity and Pediatric Extrapolation

Before initiating a pediatric clinical trial, consideration should be given to the scientific necessity of collecting data in children, including consideration for whether efficacy data from adult clinical trials could be extrapolated to establish efficacy in children ("pediatric extrapolation"). According to federal regulation, pediatric extrapolation is permissible for pediatric product development programs if the course of the disease and the product's effects are sufficiently similar in pediatric and adult populations (Food and Drug Administration 2018a; Federal Register 1994). The degree of similarity dictates how relevant the adult efficacy data may be for children and guides decisions regarding the knowledge gaps that need to be filled to establish evidence of pediatric efficacy. Reliance on adult efficacy data can limit the amount of evidence needed in children, potentially allowing for fewer or less burdensome pediatric clinical trials (Nelson 2020; Momper et al. 2020).

FDA approval of several oncologic products in children has relied upon extrapolation, including Bavencio (avelumab) for metastatic Merkel cell carcinoma, Blincyto (blinatumomab) for B-cell precursor acute lymphoblastic leukemia, and Keytruda (pembrolizumab) for classical Hodgkin lymphoma, primary mediastinal B-cell lymphoma, and microsatellite instability-high and tumor mutational burden-high cancers (Bavencio 2017; Blincyto 2014; Keytruda 2014). Each of these programs relied on efficacy data obtained from adequate and well-controlled studies in adults, along with pediatric safety and pharmacokinetic information, to support the accompanying pediatric indication. However, due to differences in the etiology, tumor biology, and natural history of pediatric and adult cancers, pediatric extrapolation has not been utilized commonly in oncology (Leong et al. 2017).

11.3.2 Prospect of Direct Benefit in Pediatric Oncology Trials

Pediatric oncology trials of investigational therapeutics typically entail exposing participants to risks that exceed the "minor increase over minimal risk" threshold. As such, these trials generally are evaluated by IRBs under 21 CFR 50.52 which specifies that the risks must be justified by the prospect of direct benefit and the balance of anticipated benefits and risks must be at least as favorable as any available alternative therapeutic options. *Direct benefit* in pediatric clinical research refers to a therapeutic benefit that arises directly from the research intervention (i.e., not from ancillary procedures included in the protocol) and accrues directly to the individual child participating in the research. FDA generally has evaluated the *prospect of direct benefit* from an investigational product based on evidence to support the proof of concept, typically derived from a compilation of multiple data sources (e.g., in vitro mechanistic studies, in vivo studies in animal models, clinical studies in adults, or prior studies in children) and supported by a strong scientific rationale and on the structure of the study intervention (e.g., enrollment population, dose selection, and duration of treatment as specified in the protocol). Rarely, substantive nonclinical evidence of antitumor activity alone may be relied upon to support the prospect of direct benefit, particularly if adults with a relevant cancer type do not exist (Food and Drug Administration 2018b). Selecting a suitable nonclinical model and ensuring adequate sample sizes, use of blinding, and appropriate endpoint selection is critical to ensure the data are valid and interpretable. Evidence from other products in the same pharmacological class or with a similar mechanism of action also can contribute to the weight of evidence (Food and Drug Administration 2019b).

Beyond a strong scientific and biologically plausible rationale for use of the product in a particular cancer, the eligibility criteria, including expression of target-specific biomarkers, are important to consider when assessing whether inhibition of a specific molecular target proven to drive a tumor provides a prospect of benefit from participation. Eligibility criteria need to specify participant characteristics (e.g., age, stage of disease, and relevant prognostic features) that are sensible based on the mechanism of action of the drug and that take into consideration the natural history of the disease and the alternative treatment options available. Appropriate dose selection also is important to ensure pediatric trial participants receive a dose that is likely to be both therapeutic and tolerable. Finally, the study duration and endpoint selection need to reflect considerations similar to those made in clinical practice for treatment duration and clinical outcome assessment, such as partial or complete response or duration of response (early-phase trials) and survival, time to progression, and progression-free survival (later stage trials). If the clinical significance of a molecularly-defined pharmacodynamic (PD) endpoint has been established, assessment of the molecular endpoint may be sufficient to make judgments regarding the potential for clinical benefit.

Nonclinical toxicology studies and prior clinical studies with the product or product class may be useful for assessing the potential short-term risks in children. Determining whether the prospect of direct benefit is sufficient to justify the risks of the intervention in the context of the alternative treatment options is complex and relies on sound scientific, clinical, and moral judgment.

11.3.2.1 Eligibility Criteria: Considerations for the Age of Enrollment

Eligibility criteria for an oncology trial should take into consideration the product's mechanism of action, the characteristics of the disease under study, and the product's anticipated safety profile. Automatic exclusion of pediatric patients may not be appropriate, particularly for cancers in which the driving tumor biology and molecular target span the age ranges distinguished legally as children versus adults. Inclusion or exclusion of pediatric patients in a clinical trial should be justified based on a clear scientific and clinical rationale guided by existing knowledge derived from nonclinical and/or clinical studies of the product or related products and the underlying biology and natural history of the disease. Pediatric enrollment should be considered when there is evidence to suggest that the potential benefits outweigh the risks in the context of the child's disease and alternative treatment options. Thoughtful consideration of pediatric enrollment helps to ensure the safety and efficacy of a product are evaluated across the population likely to use the product in clinical practice. For cancers that are similar in histology and biologic behavior in adults and adolescents (e.g., some soft tissue and bone sarcomas, central nervous system tumors, leukemias and lymphomas, and melanoma), consideration may be given to including adolescents (12 years of age and older) concurrently with adults in confirmatory trials or in early-phase trials once sufficient initial PK, efficacy, and safety data are obtained in adults, given that adult and adolescent dosing often are similar and stand-alone trials in adolescents may be challenging to conduct (Food and Drug Administration 2019c; Gore et al. 2017).

Plans to stagger enrollment of pediatric patients by chronologic age should be scientifically justified. Proof-of-concept data to support *prospect of direct benefit* generally apply to patients of all ages in whom the disease and the anticipated effectiveness of the product are expected to be similar. The anticipated safety profile of the product, however, may differ substantially based on age, particularly for products that may adversely impact growth and/or development and for neonates and children less than 2 years of age in whom maturational differences may alter the product's PK and/or effects on biomarkers related to safety (Food and Drug Administration 2014). Additional data also may be needed to establish optimal dosing for younger children due to these differences. As such, assessment of the balance of potential benefits and risks may differ based on chronologic age and may require staged trial enrollment to obtain additional data from one age group before proceeding in another, typically oldest to youngest. Additionally, in exceptional circumstances wherein more limited data are relied upon to support the potential benefits and risks, consideration may be given to first including older pediatric patients (i.e., adolescents 12 years and older) who typically have similar dosing as observed in adults and who have greater autonomy and ability to assent to participation.

11.3.2.2 Early-Phase Pediatric Oncology Trials

The ethics of early-phase pediatric oncology trials has been considered extensively in the literature (Kodish 2003; Ackerman 1995a, b; Dupont et al. 2016; Haylett 2009). The primary concern is whether these studies—which expose children to serious risks—can be considered to offer the prospect of direct therapeutic benefit given that the scientific justification is generally based on more limited evidence; the objective of the trial typically is dose-finding and toxicity assessment, with only a preliminary evaluation of activity and/or efficacy; and participants may be exposed to subtherapeutic dosing (Dupont et al. 2016; Sisk et al. 2019). IRBs and bioethicists can vary in their interpretation of *prospect* of direct benefit, ranging from possible (i.e., any chance for direct benefit is sufficient) to likely (i.e., a higher and more defined probability of benefit must exist) (Kodish 2003; Ross 2006; King 2000; Bhatnagar et al. 2021). The generally dismal response rates observed in phase 1 trials of traditional cytotoxic drugs often are highlighted as evidence against the likelihood of experiencing benefit (Kodish 2003; Ackerman 1995a). However, whether an intervention offers a prospect of direct benefit is separate from whether that prospect of benefit is of sufficient probability, magnitude, and type to justify the risks of the intervention in the context of the child's condition and alternative treatment options. For early-phase pediatric oncology trials, the population specified for enrollment generally suffers from refractory, progressive, and incurable disease, and any chance for remission or disease stabilization might be viewed as a reasonable prospect of therapeutic benefit to justify the risks to allow IRB approval. A patient and family's choice to participate in such a trial, however, must focus on serving the best interests of the child, not only taking into consideration the potential benefits and risks of the investigational product but also addressing both the child's sense of hope and altruism and the benefits of palliative care alone, potentially spending more time at home and refraining from any additional pain, discomfort, and suffering associated with trial participation (Kodish 2003; Ackerman 1995b).

The FDA has encouraged allowing inclusion of pediatric patients for whom no curative options exist in early-phase oncology trials when compelling nonclinical or early adult clinical data suggest antitumor activity and adequate information is available to mitigate patient risk (Food and Drug Administration 2019b). The FDA has provided guidance to investigators and industry sponsors regarding use of multiple expansion cohort trial designs for first-in-human oncology trials, including when inclusion of a pediatric cohort is appropriate. These trials are intended to expedite product development by allowing seamless progression to assessment of antitumor activity once a potentially effective dose is identified. Pediatric cohorts typically should enroll after a reasonably safe dose and preliminary activity have been established in adults, though substantive nonclinical evidence of activity in tumor-derived cell lines or patient-derived xenografts alone may provide sufficient justification for pediatric enrollment in exceptional circumstances. According to FDA guidance, eligibility for these trials should be restricted to patients with relapsed or refractory disease for whom no curative treatment exists (Food and Drug Administration 2018b).

11.3.2.3 Optimizing Prospect of Direct Benefit: Dose Selection and Study Design in the Era of Molecularly Targeted Products

Early-phase oncology trials of cytotoxic drugs traditionally have been designed with an emphasis on risk minimization, initiating with conservatively low dosing followed by algorithmic dose escalation based on toxicity and an assumption that the maximum tolerated dose is necessary to achieve optimal antitumor effect. Newer molecularly targeted therapies may allow for refined dosing predictions based on an understanding of the product's pharmacokinetic (PK) and pharmacodynamic (PD) (e.g., impact on specific disease biomarkers) properties, recognizing that the optimal biological dose may not necessarily be the maximally tolerated dose. Understanding exposure-response—how PK measures (i.e., parameters such as volume of distribution and clearance that reflect the body's processing of the product) are linked with PD properties (i.e., the product's effects on biomarkers or clinical outcomes for safety and efficacy)—allows for selecting a dose(s) that can provide the optimal clinical response. In cases wherein the adult and pediatric exposure-response is expected to be similar, modeling and simulation using adult PK/PD data may be used to identify an appropriate initial dose for pediatric trials with consideration of the effect of body size (Leong et al. 2017; Food and Drug Administration 2014). Pediatric PK analysis to confirm the PK estimates can be conducted during the efficacy trial, recognizing that dedicated single-dose PK studies in children generally are not allowable under the Subpart D regulations (unless existing safety information is available to characterize the risk of a single dose as imposing no more than a minor increase over minimal risk) (Roth-Cline and Nelson 2015).

Use of modeling and simulation may be most appropriate when used to identify an initial dose and then to refine the dose using PK and/or PD information collected within the context of an adaptive trial design (e.g., seamless phase 1/2 trials). In an adaptive trial design, toxicity and efficacy information collected during the trial can be incorporated and used to modify and optimize dosing within the trial itself (Thall and Cook 2004). Such approaches represent a paradigm shift from the traditional assessment of toxicity with dose escalation and may limit potential exposure to subtherapeutic dosing in early-phase oncology trials (Doussau et al. 2016). Some may argue that this approach is ethically problematic, citing concerns that therapeutic misconception may be reinforced, that the efficacy of lower (potentially less toxic) doses may be missed, and that by not prioritizing safety, participants are exposed to risks that may exceed the low probability of therapeutic benefit. This latter point raises concerns that participants may be harmed, potentially tarnishing the public's view of research and hindering the larger research community. Others have highlighted that patients with cancer often enroll in early-phase trials motivated by the hope for therapeutic benefit and argue that shifting the focus toward improving the chances of benefit through model-based adaptive trial designs that promote the potential for therapeutic benefit while limiting risks will better respect the motivations of trial participants (Sisk et al. 2019). This latter perspective may be particularly relevant when considering enrollment of children with cancer in early-phase trials given the regulatory safeguards described above which necessitate that children exposed to higher research risks must have the prospect of direct therapeutic benefit.

11.3.3 Analysis and Minimization of Risk in Pediatric Oncology Trials

When evaluating risk in pediatric clinical trials, each intervention and procedure included in the protocol needs to be assessed individually in a process known as *component analysis*. Any research intervention or procedure that does not offer the prospect of direct benefit must not exceed a "minor increase over minimal risk" (21 CFR 50.53) to participants, unless reviewed by a federal panel and allowed to proceed by the FDA Commissioner (21 CFR 50.54). Importantly, the potential benefits of one intervention or procedure cannot justify the risks presented by another, and the collective risk of all non-beneficial interventions and procedures cannot exceed the minor increase over minimal risk threshold (Institute of Medicine 2004; National Commission 1978).

Conducting a component analysis requires an understanding of how "minimal risk" and "minor increase over minimal risk" are defined and interpreted. Minimal risk is defined as risk for which the probability and magnitude of harm are no greater than what is "ordinarily encountered in daily life or during the performance of routine physical or psychological examinations or tests" (21 CFR 56.102(i)). The National Commission and the Institute of Medicine have recommended that these experiences of daily life should be interpreted in relation to those of an average healthy child (Institute of Medicine 2004; National Commission 1978). Physical examination, chest X-ray, venipuncture, and vision testing are examples of procedures that constitute minimal risk (Institute of Medicine 2004). A minor increase over minimal risk refers to risk that extends beyond the narrow boundaries of minimal risk but poses "no significant threat to the child's health or well-being" (National Commission 1978). For research that exposes children to this level of risk, the child must either have or be at high risk for a disorder or condition and the research must be "likely to yield generalizable knowledge about the [child's] disorder or condition that is of vital importance for the understanding or amelioration of the [child's] disorder or condition" (21 CFR 50.53). Lumbar puncture, bone marrow aspirate, and urine collection via catheter are examples of procedures that constitute a minor increase over minimal risk (Institute of Medicine 2004).

Interventions or procedures that often require special consideration when conducting a component protocol analysis include use of placebo, biopsies, and nontherapeutic procedural sedation. While pediatric oncology trials generally do not include a placebo arm, the risks of a placebo and the risk of withholding any established effective therapies would be considered as part of a component analysis. Because participants in a placebo arm do not have a prospect of therapeutic benefit directly from the placebo, the overall risks to which they are exposed cannot exceed a minor increase over minimal risk. Protocol-specified biopsies that are normally performed in the context of clinical care or that are important for appropriate treatment stratification are considered to offer a prospect of direct benefit. Biopsies performed solely for research purposes, however, do not offer the prospect of direct benefit and so cannot exceed the minor increase over minimal risk threshold unless reviewed by a federal panel (Anderson et al. 2004). Similarly, use of sedation to perform research-only procedures must fall within the minor increase over minimal risk threshold. In March 2015, the FDA convened a meeting of the Pediatric Ethics Subcommittee of the Pediatric Advisory Committee to discuss whether nontherapeutic procedural sedation could be considered to fall within this risk threshold. The subcommittee was unable to reach consensus but did agree on several recommendations for risk reduction if an IRB were to allow nontherapeutic procedural sedation under this category. Their recommendations emphasize the need for qualified providers, rigorous scientific justification, and potential exclusion of children with conditions that may place them at higher risk (Food and Drug Administration 2015).

Every effort should be made to minimize risks and burden for children involved in research. Study interventions and procedures should be limited to only those which are necessary to meet an important scientific objective and should be aligned with clinical care when feasible to reduce research burden. For example, the number and frequency of imaging studies should be restricted to only those necessary, taking into consideration the risks associated with radiation and contrast agents. Blood sampling frequency and volumes also should be limited, particularly given the added potential hematologic toxicities of oncologic therapeutics and the risks associated with accessing and maintaining sterility associated with a central line (Howie 2011; Cole et al. 2006). When PK analysis is necessary, a population PK (PopPK) approach is particularly appropriate in children because it allows for infrequent (i.e., sparse) blood sampling compared to the rich sampling associated with traditional PK analyses. The volume of blood sampling potentially can be minimized with use of micro-volume drug assays, particularly for neonates (Food and Drug Administration 2019d).

Pediatric patients should be treated in facilities appropriate to address the unique care needs of the pediatric population (Food and Drug Administration 2019b). Safety monitoring during a clinical trial is critical to ensure adverse product effects are appropriately identified and managed. Potential risks that are unique to children may not be detected in nonclinical toxicology studies or studies in adults, including adverse effects on growth and development or related to differences in how a product is absorbed, distributed, metabolized, or excreted due to continuing maturation of these processes, especially in neonates and children less than 2 years of age (Food and Drug Administration 2014). IRBs and independent safety assessment or data monitoring committees should include appropriate pediatric oncology and pediatric ethics expertise (Food and Drug Administration 2006).

11.4 Parental Permission and Child Assent

As described above, respect for persons, including an individual's autonomy and right to provide informed and voluntary consent, is one of the three basic principles guiding ethical research in humans (National Commission 1979). Obtaining parental permission for a child's participation in research serves to respect and protect this vulnerable population, and obtaining child assent serves to respect the child's developing autonomy (Institute of Medicine 2004).

For research involving an FDA-regulated product, the process and documentation of parental permission must be in accordance with regulations found under Subparts B and D of 21 CFR 50, unless a waiver is granted. An IRB may consider a waiver of parental permission for (1) life-threatening situations in which immediate use of an investigational product is deemed necessary to save the life of the child, no other therapies are available, and time is not sufficient to obtain parental permission (21 CFR 50.23), (2) research in an emergency setting (21 CFR 50.24), and (3) research involving no more than minimal risk when specific criteria are met (Food and Drug Administration 2017).

Adequate provisions also must be in place for soliciting the child's assent to participate in research (21 CFR 50.55). Federal regulations define assent as "a child's affirmative agreement to participate in research" and further specify that "mere failure to object should not, absent affirmative agreement, be construed as assent" (21 CFR 50.3(n)). The precise age at which assent can be achieved is difficult to define and must take into consideration the variable maturity and decision-making capacity and psychological state of children involved in the research. For reference, the National Commission recommended that assent be required for children 7 years of age and older (National Commission 1978), though others have suggested based on empirical data that age 9 or 10 years is an appropriate threshold for IRBs to begin expecting child involvement in decision-making for cancer clinical trials (Joffe et al. 2006). IRBs are given considerable discretion in determining if assent is required and how assent is obtained and documented. An IRB can waive the requirement for child assent if (1) the child is not capable of assent, (2) the clinical investigation offers a prospect of direct benefit important to the health or well-being of the child and is available only in the context of the trial, or (3) for the same reasons listed above under which parental permission can be waived. Regardless, all children participating in a trial should receive developmentally appropriate information about the study and their role and should be invited to share their views on study participation over time, taking into consideration their emerging autonomy and capacity with age (Joffe et al. 2006). Parental permission and child assent should be considered an ongoing process and not merely a one-time event (Institute of Medicine 2004).

Research in pediatric oncology presents several unique challenges to the process of obtaining permission and assent. Oncology research often is integrated with clinical care, so investigators must balance their role as a scientist and clinician and help families navigate the distinction between research and clinical care (Kodish 2003). Thoughtful discussion of the comparative advantages and disadvantages of participating in a trial or opting for alternatives, including palliative care, can help to avoid what has been coined *therapeutic misconception*, or belief that the purpose of the research is treatment (Institute of Medicine 2004). When discussing the potential for trial participation, investigator's must take into consideration the emotionally charged context of childhood cancer and a family's potential feelings of denial, guilt, helplessness, or hope for outcomes that are no longer appropriate to the child's condition which may impact their ability to consider trial participation in a way that truly reflects their values and goals (Ackerman 1995b).

11.5 Conclusions

Despite major therapeutic advances, cancer remains the leading cause of childhood death from disease (Heron 2013). Clinical investigation of promising new therapeutics will be necessary to continue the remarkable progress in the treatment of childhood cancer that has been witnessed over the preceding decades. Advances in biomedical science and technology will undoubtedly continue to improve our understanding of cancer biology and allow more targeted product development. Ensuring children with cancer benefit from these scientific advances will require thoughtful consideration for their enrollment in clinical trials that is grounded on the ethical principles that guide research in humans—respect for persons, beneficence, and justice—and that accounts for the additional safeguards necessary to protect children because they are unable to provide informed consent to research participation. Clinicians, investigators, industry sponsors, regulators, and IRBs must make every effort to limit the risks and burden to which children are exposed, enhance the potential benefits they may experience, and communicate clearly these potential benefits and risks to children and their families so they may make decisions about participating in research that are well informed and reflective of their values and goals.

References

Ackerman TF (1995a) Ethical issues: phase I pediatric oncology trials. J Pediatr Oncol Nursing 12:143–145

Ackerman TF (1995b) The ethics of phase I pediatric oncology trials. IRB 17:1–5

Adamson PC (2015) Improving the outcome for children with cancer: development of targeted new agents. CA Cancer J Clin 65(3):212–220. https://doi.org/10.3322/caac.21273

Anderson BD, Adamson PC, Weiner SL, McCabe MS, Smith MA (2004) Tissue collection for correlative studies in childhood cancer clinical trials: ethical considerations and special imperatives. J Clin Oncol 22(23):4846–4850. https://doi.org/10.1200/JCO.2004.02.138

Bavencio (2017) Bavencio (avelumab) labeling. https://www.accessdata.fda.gov/drugsatfda_docs/label/2017/761049s000lbl.pdf

Beecher HK (1966) Ethics and clinical research. N Engl J Med 274(24):1354–1360. https://doi.org/10.1056/NEJM196606162742405

Bhatnagar M, Sheehan S, Sharma I, Baer G, Green D, McCune S et al (2021) Prospect of direct benefit in pediatric trials: practical challenges and potential solutions. Pediatrics 147(5):e2020049602. https://doi.org/10.1542/peds.2020-049602

Blincyto (2014) Blincyto (blinatumomab) labeling. https://www.accessdata.fda.gov/drugsatfda_docs/label/2020/125557s017lbl.pdf

Cole M, Boddy AV, Kearns P, Teh KH, Price L, Parry A et al (2006) Potential clinical impact of taking multiple blood samples for research studies in paediatric oncology: how much do we really know? Pediatr Blood Cancer 46(7):723–727. https://doi.org/10.1002/pbc.20463

de Vries MC, Houtlosser M, Wit JM et al (2011) Ethical issues at the interface of clinical care and research practice in pediatric oncology: a narrative review of parents' and physicians' experiences. BMC Med Ethics 12:1–11

Doussau A, Geoerger B, Jimenez I, Paoletti X (2016) Innovations for phase I dose-finding designs in pediatric oncology clinical trials. Contemp Clin Trials 47:217–227. https://doi.org/10.1016/j.cct.2016.01.009

Dupont JC, Pritchard-Jones K, Doz F (2016) Ethical issues of clinical trials in paediatric oncology from 2003 to 2013: a systematic review. Lancet Oncol 17(5):e187–e197. https://doi.org/10.1016/S1470-2045(16)00142-X

Federal Register [59 FR 64240-64250] (1994) Human drugs: pediatric use subsection of professional labeling requirements

Food and Drug Administration (2001) Additional safeguards for children in clinical investigations of food and drug administration-regulated products. Fed Regist 66(79):20589–20600

Food and Drug Administration (2006) Guidance for clinical trial sponsors: establishment and operation of clinical trial data monitoring committees. https://www.fda.gov/media/75398/download

Food and Drug Administration (2013) Additional safeguards for children in clinical investigations of food and drug administration-regulated products. Fed Regist 78(38):12937–12951

Food and Drug Administration (2014) Guidance for industry: general clinical pharmacology considerations for pediatric studies for drugs and biological products. https://www.fda.gov/regulatory-information/search-fda-guidance-documents/general-clinical-pharmacology-considerations-pediatric-studies-drugs-and-biological-products

Food and Drug Administration (2015) Pediatric procedural sedation. Minutes of the Pediatric Ethics Subcommittee of the Pediatric Ethics Advisory Committee, 23 Mar 2015. http://wayback.archive-it.org/7993/20180127092544/https://www.fda.gov/downloads/AdvisoryCommittees/CommitteesMeetingMaterials/PediatricAdvisoryCommittee/UCM510177.pdf.

Food and Drug Administration (2017) IRB waiver or alteration of informed consent for clinical investigations involving no more than minimal risk to human subjects: guidance for sponsors, investigators, and institutional review boards. https://www.fda.gov/media/106587/download

Food and Drug Administration (2018a) Guidance for industry: E11 (R1) addendum: clinical investigation of medicinal products in the pediatric population. https://www.fda.gov/regulatory-information/search-fda-guidance-documents/e11r1-addendum-clinical-investigation-medicinal-products-pediatric-population. Accessed 11 May 2019

Food and Drug Administration (2018b) Guidance for industry: expansion cohorts: use in first-in-human clinical trials to expedite development of oncology drugs and biologics. https://www.fda.gov/media/115172/download

Food and Drug Administration (2019a) FDARA implementation guidance for pediatric studies of molecularly targeted oncology drugs: Amendments to Sec. 505B of the FD&C Act Guidance for Industry. https://www.fda.gov/media/133440/download

Food and Drug Administration (2019b) Cancer clinical trial eligibility criteria: minimum age for pediatric patients

Food and Drug Administration (2019c) Guidance for industry: considerations for the inclusion of adolescent patients in adult oncology clinical trials. https://www.fda.gov/media/113499/download

Food and Drug Administration (2019d) Population pharmacokinetics guidance for industry. https://www.fda.gov/media/128793/download

Gore L, Ivy SP, Balis FM, Rubin E, Thornton K, Donoghue M et al (2017) Modernizing clinical trial eligibility: recommendations of the American Society of Clinical Oncology-Friends of Cancer Research Minimum Age Working Group. J Clin Oncol 35(33):3781–3787. https://doi.org/10.1200/JCO.2017.74.4144

Haylett WJ (2009) Ethical considerations in pediatric oncology phase I clinical trials according to the Belmont report. J Pediatr Oncol Nurs 26(2):107–112. https://doi.org/10.1177/1043454208328764

Heron M (2013) Deaths: leading causes for 2010. Natl Vital Stat Rep 62(6):1–96

Howie SR (2011) Blood sample volumes in child health research: review of safe limits. Bull World Health Organ 89(1):46–53. https://doi.org/10.2471/BLT.10.080010

Institute of Medicine (2004) Committee on clinical research involving children, ethical conduct of clinical research involving children. National Academies Press, Washington, DC

Joffe S, Fernandez CV, Pentz RD, Ungar DR, Mathew NA, Turner CW et al (2006) Involving children with cancer in decision-making about research participation. J Pediatr 149(6):862–868. https://doi.org/10.1016/j.jpeds.2006.08.027

Keytruda (2014) Keytruda (pembrolizumab) labeling. https://www.accessdata.fda.gov/drugsatfda_docs/label/2020/125514s084lbl.pdf

King NM (2000) Defining and describing benefit appropriately in clinical trials. J Law Med Ethics 28(4):332–343

Kodish E (2003) Pediatric ethics and early-phase childhood cancer research: conflicted goals and the prospect of benefit. Account Res 10(1):17–25. https://doi.org/10.1080/08989620300502

Leong R, Zhao H, Reaman G, Liu Q, Wang Y, Stewart CF et al (2017) Bridging adult experience to pediatrics in oncology drug development. J Clin Pharmacol 57(Suppl 10):S129–S135. https://doi.org/10.1002/jcph.910

Momper JD, Heinrichs MT, Krudys K, Griebel D, Kumar S, Kim I et al (2020) Extrapolation of adult efficacy to pediatric patients with chemotherapy-induced nausea and vomiting. J Clin Pharmacol 60(6):775–784. https://doi.org/10.1002/jcph.1577

National Commission (1978) National Commission for the protection of human subjects of biomedical and behavioral research. Research involving children: report and recommendations. Fed Regist 43(9):2083–2114

National Commission (1979) National Commission for the protection of human subjects of biomedical and behavioral research. The Belmont report: ethical principles and guidelines for the protection of human subjects of research, 18 Apr 1979. https://www.hhs.gov/ohrp/regulations-and-policy/belmont-report/read-the-belmont-report/index.html Accessed 11 May 2019

Nelson RM (2020) The use of pediatric extrapolation to avoid unnecessary pediatric clinical trials. Am J Bioethics 20(4):114–116. https://doi.org/10.1080/15265161.2020.1730489

Ross L (2006) Phase I research and the meaning of direct benefit. J Pediatr 149(1 Suppl):S20–S24. https://doi.org/10.1016/j.jpeds.2006.04.046

Roth-Cline M, Nelson R (2014) The ethical principle of scientific necessity in pediatric research. Am J Bioethics 14(12):14–15. https://doi.org/10.1080/15265161.2014.964874

Roth-Cline M, Nelson RM (2015) Ethical considerations in conducting pediatric and neonatal research in clinical pharmacology. Curr Pharm Des 21(39):5619–5635. https://doi.org/10.2174/1381612821666150901105146

Roth-Cline M, Gerson J, Bright P, Lee CS, Nelson RM (2011) Ethical considerations in conducting pediatric research. Handb Exp Pharmacol 205:219–244. https://doi.org/10.1007/978-3-642-20195-0_11

Sisk BA, Dubois J, Hobbs BP, Kodish E (2019) Reprioritizing risk and benefit: the future of study design in early-phase cancer research. Ethics Hum Res 41(6):2–11. https://doi.org/10.1002/eahr.500033

Thall PF, Cook JD (2004) Dose-finding based on efficacy-toxicity trade-offs. Biometrics 60(3):684–693. https://doi.org/10.1111/j.0006-341X.2004.00218.x

U.S. Government Printing Office (1949) Trials of War Criminals before the Nuremberg Military Tribunals under Control Council Law No. 10, pp 181–182

Future Directions

12

Jorge DiMartino

Contents

Advances in the treatment of childhood cancer have transformed a uniformly fatal disease into one in which the majority of patients will eventually survive. While this is undoubtedly one of the great successes of twentieth-century medicine, there is still much work to be done. Approximately 1800 children and adolescents in the USA will die of cancer in 2021, making it the leading cause of death from disease in this age group (Siegel et al. 2021; Cunningham et al. 2018). Moreover, although 84% of children diagnosed with cancer between 2010 and 2016 will survive 5 years or more, many of these survivors will carry the burden of their treatment into adulthood. Long-term sequelae of high-dose chemotherapy and radiation are still being defined but already encompass not only secondary malignancies but also endocrine dysfunction, metabolic syndrome, cognitive defects, and other health impacts leading to a shorter life expectancy and reduced quality of life in childhood cancer survivors as compared to adults of a similar age. The psychological impacts of surviving childhood cancer and its treatment are no less onerous, with higher incidence of depression and anxiety-related diagnoses. Addressing the needs of current long-term survivors is of the utmost importance and will require ongoing investment in research and multidisciplinary care. The objective of pediatric oncology drug development in the twenty-first century is to ensure that future patients have therapeutic options that are at least as, if not more, efficacious than current drugs that constitute standard of care but importantly with less potential for acute and chronic toxicities. Achieving this objective will require advances on multiple fronts:

- Increased research focused on identifying the molecular drivers of childhood cancer.
- Improved tools and expanded resources and industry interest to discover and develop therapeutic targeting of these drivers.
- Addressing the logistical barriers to developing drugs for a limited population of patients.

As discussed in Chap. 2, there is some overlap between targets that have been implicated as drivers of adult cancers and those that play a role

J. DiMartino (✉)
Clinical Development, Kronos Bio Inc.,
San Mateo, CA, USA
e-mail: Jorge.dimartino@kronosbio.com

J. DiMartino et al. (eds.), *Pediatric Cancer Therapeutics Development*, Pediatric Oncology,
https://doi.org/10.1007/978-3-031-06357-2_12

in childhood cancers. For example, children with Ph+ ALL have been the beneficiaries of drugs such as imatinib that were originally developed for adults with CML based on the shared dependency on the BCR-ABL gene fusion. While enhanced efforts to extend approval for use of targeted drugs to children with the same cancer indication is critical, reliance on the repurposing of drugs developed for adults for childhood cancer indications should not be the only or even the major strategy to bring novel therapies to children with cancer. For one thing, certain types of druggable targets, such as activated tyrosine kinases, that are more common in adult tumors are far less frequent in even the most common pediatric tumors. In general, pediatric tumors have a simpler mutational landscape than their adult counterparts, often relying predominantly on a single foundational genomic event such as MYCN amplification in neuroblastoma or translocations leading to transcription factor fusions like EWS-FLI1 in Ewing sarcoma. Alternatively, loss-of-function mutations in components of the SWI/SNF nucleosome remodeling complex can lead to malignant rhabdoid tumor with few or no additional mutations required. This highlights a recurring theme that distinguishes pediatric tumors from adult malignancies: in the former, mutations affecting the regulation of gene expression, including epigenetic regulators and master transcription factors, are more common (Brien et al. 2019). Unlike the mutations that accumulate over a lifetime to drive the common epithelial malignancies of adults, a single mutation or genomic rearrangement altering a single transcriptional regulatory protein can reprogram cell identity and perturb control of growth and survival pathways. Better understanding this and other peculiarities of childhood cancer biology needs to point the way to targets that can be pursued specifically or primarily with pediatric malignancies in mind.

The relative importance of transcription factors and chromatin regulators as therapeutic targets in childhood cancer highlights the need for innovative drug discovery approaches for this very challenging class of targets. The great successes of target-based drug discovery over the past 20 years have been almost exclusively enzymes (primarily protein kinases) and cell surface receptors. While it has by no means been easy to identify potent and selective inhibitors of these targets, they do share certain features that make them far more tractable than transcriptional regulators. Specifically, they can retain their three-dimensional structure and function as purified proteins, making them amenable to traditional screening platforms and functional assays to drive medicinal chemistry campaigns. Many chromatin modifiers and reader proteins also retain their structure as purified proteins; however, recapitulating their enzymatic function is complicated by the context-dependent nature of their key substrates (e.g., nucleosomes). Transcription factors present a unique challenge for drug discovery in that, with few exceptions, they lack obvious features for specific interactions with small molecules. This is because, with the exception of their DNA-binding domains, which are structured, transcription factors are mostly disordered, i.e., they only adopt a functional conformation in their native nuclear context. Screening approaches to identify binders and modulators of transcription factors must take this into account. In addition, functional assays to drive hit validation and medicinal chemistry efforts will need to recapitulate the context-dependent gene expression changes mediated by the transcription factor target. The importance of this target class is not limited to childhood cancers, and a number of innovative biotechnology companies are actively engaged in overcoming these technical hurdles. It will be incumbent on clinical investigators, patient advocates, and regulators who work with pediatric cancer patients to make these companies aware of the need to engage as early as possible in planning and executing trials in children when appropriate.

Assuming continued progress in the identification of molecular drivers of childhood cancer and in the ability to generate drug candidates against them, the feasibility of evaluating new agents in children remains a major hurdle. Ironically, it is the very success of the current standard of care regimens, combined with the relative rarity of pediatric cancer as a whole, that limits the opportunity to evaluate novel therapies, at least via the conventional approaches developed and utilized in the past half-century. The delay in initial pediatric investigation of new cancer drugs, recently highlighted by the observation of the mean lag time between first-in-human and first-in-child studies of greater than 6 years, has had profound downstream effects on cancer drug development for children. Delays in identifying a signal of activity of a new agent and rational proof of concept negatively impact the historical pediatric cancer drug development paradigm and successful incorporation of new active agents into proven effective combination regimens (Neel et al. 2019). The success of large, randomized clinical trials leading to improved patient outcomes was built on large, multicenter, cooperative group trials with the overwhelming majority of eligible pediatric cancer patients participating. This is in stark contrast to adult oncology in which trial participation rates are in the low single digits. Nevertheless, participation in pediatric oncology trials, both frontline and early phase salvage trials for recurrent and refractory disease, is declining (Faulk et al. 2020; Nooka et al. 2016) at the same time that the number of novel agents is increasing rapidly. Moreover, genomic characterization and biomarker-enriched clinical trial strategies in what were once considered common childhood cancers result in decreasing eligible study populations.

As detailed in Chap. 10, recent changes in the legislation governing pediatric cancer drug development in both the USA and the EU are significantly transforming the regulatory environment and require a coordinated, rational approach to implementation to assure that any possible unintended consequences of well-intentioned regulatory requirements do not negatively impact an already stressed system. Sponsors seeking marketing authorization in the USA and EU are now required to propose plans for developing their agents in pediatric populations, from early studies to define dose, tolerability, and signals of activity in the USA as a result of the amended PREA provisions of Sec. 504 of FDARA to more complete pediatric development plans in the EU as a result of the Paediatric Regulation and the elimination of some class waivers. Previously, sponsors could request waivers on the basis that the intended tumor type for adult development (e.g., non-small cell lung cancer) does not exist in children making studies impossible. More recently, with the advent of molecularly targeted agents, sponsors are required to consider whether the target of the drug is relevant to a pediatric tumor. As a result, there may be multiple targeted agents in the same class (i.e., against the same target) or against multiple targets relevant to the same tumor type, all proposing parallel development plans to enroll dozens or hundreds of patients in indications where there may be only a handful of eligible patients each year. This somewhat anticipated yet unintended consequence has been addressed by the FDA in its FDARA Implementation Guidance (United States Food and Drug Administration 2021) which addresses the problem with multiple same-in-class agents and the patient population constraints associated with rare diseases. Specific advice is provided to sponsors to plan for waiver requests for agents with the same mechanism of action directed at the same molecular target unless there is evidence of improved activity or effectiveness in a particular cancer, improved toxicity profile, preferential PK parameters including CNS penetration of an agent, preferred routes of administration, and superior pediatric-appropriate formulations. To date, Initial Pediatric Study Plans incorporating planned waiver requests have been agreed to by the FDA for multiple same-in-class products, including PD-1/PD-L1 axis inhibitors, PI3K delta isoform inhibitors, BTK inhibitors, EGFR inhibitors, anti-CD20 antibodies, and others. Unlike in adult oncology, where sponsors contract with individual hospitals and investigators to conduct trials, pediatric patients are treated at a relatively limited number of specialized institutions in association with academic cooperative groups and clinical trial networks. Consequently, the timelines associated with opening and attempting to enroll patients in multiple competing studies almost ensure that the results will be irrelevant by the time duplicative studies are completed. This is a situation that does not suit the needs of patients or sponsors and could actually threaten any progress in pediatric development opportunities afforded by legislative change.

Potential solutions to address what might have the potential to become a bottleneck in pediatric drug development include policy changes that acknowledge the current massive volume of drugs in development, in relation to the limited availability of patients, while still protecting the safety and autonomy of these patients, as well as multi-stakeholder discussion and consideration of optimal development strategies while avoiding needless competition and duplication. Coordinated approaches to the alignment of industry sponsors with clinical trial networks globally in decision-making as to prioritization of new molecules in specific disease conditions are being addressed by the ACCELERATE Platform. The international multi-stakeholder organization ACCELERATE was created to advance the timely investigation of new anticancer drugs (Pearson et al. 2016; Karres et al. 2020). By creating a framework that promotes scientific transparency and precompetitive information sharing, ACCELERATE has enhanced communication and understanding between academia, industry, patient advocates, and regulators. It has promoted a mechanism-of-action (MoA)-driven drug development approach by aligning publicly accessible databases of molecular targets relevant to pediatric cancer with drug pipelines and MoA-based opportunities and prioritization and conduct of early phase trials, informed, when appropriate, by data from preclinical investigations in pediatric-specific tumor models within the context of Paediatric Strategy Forums. From 2017 to 2020, five forums were held with topics ranging from the use of ALK inhibitors to combinations with immune checkpoint inhibitors as well as disease-focused forums around B-cell malignancies and AML. Each forum included participation from multiple industry sponsors and discussion of multiple development compounds from their respective pipelines, demonstrating the value of creating a safe space for information sharing. These initiatives have facilitated prioritization of new targeted molecules and a focused and sequential strategy for drug development when multiple, new potential agents may warrant pediatric investigation. Much of ACCELERATE's success has resulted from closer alignment between the European Medicines Agency and the US Food and Drug Administration (Reaman et al. 2020; Karres et al. 2021) and identification by clinical investigators and parent/patient advocates of pressing unmet clinical needs across the continuum of pediatric cancer through multi-stakeholder collaboration.

Early engagement between all stakeholders in development of new drugs is critical, and multiple parallel, complementary approaches will be required to optimize the evaluation of these drugs in children with cancer. Innovative clinical trial designs including master or platform trials prominent in oncology drug development (Burd et al. 2020; Barker et al. 2009) are beginning to make headway in the pediatric oncology space including the Pediatric Acute Leukemia (PedAL) trial, sponsored by the Leukemia & Lymphoma Society, NCI, and the Children's Oncology Group (NCT04726241). Other pediatric-focused trials using cancer genomic data to direct treatment choices include MATCH (described in Chap. 10) as well as the Genomic Assessment Informs Novel Therapy (GAIN) trial at the Dana-Farber Cancer Institute/Boston Children's Hospital (NCT02520713) and the European Proof-of-Concept Therapeutic Stratification Trial of Molecular Anomalies in Relapsed or Refractory Tumors (ESMART, NCT02813135). Interpretation of data from these innovative trials will require adaptive Bayesian strategies (Ye et al. 2020), expanded use of extrapolation, more rapid dose optimization, and the use of real-world evidence supported by adequately validated real-world data (United States Food and Drug Administration 2018) for use in constructing synthetic controls in rare populations. In addition to potentially streamlining the process of evaluating novel agents in pediatric cancer, these platform trials afford multiple sponsors the opportunity to meet regulatory requirements and accelerate timelines for developing multiple drugs simultaneously. This necessitates early discussion between investigators, sponsors, and regulators. Amplifying the patient advocate voice through inclusion across the drug development continuum will lead to better, patient-centric trials. By these means, children and adolescents with cancer can maximally and rapidly benefit from innovative products, to improve disease outcomes and reduce the burden of treatment sequelae. This evolving landscape of global, multi-institutional, and industry-academia collaboration informed by patients and their advocates intensifies the importance of collaboration that resulted in pediatric oncology becoming the success story that it is today and how it must move into the future.

References

Barker AD, Sigman CC, Kelloff GJ, Hylton NM, Berry DA, Esserman LJ (2009) I-SPY 2: an adaptive breast cancer trial design in the setting of neoadjuvant chemotherapy. Clin Pharmacol Ther 86(1):97–100. https://doi.org/10.1038/clpt.2009.68. Epub 2009 May 13

Brien GL, Stegmaier K, Armstrong SA (2019) Targeting chromatin complexes in fusion protein-driven malignancies. Nat Rev Cancer 19(5):255–269. https://doi.org/10.1038/s41568-019-0132-x

Burd A, Levine RL, Ruppert AS, Mims AS, Borate U, Stein EM, Patel P, Baer MR, Stock W, Deininger M, Blum W, Schiller G, Olin R, Litzow M, Foran J, Lin TL, Ball B, Boyiadzis M, Traer E, Odenike O, Arellano M, Walker A, Duong VH, Kovacsovics T, Collins R, Shoben AB, Heerema NA, Foster MC, Vergilio JA, Brennan T, Vietz C, Severson E, Miller M, Rosenberg L, Marcus S, Yocum A, Chen T, Stefanos M, Druker B, Byrd JC (2020) Precision medicine treatment in acute myeloid leukemia using prospective genomic profiling: feasibility and preliminary efficacy of the Beat AML Master Trial. Nat Med 26(12):1852–1858. https://doi.org/10.1038/s41591-020-1089-8. Epub 2020 Oct 26

Cunningham RM, Walton MA, Carter PM (2018) The major causes of death in children and adolescents in the United States. N Engl J Med 379(25):2468–2475. https://doi.org/10.1056/NEJMsr1804754

Faulk KE, Anderson-Mellies A, Cockburn M, Green AL (2020) Assessment of enrollment characteristics for Children's Oncology Group (COG) upfront therapeutic clinical trials 2004-2015. PLoS One 15(4):e0230824. https://doi.org/10.1371/journal.pone.0230824

Karres D, Lesa G, Ligas F, Annunen P, van Dartel M, Demolis P et al (2020) Can a multi-stakeholder prioritisation structure support regulatory decision making? A review of Paediatric oncology strategy forums reflecting on challenges and opportunities of this concept. Clin Pharmacol Ther. https://doi.org/10.1002/cpt.1939

Karres D et al (2021) Common commentary on paediatric oncology drug development. Ther Innov Regul Sci. https://doi.org/10.1007/s43441-021-00339-z

Neel DV, Shulman DS, DuBois SG (2019) Timing of first-in-child trials of FDA-approved oncology drugs. Eur J Cancer 112:49–56. https://doi.org/10.1016/j.ejca.2019.02.011. Epub 2019 Mar 28

Nooka AK, Behera M, Lonial S, Dixon MD, Ramalingam SS, Pentz RD (2016) Access to Children's Oncology Group and Pediatric Brain Tumor Consortium phase 1 clinical trials: racial/ethnic dissimilarities in participation. Cancer 122(20):3207–3214. https://doi.org/10.1002/cncr.30090. Epub 2016 Jul 12

Pearson AD, et al., On behalf of Members of Working Group 1 of the Paediatric Platform of ACCELERATE. Implementation of mechanism of action biology-driven early drug development for children with cancer. Eur J Cancer. 2016;62:124–131.

Reaman G et al (2020) Accelerating the global development of pediatric cancer drugs: a call to coordinate the submissions of pediatric investigation plans and pediatric study plans to the European Medicines Agency and US Food and Drug Administration. J Clin Oncol 38(36):4227–4230. https://doi.org/10.1200/JCO.20.02152

Siegel RL, Miller KD, Fuchs HE, Jemal A (2021) Cancer statistics, 2021. CA Cancer J Clin 71(1):7–33. https://doi.org/10.3322/caac.21654. Epub 2021 Jan 12. Erratum in: CA Cancer J Clin. 2021;71(4):359

United States Food and Drug Administration. Framework for the FDA's real world evidence program. 2018. https://www.fda.gov/media/120060/download. Accessed 28 Nov 2021

United States Food and Drug Administration. Guidance for industry: FDARA implementation guidance for pediatric studies of molecularly targeted oncology drugs: amendments to Sec. 505B of the FD&C Act. 2021. https://www.fda.gov/media/133440/download. Accessed 29 Nov 2021

Ye JY et al (2020) A Bayesian approach in design and analysis of pediatric cancer clinical trials. Pharm Stat 19(6):814–826. https://doi.org/10.1002/pst.2039

GPSR Compliance

The European Union's (EU) General Product Safety Regulation (GPSR) is a set of rules that requires consumer products to be safe and our obligations to ensure this.

If you have any concerns about our products, you can contact us on ProductSafety@springernature.com

In case Publisher is established outside the EU, the EU authorized representative is:

Springer Nature Customer Service Center GmbH
Europaplatz 3
69115 Heidelberg, Germany

Batch number: 10732801

Printed by Printforce, the Netherlands